1989

PATHOLOGY
ANNUAL
PART 2

1989

PATHOLOGY ANNUAL

PART 2 / VOLUME 24

Series Editors

PAUL PETER ROSEN, M.D.

Attending Pathologist and Member,
Memorial Sloan-Kettering Cancer Center; Professor of Pathology,
Cornell University Medical College, New York, New York

ROBERT E. FECHNER, M.D.

Professor and Director, Division of Surgical Pathology,
University of Virginia Health Sciences Center, Charlottesville, Virginia

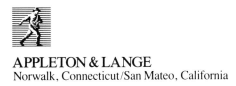

APPLETON & LANGE
Norwalk, Connecticut/San Mateo, California

0-8385-7713-X

Notice: The author(s) and publisher of this volume have taken care that
the information and recommendations contained herein are accurate and
compatible with the standards generally accepted at the time of publication.

Copyright © 1989 by Appleton & Lange
A Publishing Division of Prentice Hall

89 90 91 92 93 / 10 9 8 7 6 5 4 3 2 1

Prentice-Hall International (UK) Limited, *London*
Prentice-Hall of Australia Pty. Limited, *Sydney*
Prentice-Hall Canada, Inc., *Toronto*
Prentice-Hall Hispanoamericana, S.A., *Mexico*
Prentice-Hall of India Private Limited, *New Delhi*
Prentice-Hall of Japan, Inc., *Tokyo*
Simon & Schuster Asia Pte. Ltd., *Singapore*
Editora Prentice-Hall do Brasil Ltda., *Rio de Janeiro*
Prentice-Hall, *Englewood Cliffs, New Jersey*

ISBN: 0-8385-7713-X
ISSN: 0079-0184

Production Editor: Charles F. Evans

PRINTED IN THE UNITED STATES OF AMERICA

Contributors

Jacki Abrams, M.D.
Assistant Professor of Pathology, Baylor College of Medicine, Houston, Texas

Debra A. Bell, M.D.
Assistant Professor of Pathology, Harvard Medical School; and Assistant Pathologist, the James Homer Wright Pathology Laboratories of Massachusetts General Hospital, Boston, Massachusetts

Philip B. Clement, M.D.
Departments of Pathology, Vancouver General Hospital and the University of British Columbia

Harvey Cramer, M.D.
Staff Pathologist, St. Joseph's Health Center of London, Ontario, Canada

John D. Crissman, M.D.
Senior Staff Pathologist, Department of Pathology, Henry Ford Hospital, Detroit, Michigan

Louis P. Dehner, M.D.
Division of Surgical Pathology, Department of Laboratory Medicine and Pathology, University of Minnesota, Minneapolis, Minnesota

Adel El-Naggar, M.D.
Division of Pathology, University of Texas M.D. Anderson Cancer Center, Houston, Texas

Ben J. Glasgow, M.D.
Resident in Pathology, Department of Pathology, UCLA School of Medicine, Los Angeles, California

David R. Kelly, M.D.
Department of Pathology and Laboratory Medicine, the Children's Hospital, Birmingham, Alabama

Lester J. Layfield, M.D.
Assistant Professor of Pathology and Director of the Fine Needle Aspiration Service, Department of Pathology, UCLA School of Medicine, Los Angeles, California

J.T. Lie, M.D., F.A.C.C., F.A.C.A., F.A.R.A.
Professor of Pathology, Mayo Medical School and Mayo Graduate School of Medicine; Consultant in Pathology and Cardiovascular Diseases and Internal Medicine, Mayo Clinic and Mayo Foundation, Rochester, Minnesota

Chan K. Ma, M.D.
Senior Staff Pathologist, Department of Pathology, Henry Ford Hospital, Detroit, Michigan

Juan Carlos Manivel, M.D.
Division of Surgical Pathology, Department of Laboratory Medicine and Pathology, University of Minnesota, Minneapolis, Minnesota

Donia McLemore, H.T.L. (A.S.C.P.)
Divison of Pathology, University of Texas M.D. Anderson Cancer Center, Houston, Texas

Guido Pettinato, M.D.
Department of Pathology, 2nd Medical School, University of Naples, Italy

Paul Peter Rosen, M.D.
Attending Pathologist, Department of Pathology, Memorial Sloan-Kettering Cancer Center, New York, New York

Michael L. Rutledge, M.D.
Division of Pathology, University of Texas M.D. Anderson Cancer Center; and Instructor, Department of Pathology, Baylor College of Medicine, Houston, Texas

Robert E. Scully, M.D.
Professor of Pathology, Harvard Medical School, and the James Homer Wright Pathology Laboratories of Massachusetts General Hospital, Boston, Massachusetts

Elvio G. Silva, M.D.
Division of Pathology, University of Texas M.D. Anderson Cancer Center, Houston, Texas

Steven G. Silverberg, M.D.
Professor of Pathology and Director of Anatomic Pathology, the George Washington University Medical Center, Washington, D.C.

Dale C. Snover, M.D.
Associate Professor and Associate Director of Anatomic Pathology,
Department of Laboratory Medicine and Pathology, University of Minnesota
Medical School, Minneapolis, Minnesota

James A. Strauchen, M.D.
Professor of Pathology and Neoplastic Disease, Mount Sinai School of
Medicine, New York, New York

Daniel W. Visscher, M.D.
Senior Staff Pathologist, Department of Pathology, Henry Ford Hospital,
Detroit, Michigan

Lester E. Wold, M.D.
Department of Surgical Pathology, Mayo Clinic-Methodist Hospital,
Rochester, Minnesota

Robert H. Young, M.D.
Department of Pathology, Harvard Medical School; and the James Homer
Wright Laboratories of Massachusetts General Hospital

Richard J. Zarbo, M.D.
Senior Staff Pathologist, Department of Pathology, Henry Ford Hospital,
Detroit, Michigan

Contents

Benign and Borderline Serous Lesions of the Peritoneum in Women

Debra A. Bell and Robert E. Scully

Lesions mimicking the full spectrum from normal fallopian tube epithelium through various forms of serous neoplasia of the female genital tract have been reported to involve the peritoneal surfaces, either as primary peritoneal proliferations or as implants from female genital sites. The histological appearance of these lesions ranges from the simple glandular tubal–epithelial inclusions of endosalpingiosis to epithelial implants that resemble serous borderline tumors (SBTs) to serous carcinomas. Although a number of articles have described the involvement of the peritoneum by either primary peritoneal or metastatic ovarian serous carcinoma,[1–5] the histological appearance and clinical features of the more benign-appearing serous proliferations of the peritoneum have received less attention. In this article, we review the clinicopathologic features of endosalpingiosis, serous neoplasia of the peritoneum, and peritoneal "implants" associated with SBTs with an emphasis on the histological features that differentiate among these entities.

ENDOSALPINGIOSIS

Endosalpingiosis is defined as the presence of glandular inclusions lined by tubal-appearing epithelium located in the superficial layers of the peritoneum or in pelvic or para-aortic lymph nodes.[6–16]

Endosalpingiosis has been reported in women ranging in age from 12 to 66 years, with a peak frequency in the third and fourth decades of life.[6–16] The majority of these women have clinical or pathologic evidence of tubal disease such as chronic salpingitis with or without hydrosalpinx, prior tubal pregnancies, or salpingitis isthmica nodosum.[8–10,13,14] Endosalpingiosis has also been identified in up to 56 percent of women with stage II or III ovarian serous borderline tumors[6,7,9,12,13]; it has been noted likewise in association with benign[9,13,16] and, more rarely, malignant[9] serous tumors of the ovary.

On gross examination, endosalpingiosis can occasionally be appreciated as fine granularity or small cysts on the peritoneal surfaces[8,10–16]; in some cases, it is associated with pelvic fibrous adhesions, which may be related to tubal inflammatory disease. Histological examination discloses the presence of single smoothly contoured, round or oval glands, or clusters of them beneath the serosa of the uterus or fallopian tubes (Fig. 1), the pelvic or extrapelvic parietal peritoneum, or the peritoneal surfaces of the omentum. The glands are lined by one to two layers of columnar cells that are commonly ciliated. Less often, the lining epithelium is identical to that of the fallopian tube, containing ciliated cells, secretory nonciliated cells, and peg-shaped intercalated cells (Fig. 2). The nuclei are generally round, oval or pencil-shaped, uniform, basally oriented, and show no cytological atypicality. Rarely, blunt papillae with prominent fibrovascular cores lined by similar epithelial cells are present within the

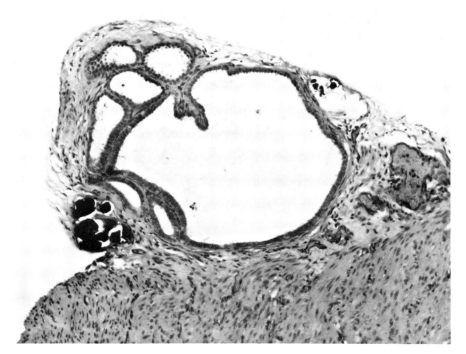

Figure 1. Endosalpingiosis, uterine serosa. A cluster of smoothly contoured round-to-oval glands lined by a single layer of columnar cells is present beneath the serosa. Psammoma bodies are present in the stroma adjacent to the glands.

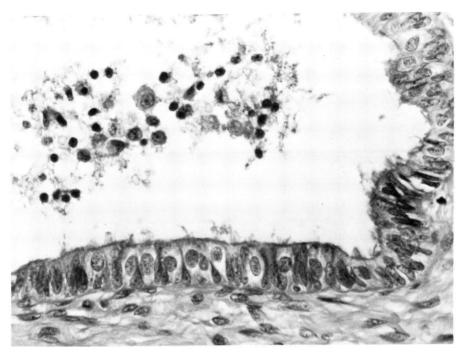

Figure 2. Endosalpingiosis. A smoothly contoured gland is lined by fallopian tube-like epithelium containing ciliated cells, secretory nonciliated cells, and peg-shaped intercalated cells.

glands. Mitotic figures are usually absent. Psammoma bodies are often present in the glands, in the stroma beneath the epithelium of the glands, or unassociated with epithelial cells. The glands are usually surrounded by several layers of delicate connective tissue infiltrated with scattered lymphocytes. In occasional cases, many of the glands are rimmed by a dense lymphocytic infiltrate.[6–16]

Although few reports with long-term follow-up are available, Zinsser and Wheeler[9] reported that subsequent tumor did not develop in any of their 16 patients with endosalpingiosis, who were followed from 1 to 6 years.

The histological differential diagnosis of endosalpingiosis includes endometriosis, mesothelial hyperplasia, peritoneal inclusion cysts, implants of ovarian SBTs, primary peritoneal SBTs, and metastatic adenocarcinoma. Although the cellular features of the glandular epithelium in endosalpingiosis and endometriosis may be similar, the obvious periglandular endometrial stroma that is usually identified in endometriosis in premenopausal women is not apparent in endosalpingiosis. In contrast, it may be difficult to distinguish these entities in postmenopausal women, when no endometrial stroma is discernible in endometriosis due to atrophy and fibrosis. The presence of stroma around some of the glands should not preclude a diagnosis of endosalpingiosis if typical endosalpingiotic glands without stroma are present as well, since endosalpingiosis and endometriosis are commonly found in continuity or in adjacent tissue.[9] In mesothelial hyperplasia, the normally flat mesothelial cells become cuboidal with uniform vesicular nuclei, and cords and gland-like spaces lined by such cells may be embedded in reparative fibrous tissue, often arranged in rows parallel to the surface (Fig. 3).[18,19] The cells lining these spaces are typically not columnar and are not ciliated. Peritoneal inclusion cysts are lined by one to several layers of flat-to-cuboidal mesothelial cells separated by fibrous septa. Focally the cysts may be lined by columnar cells characteristic of endosalpingiosis; however, this is considered evidence of tubal metaplasia of the lining mesothelium. The lining cells may also undergo squamous metaplasia.[17] Endosalpingiosis may be differentiated from implants of ovarian SBTs and primary peritoneal SBTs by both architectural and cytological features. The papillarity, tufting, and especially detached buds of epithelial cells that are characteristic of serous borderline tumors are not seen in endosalpingiosis; also, the cells of endosalpingiosis show little or no cytological atypia. Endosalpingiosis can be distinguished from metastatic adenocarcinoma by the regular arrangement of simple glands in a noninfiltrative pattern and by the absence of cytological atypia or a significant stromal response. Cilia may be prominent in endosalpingiosis and are very rare in metastatic adenocarcinoma.[9]

The histogenesis of endosalpingiosis remains in dispute. Theories of its origin are similar to those that have been suggested for the origin of endometriosis.[8–10] It has been suggested that endosalpingiosis results from direct extension of proliferating tubal epithelium to surrounding tissue, from implantation of sloughed tubal epithelium into the peritoneal cavity, from "müllerian" metaplasia of the coelomic epithelium, or from lymphatic or hematogenous

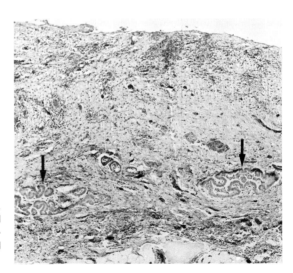

Figure 3. Mesothelial hyperplasia. Gland-like spaces containing focal papillary projections lined by cuboidal cells (*arrows*) are arranged in a row parallel to the surface.

spread to lymph nodes. The two most widely accepted theories currently are that of müllerian metaplasia, which would also explain the common co-existence of endosalpingiosis and endometriosis, and that of peritoneal implantation by sloughed tubal epithelium, which would explain in part the strong association between endosalpingiosis and inflammation of the fallopian tubes.[9]

SEROUS BORDERLINE NEOPLASIA OF THE PERITONEUM

Rare cases of endosalpingiosis with epithelial proliferation and significant degrees of cytological atypia have been reported[9,11,20] and we have observed a small number of such cases as well.[21] In this disorder, the glands are lined by stratified, tufted, columnar epithelial cells that show moderate nuclear atypia and hyperchromasia. These lesions may be impossible to distinguish from implants of ovarian SBTs except that no tumor is present in the ovaries or that their surfaces are minimally involved by tumor.[21–23] Lesions of this type have been termed "atypical endosalpingiosis" by some authors[9,11,20] and serous borderline tumor of the peritoneum by others.[21,22]

We have encountered 13 patients with SBTs of the peritoneum for whom long-term follow-up is available.[21] These 13 women ranged in age from 19 to 53 years (mean, 30 years) and 77 percent of them were younger than 35 years of age. Their most common presenting complaint was infertility. The gross appearance of the lesions was described as peritoneal granularity or fibrous adhesions in 11 cases and as a peritoneal mass or plaque in 1 patient each. The tumor involved the pelvic peritoneum in ten patients and the extrapelvic peritoneum as well in three patients. No ovarian involvement was present in six women and minimal surface involvement was present in seven of them. Ten of the women were treated by removal of their reproductive organs and three women had only a peritoneal or ovarian biopsy without further therapy.

Histologically, the lesions had microscopic features identical to those of implants of ovarian SBTs without invasion of underlying tissue (Figs. 4 through 6). Both predominantly epithelial and desmoplastic lesions were present in seven women, epithelial lesions alone were present in five women, and only desmoplastic tumor was identified in one woman. The epithelium in all of the cases showed mild or moderate atypia (Fig. 5). Significant associated pathologic findings were endosalpingiosis in 11 women (Fig. 6), hydrosalpinx in 5, evidence of chronic salpingitis in 3, endometriosis in 3, and co-existing benign ovarian serous cystadenomas in 2 patients.

The prognosis is excellent; 12 patients had no evidence of disease from 4.7 to 11.6 years after presentation and 1 patient was alive and well 2 years after resection of a recurrence that occurred 8 years after initial diagnosis.

The histological differential diagnosis of SBTs of the peritoneum as well as implants of ovarian SBTs includes endosalpingiosis and florid papillary mesothelial hyperplasia. Solid papillary appearing sheets of polygonal mesothelial

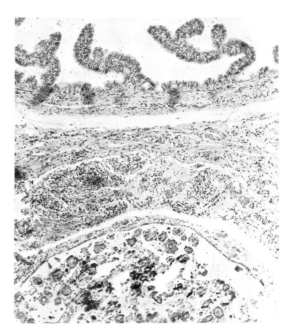

Figure 4. Serous borderline tumor of the peritoneum, epithelial lesion. Fine papillae and detached cell clusters similar to those seen in an implant of an ovarian serous borderline tumor are present in a smoothly contoured submesothelial invagination in the mesosalpinx. No stromal response is present.

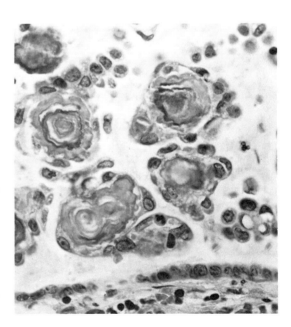

Figure 5. Serous borderline tumor of the peritoneum, epithelial lesion (higher power of Figure 4). Polygonal-to-cuboidal cells showing moderate nuclear atypia and delicate cytoplasm are present surrounding psammoma bodies and in detached cell clusters in an invagination lined by a single layer of cuboidal cells.

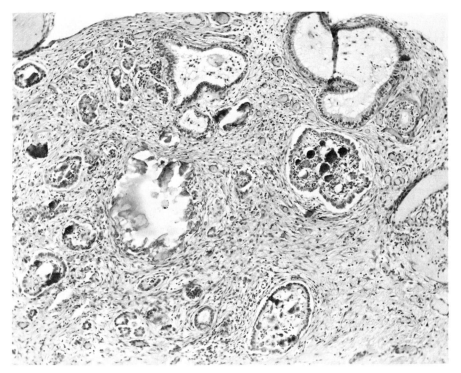

Figure 6. Serous borderline tumor of the peritoneum, desmoplastic lesion. Glands and papillae are present in a plaque of reactive fibrous tissue plastered on the peritoneal surface. Simple glands lined by a single layer of columnar cells (endo-salpingiosis) are present (*upper right*) as well as numerous psammoma bodies.

cells, papillary projections with delicate or hyalinized fibrovascular cores lined by a single layer of cuboidal mesothelial cells (Fig. 3), and small irregular nests and solid cell clusters embedded in reparative fibrous stroma (Fig. 7) may be seen in florid mesothelial hyperplasia.[18] This reactive process can generally be distinguished from borderline serous neoplasia based on the appearance of the cells lining the glands and papillae, which are usually columnar with delicate cytoplasm in serous borderline tumors whereas the cells in nests and lining papillae in mesothelial hyperplasia are cuboidal with uniform nuclei and abundant eosinophilic cytoplasm. Psammoma bodies may be seen in either lesion, although they are usually more numerous in peritoneal SBTs or implants of SBTs (Fig. 6). The features that differentiate endosalpingiosis from borderline serous neoplasia have already been discussed in detail in the section on endosalpingiosis.

The excellent prognosis of peritoneal SBTs, even when they are untreated, indicates that conservation of the reproductive organs should be considered in these young women after careful clinical evaluation to exclude a primary ovarian SBT has been performed.

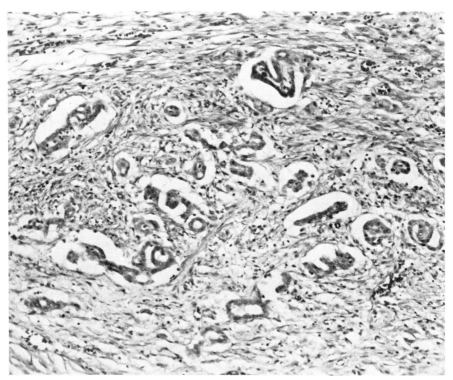

Figure 7. Florid mesothelial hyperplasia. Small gland-like spaces and solid nests of mesothelial cells are present in a reactive fibrous stroma. The cells are arranged in a somewhat poorly defined row parallel to the overlying surface and are cuboidal or polygonal with uniform nuclei.

PERITONEAL IMPLANTS OF SEROUS BORDERLINE TUMORS

The category of borderline tumors was created to identify a subgroup of malignant common epithelial ovarian tumors that have an unusually good prognosis.[24] Ovarian serous borderline tumors are defined by the World Health Organization (WHO) as serous neoplasms that show epithelial proliferation greater than that seen in serous cystadenomas, but in which "destructive" invasion of the stroma of the primary ovarian tumor is absent. The diagnosis is based on histological examination of the ovarian tumor irrespective of whether spread beyond the ovary has occurred.[25] These tumors have an excellent prognosis when confined to the ovary[26–38]; however, 30 to 40 percent of patients with peritoneal implants ultimately die of their disease.[27,29] Because both the presence of implants[6,7,26–40] and their histological features[17–19] strongly correlate with prognosis and may affect therapeutic decisions, it is important to distinguish these lesions from benign or reactive peritoneal lesions, which are often also present in patients with ovarian SBTs.[6,7,37]

SBTs account for 21 to 33 percent of malignant serous tumors of the ovary.[29,32,41,42] They often occur in young women, with a peak frequency in the fourth and fifth decades.[7,27,31,35,37,41,43] Forty-one to 84 percent of the tumors are confined to the ovary or ovaries at the time of presentation (stage I); 7 to 22 percent have spread to the serosa of the uterus, fallopian tubes, or pelvic parietal peritoneum (stage II); 4 to 40 percent have extended to the upper abdomen (stage III); and only very rare cases have spread beyond the abdominal cavity (stage IV).[26–38]

Ovarian SBTs are usually endophytic, cystic tumors (serous cystadenomas of borderline malignancy), although occasionally they grow only on the ovarian surface (serous surface papillomas of borderline malignancy); often the tumor is both endophytic and exophytic.[44] Both ovaries are involved in 28 to 50 percent of the cases.[27–30,32,33,35,37]

Histological examination reveals that the cysts and papillae are lined by stratified, columnar cells that show varying degrees of nuclear atypia and typically only minimal or slight mitotic activity (Figs. 8 and 9) Epithelial tufting and varying numbers of small, apparently detached buds of epithelial cells are typically present (Fig. 9). "Destructive" invasion of the stroma, characterized by cellular nests and glands with irregular contours haphazardly distributed in a myxoid, hyaline, or desmoplastic stroma, is absent.

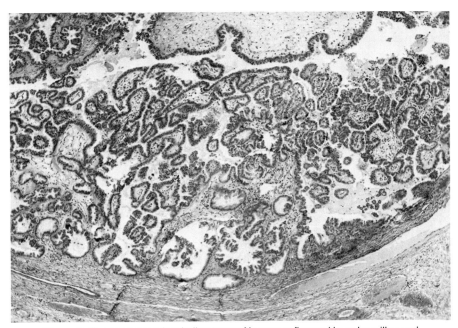

Figure 8. Ovarian serous borderline tumor. Numerous fine and broad papillae and detached clusters of cells are present in a cyst. Destructive invasion of the stroma is not present. *(From Bell DA, et al, 1988, with permission.[45])*

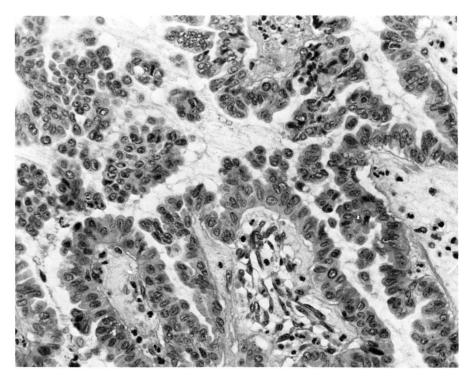

Figure 9. Ovarian serous borderline tumor. The papillae are lined by stratified and tufted columnar cells with moderate nuclear atypicality. Numerous apparently detached buds of epithelial cells are also present. *(From Bell DA, et al, 1988, with permission.[45])*

Although stromal invasion must not be identified in the ovarian tumor for inclusion in the borderline category, extraovarian peritoneal implants of SBTs may be superficial and noninvasive or may invade underlying normal tissue.[6,7,39,40] Two types of noninvasive implants have been described, based on whether the neoplastic cells or their stroma predominates[6,7]. The epithelial noninvasive implant is characterized by epithelial proliferations similar to those seen in the primary tumor but located on the surface of the peritoneum or in smoothly contoured submesothelial invaginations. Little or no stromal response is present (Fig. 10). The papillae are lined by stratified and tufted epithelial cells that usually show mild-to-moderate cytological atypia, but occasionally the atypicality is severe. Mitotic activity is absent or minimal. Psammoma bodies are often seen (Figs. 11 and 12). The desmoplastic noninvasive implant, in contrast, is characterized by a predominant, marked, stromal proliferation that compresses and distorts glands and papillae, but is plastered on the peritoneal surfaces and does not invade underlying tissue (Fig. 13). The glands, although compressed, usually have smooth outlines and are lined by stratified and tufted columnar epithelial cells (Fig. 14). Gland spaces containing papillae are seen;

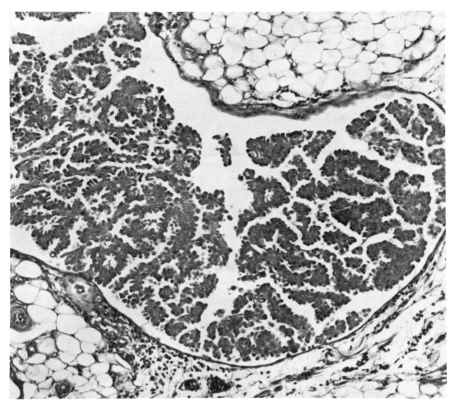

Figure 10. Epithelial noninvasive implant, omentum. Fine papillae are present in a smoothly contoured submesothelial invagination. Little or no stromal response is present.

less often solid nests of cells, or single cells are trapped in the fibrotic stroma. The epithelial cells usually show mild-to-moderate cytological atypia although rarely severe atypia is present (Fig. 15) and mitotic figures are absent or infrequent. Psammoma bodies are often present. The stroma is usually dense and contains an inflammatory infiltrate of polymorphonuclear leukocytes; necrosis, fibrin deposition, and recent hemorrhage are often present, especially near the peritoneal surface of the implant.

Invasive implants are characterized by an irregular infiltration of epithelium into underlying normal tissue (Figs. 16 and 17).[6,7] Papillae or glands with irregular contours and sometimes extensive intraglandular bridging are embedded in a myxoid or desmoplastic stroma that usually contains only scattered lymphocytes. The glands and papillae are lined by cuboidal-to-columnar epithelial cells, which often show severe cytological atypia. Scattered mitotic figures are commonly identified (Fig. 18).

The prognostic significance of the presence of extraovarian implants of

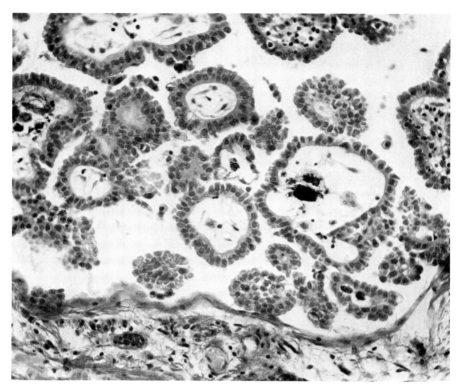

Figure 11. Epithelial noninvasive implant, omentum. The papillae are lined by stratified and tufted columnar epithelial cells similar to those seen in a primary ovarian serous borderline tumor. Apparently detached clusters of similar cells are also present.

SBTs has been confirmed in numerous studies: the death rate is near 0 for patients with tumors confined to the ovary, in contrast to 0 to 20 percent for patients with pelvic implants and 14 to 50 percent for those with tumor implants in the upper abdomen.[7,27,29,30,32,34,36,37] Several studies have shown a strong correlation between the histological features of the implants and prognosis.[6,7] In our study of 56 women with extraovarian peritoneal implants of ovarian SBTs and a mean follow-up time of 6.6 years and a median follow-up of 6.0 years,[7] we found that 4 of the 6 patients with invasive implants died of tumor and 1 was alive with widespread disease; in contrast only 3 of the 50 patients with noninvasive implants died of tumor. Similarly, McCaughey and co-workers[6] found that of their 5 patients with invasive implants, 4 died of tumor and 1 was alive with widespread disease, whereas only 2 of the 13 patients with noninvasive implants died of tumor. On the other hand, Bostwick and co-workers[37] and Michael and Roth[39] found no differences in survival between patients with invasive implants and those with noninvasive implants. The discrepancies among these findings are probably due to differences in classification of noninvasive implants of the desmoplastic type, which may have been considered invasive by the latter groups of investigators.[37–39]

We also noted a strong correlation between severe cytological atypia and an adverse prognosis in our study[7]; 5 of 12 patients with severely atypical implants died of tumor in contrast to only 2 of 44 patients with no greater than moderate atypia. The presence of mitotic activity was a statistically significant predictor of an adverse prognosis as well.

Because of this strong correlation between the histological features of implants and prognosis and because implants may vary in their features from one area to another, extensive sampling and careful microscopic evaluation of peritoneal implants in cases of stages II and III ovarian serous borderline tumors is recommended.[6,7]

The presence of gross residual tumor, as assessed by the surgeon, was also shown to be associated with an adverse clinical outcome in our study, although this association was not statistically significant when the histologically sampled

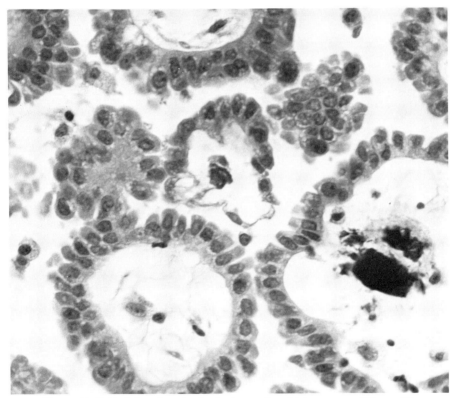

Figure 12. Epithelial noninvasive implant, omentum (higher power of Figure 11). The lining cells are columnar, stratified and show mild-to-moderate nuclear atypia. Detached clusters of similar cells are present.

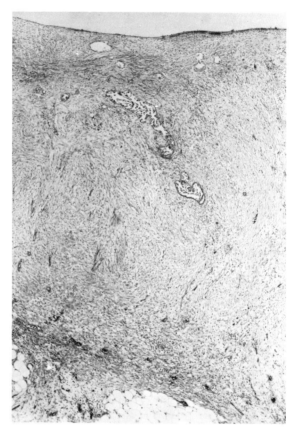

Figure 13. Desmoplastic noninvasive implant, omentum. Glands and papillae are present in a predominant, marked fibrous stroma that is present as a plaque on the surface of the omentum (*left lower corner*) and does not invade underlying tissue. The glands are not arranged parallel to the overlying surface.

implants were all of the noninvasive type.[7] Nation and Krepart[36] and Bostwick and co-workers[37] reported similar findings, but Tasker and Langley[33] could not establish a relation between the amount of residual disease and prognosis. The findings of most of these studies suggest that every effort should be made to resect as much tumor as possible.

The therapy of patients with ovarian SBTs and peritoneal implants has been a source of controversy. Several retrospective reviews of these tumors, including our own,[7] have failed to show a relation between the administration of postoperative therapy of any type and survival.[35,37] The recent recognition of the previously discussed adverse prognostic factors, however, may allow identification of a high risk group of patients who might benefit from additional treatment. The results of our study would indicate that patients with implants characterized by invasion or severe cellular atypia have a poor prognosis and may benefit from aggressive therapy. In contrast, patients without these risk factors have an excellent prognosis and do not need additional therapy, which may cause complications and, occasionally, the death of the patient.

The recent data regarding the prognostic significance of the histological features of the peritoneal implants of SBTs have prompted McCaughey and co-workers[6] to suggest that these tumors should be classified based on the histological appearance of the implants, rather than the appearance of the ovarian tumor as defined in the WHO classification.[25] These authors recommend that borderline appearing ovarian tumors with invasive implants should be designated serous cystadenocarcinomas and only those with noninvasive implants should be retained in the borderline category. We disagree with this proposal on several grounds. First, exclusion of patients with invasive implants, most of whom have an unfavorable prognosis, from the borderline category would make it impossible to determine the biologic behavior of ovarian SBTs. Secondly, this approach would make it theoretically impossible to diagnose a borderline tumor without extensive sampling of the peritoneum. Nevertheless, it is important to subclassify patients with ovarian SBTs and extraovarian disease into low and high risk groups based on the presence of invasion or severe cytological atypicality in the implants.

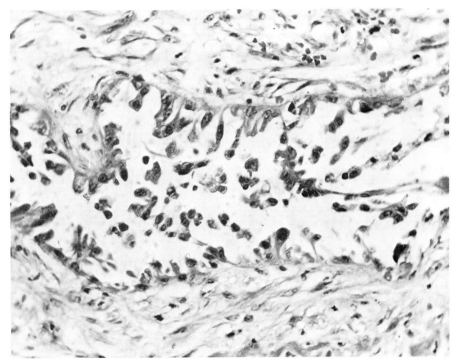

Figure 14. Desmoplastic noninvasive implant, omentum (higher power of Figure 13). A gland lined by moderately atypical, stratified, and tufted columnar cells and rare hobnail cells is present in loose fibrous stroma.

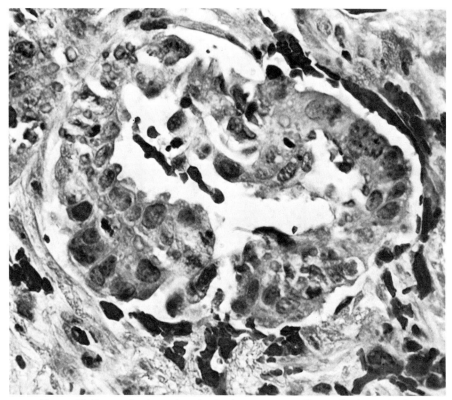

Figure 15. Desmoplastic noninvasive implant, omentum. Nests of polygonal cells with severe nuclear atypia and delicate cytoplasm are present in a fibrous stroma. Several mitotic figures are apparent (*center*). *(From Bell DA, et al, 1988, with permission.[45])*

The acknowledged capability of the extraovarian pelvic peritoneum to give rise to müllerian types of borderline and invasive tumors and the indolent biologic behavior of SBTs with extraovarian implants has led to speculation that the so-called peritoneal implants of ovarian SBTs are not true metastatic deposits but reflect co-existent primary multicentric neoplasia of the extraovarian mesothelium. The evidence for multicentric tumorigenesis has been presented in detail by Russell.[28] Despite this evidence, it is not possible to be certain whether extraovarian peritoneal serous neoplasia co-existing with ovarian serous borderline tumors is primary or secondary. It is unlikely, however, that this differentiation is important from a practical standpoint, since the significant determinants from the viewpoint of prognosis and therapy are the presence of implants, their extent, and their histological appearance rather than their site of origin.

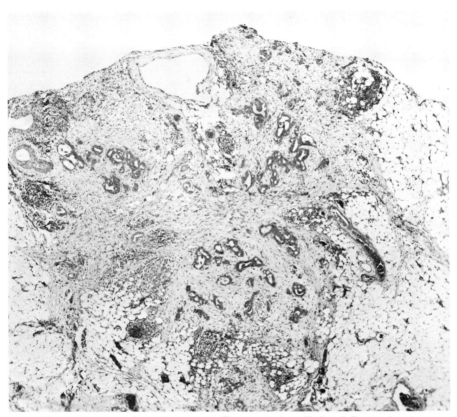

Figure 16. Invasive implant, omentum. The neoplastic epithelium infiltrates deeply into the underlying normal omentum with an irregular margin.

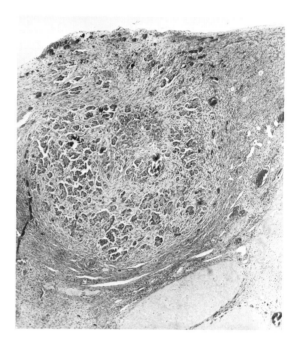

Figure 17. Invasive implant, contralateral ovary. Neoplastic epithelium extends deeply into normal ovarian cortex.

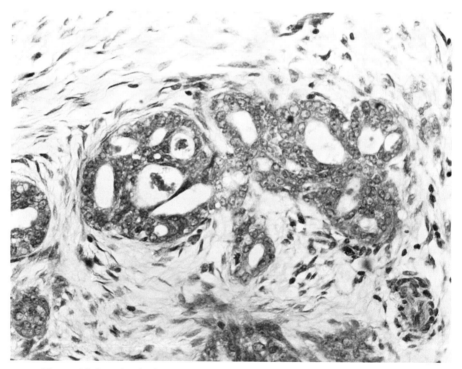

Figure 18. Invasive implant, omentum. Irregularly shaped glands with extensive intraglandular bridging lined by epithelial cells with severe cytological atypia are present in a myxoid stroma. Mitotic figures are seen (*upper center*).

REFERENCES

1. Foyle A, Al-Jabi M, McCaughey WTE: Papillary peritoneal tumors in women. Am J Surg Pathol 5:241, 1981
2. White PF, Merino MJ, Barwick KW: Serous surface papillary carcinoma of the ovary: A clinical, pathologic, ultrastructural, and immunohistochemical study of 11 cases. Pathol Annu 20(Pt 1):403, 1985
3. Goonerate S, Sassone M, Blaustein A, et al: Serous surface papillary carcinoma of the ovary: A clinicopathologic study of 16 cases. Int J Gynecol Pathol 1:258, 1982
4. McCaughey WTE: Papillary peritoneal neoplasms in females. Pathol Annu 20(Pt 2):387, 1985
5. McCaughey WTE, Kannerstein M, Churg J: Tumors and pseudotumors of the serous membranes. Atlas of Tumor Pathology, 2nd Series, Fascicle 20. Armed Forces Institute of Pathology, Washington, DC, 1985
6. McCaughey WTE, Kirk ME, Lester W, Dardick I: Peritoneal epithelial lesions associated with proliferative serous tumours of ovary. Histopathology 8:195, 1984
7. Bell DA, Weinstock MA, Scully RE: Peritoneal implants of ovarian serous borderline tumors: Histologic features and prognosis. Cancer 62:2212, 1988
8. Shen SC, Bansal M, Purrazzella R, et al: Benign glandular inclusions in lymph nodes, endosalpingiosis, and salpingitis isthmica nodosa in a young girl with clear cell adenocarcinoma of the cervix. Am J Surg Pathol 7:293, 1983
9. Zinsser KR, Wheeler JE: Endosalpingiosis in the omentum: A study of autopsy and surgical material. Am J Surg Pathol 6:109, 1982
10. Holmes MD, Levin HS, Ballard LA Jr: Endosalpingiosis. Cleve Clin Q 48:345, 1981
11. Dallenbach-Hellweg G: Atypical endosalpingiosis: A case report with consideration of the differential diagnosis of glandular subperitoneal inclusions. Pathol Res Pract 182:180, 1987
12. Burmeister RE, Fechner RE, Franklin RR: Endosalpingiosis of the peritoneum. Obstet Gynecol 34:310, 1969
13. Sinykin MB: Endosalpingiosis. Minn Medicine 43:759, 1960
14. Schuldenfrei R, Janovski NA: Disseminated endosalpingiosis associated with bilateral papillary serous cystadenocarcinoma of the ovaries. A case report. Am J Obstet Gynecol 84:382, 1962
15. Bryce RL, Barbatis C, Charnock M: Endosalpingiosis in pregnancy. Case report. Br J Obstet Gynecol 89:166, 1982
16. Tutschka BG, Lauchlan SC: Endosalpingiosis. Obstet Gynecol 55:57s, 1980
17. Ross MJ, Welch WR, Scully RE: Multilocular peritoneal inclusion cysts (so-called cystic mesothelioma): A report of twenty-five cases and review of the literature. Cancer (in press)
18. McCaughey WTE, Al-Jabi M: Differentiation of serosal hyperplasia and neoplasia in biopsies. Pathol Annu 21(pt.1):271, 1986
19. Rosai J, Dehner LP: Nodular mesothelial hyperplasia in hernia sacs. A benign reactive condition simulating a neoplastic process. Cancer 35:165, 1975
20. Fievez M, Lambot P, Dewin B: Endosalpingiose du peritoine et salpingite chronique. Arch Anat Cytol Pathol 31:355, 1983
21. Bell DA, Scully RE: Serous borderline tumors of the peritoneum. Lab Invest 5A, 1987

22. Genadry R, Poliakoff S, Rotmensch J, et al: Primary, papillary peritoneal neoplasia. Obstet Gynecol 58:730, 1981

23. Russell P: The pathological assessment of ovarian neoplasms. I. Introduction to the common "epithelial" tumours and analysis of benign "epithelial" tumours. Pathology 11:5, 1979

24. Scully RE: Common epithelial tumors of borderline malignancy (carcinomas of low malignant potential). Bull Cancer (Paris) 3:228, 1982

25. Serov SF, Scully RE, Sobin LH: International Histological Classification of Tumours No. 9. Histological Typing of Ovarian Tumours. Geneva, World Health Organization, 1973

26. Julian CG, Woodruff JD: The biologic behavior of low-grade papillary serous carcinoma of the ovary. Obstet Gynecol 6:860, 1972

27. Katzenstein AA, Mazur MT, Morgan TE, Kao M-S: Proliferative serous tumors of the ovary. Histologic features and prognosis. Am J Surg Pathol 2:339, 1978

28. Russell P: The pathological assessment of ovarian neoplasms. II. The proliferating "epithelial" tumours. Pathology 11:251, 1979

29. Russell P, Merkur H: Proliferating ovarian "epithelial" tumours: A clinico-pathological analysis of 144 cases. Aust NZ J Obstet Gynaecol 19:45, 1979

30. Tang M, Lian L, Lui T: The characteristics of ovarian serous tumors of borderline malignancy. Chin Med J 93:459, 1980

31. Chenevart P, Gloor E: Cystadenomes sereux et muqueux de l'ovaire a la limite de la malignite. Schweiz Med Wschr 110:531, 1980

32. Nikrui N: Survey of clinical behavior of patients with borderline epithelial tumors of the ovary. Gynecol Oncol 12:107, 1981

33. Tasker M, Langley FA: The outlook for women with borderline epithelial tumours of the ovary. Br J Obstet Gynaecol 92:969, 1985

34. Barnhill D, Heller P, Brzozowski P, et al: Epithelial ovarian carcinoma of low malignant potential. Obstet Gynecol 65:53, 1985

35. Kliman L, Rome RM, Fortune DW: Low malignant potential tumors of the ovary: A study of 76 cases. Obstet Gynecol 68:338, 1986

36. Nation JG, Krepart GV: Ovarian carcinoma of low malignant potential: Staging and treatment. Am J Obstet Gynecol 154:290, 1986

37. Bostwick DG, Tazelaar HD, Ballon SC, et al: Ovarian epithelial tumors of borderline malignancy. A clinical and pathologic study of 109 cases. Cancer 58:2052, 1986

38. Aalto ML, Clooan Y: Periodic acid-Schiff as a prognostic indicator in serous and mucinous ovarian tumors. Int J Gynaecol Obstet 24:27, 1986

39. Michael H, Roth LM: Invasive and noninvasive implants in ovarian serous tumors of low malignant potential. Cancer 57:1240, 1986

40. Russell P: Borderline epithelial tumours of the ovary: A conceptual dilemma. Clin Obstet Gynecol 11:259, 1984

41. Aure JC, Høeg K, Kolstad P: Clinical and histological studies of ovarian carcinoma. Long-term follow-up of 990 cases. Obstet Gynecol 37:1, 1971

42. Santesson L., Kottmeier HL: General classification of ovarian tumours. In Gentil F, Janqueira AC (eds): Ovarian Cancer. UICC Monograph Series, Volume 11. New York, Springer-Verlag, 1968, pp 1–8

43. Bjorkholm E, Pettersson F, Einhoen N, et al: Long-term follow-up and prognostic factors in ovarian carcinoma. The Radiumhemmet series 1958 to 1973. Acta Radiol Oncol 21:413, 1982

44. Scully RE: Tumors of the ovary and maldeveloped gonads. Atlas of Tumor Pathology, 2nd series, Fascicle 16. Washington, DC, Armed Forces Institute of Pathology, 1979
45. Bell DA, Rutgers JK, Scully RE: Ovarian epithelial tumors of borderline malignancy. In Damjanov I (ed): Progress in Reproductive and Genitourinary Pathology. New York, Field & Wood, 1989

Fine-Needle Aspiration in the Management of Breast Masses

Lester J. Layfield, Ben J. Glasgow, and Harvey Cramer

The management of recently discovered breast masses represents a significant clinical challenge and over 560,000 open breast biopsies are performed annually.[144] Standard clinical management dictates open biopsy of most recently discovered breast masses with 80 percent of resultant biopsies being benign.[144] Fine-needle aspiration cytology (FNA) may have a role in obviating some of these biopsies but its use in the United States has been hampered by concerns regarding diagnostic accuracy. False-negative rates are reported to be as high as 48 percent.[34,99,129,139] Some authors question the value of a negative cytology[18,40,41,138]; others recommend that all masses with benign cytological diagnoses be excised under local anesthesia.[2,64,93,106] The false-positive rates have ranged from 0 to 11 percent[6,91,106] and have resulted in controversy regarding the need for confirmatory open biopsy or premastectomy frozen section.[2,8,15,30,37,42,44,66-68,82,88,106,129,136,141,149] Several studies[19,30,73,104,125] have suggested that relatively few lesions are responsible for the majority of erroneous cytological diagnoses and increased awareness of the variable cytological appearances of these entities may improve the overall accuracy of FNA.

The combination of palpation, mammography, and FNA has been suggested as a diagnostic "triplet" to guide management of breast lesions.[10,26,53,59,77,78,80,124,132,135] Using this approach, breast lesions with three positive components of the triplet would undergo therapy while those patients with three negative studies could be clinically followed without open biopsy. Patients with other triplet combinations would undergo open biopsy. We reviewed the UCLA experience of 250 breast lesions that underwent FNA and subsequent open biopsy and reviewed 83 published series (63,000 breast aspirates) in an attempt to delineate diagnostic problems of breast FNA.

METHODS AND RESULTS

Between January 1981 and July of 1986 approximately 600 FNAs of palpable breast nodules were performed at the UCLA Medical Center using the technique of Zajicek.[87,151] Each lesion was aspirated two to three times; the material smeared on glass slides and air-dried or fixed in 95 percent ethanol for May-Grunwald-Giemsa or Papanicolau staining respectively. Histological follow-up was available for 250 of the cytological specimens.

Correlation between the cytological and histological findings is shown in Table 1. One hundred and forty-two lesions were histologically malignant cases and the remaining 108 cases were benign neoplastic, inflammatory, or proliferative lesions (Table 2). One hundred and twenty-two of the 142 histologically proven carcinomas (86 percent) were correctly identified as carcinoma by cytological examination. Eleven histologically proven carcinomas were cytologically suspicious for malignancy and seven were cytologically benign. Seven of the 250 FNAs were not satisfactory for evaluation. Two of these patients had breast carcinoma on surgical biopsy. The overall false-negative rate for FNA of breast lesions, including unsatisfactory aspirates, was 3.6 percent (2.9 percent excluding unsatisfactory specimens). A single false-positive diagnosis of carcinoma was made resulting in a false-positive rate of 0.4 percent. An intraoperative frozen section diagnosis of fat necrosis negated the need for further therapy. One additional case diagnosed on FNA as poorly differentiated carcinoma proved to be lymphocyte-depleted Hodgkin's disease on frozen section examination. The frozen section interpretation averted inappropriate therapy in this patient.

Correlation of lesion size at pathologic examination with cytological and histological diagnoses revealed that breast masses over 4 cm in diameter were more likely to be associated with false-negative diagnoses than were lesions 1 to 3 cm in diameter (Table 3).

TABLE 1. CYTOLOGICAL–HISTOLOGICAL CORRELATION OF THE 250 FINE-NEEDLE ASPIRATION CYTOLOGIES OF BREAST PERFORMED AT UCLA

	Histology				
	Benign		*Malignant*		
Cytology	*no.*	*(%)*	*no.*	*(%)*	Total
Benign	93	(93)	7	(7)	100
Suspicious	9	(45)	11	(55)	20
Malignant	1	(0.8)	122	(99.2)	123
Inadequate	5	(71)	2	(29)	7
Total	108	(43)	142	(57)	250

TABLE 2. CYTOLOGICAL CORRELATION WITH FINAL HISTOLOGICAL DIAGNOSIS FOR THE 250 FNAS PERFORMED AT UCLA

Cytological Diagnosis	Histological Findings on Open Biopsy														
	Lob[a]	Duc	LY	ML	FD	FA	FN	Pap	Hem	Mas	Lip	Gyn	Abs	Lya	CP
Ca[a]	9	109	1				1								
LY		2													
ML				1											
FD	1	5		1	44	9	1				1		1		
FA					5	12									1
FN							5								
Pap					1			2							
Hem					1				1						
Mas					1					1					
Lip											1				
Gyn												3			
Lac					1										
Nec					1										
NDC														1	
Sus	3	8			5	1	1			1				1	
Ina	1	1			3	1	1								

[a]Ca = carcinoma; LY = lymphoma; ML = melanoma; FD = fibrocystic disease; FA = fibroadenoma; FN = fat necrosis; Pap = papilloma; Hem = hematoma; Mas = mastitis; Lip = lipoma; Gyn = gynecomastia; Lac = lactational change; Nec = necrosis; NDC = no diagnostic change; Sus = suspicious; Ina = inadequate; Lob = lobular carcinoma; Duc = ductal carcinoma; Abs = abscess; Lya = lymphangioma; CP = benign cystosarcoma phyllodes.

SOURCES OF DIAGNOSTIC ERROR

Diagnostic errors in FNA may be caused by technical and interpretative mistakes. Technical difficulties generally result in an unsatisfactory specimen or a suboptimal preparation and usually are associated with false-negative diagnoses. Proper

TABLE 3. LESION SIZE AND DIAGNOSTIC ACCURACY

Cytology	Total Cases in Category	Mean Diameter of Lesions (S.D.)	Number of Cases Where Diameter Was Recorded
FNA positive	123	3.1(+/−0.4)	101
Malignant histology	122	3.1(+/−0.4)	100
Benign histology	1	4.5	1
FNA negative	100	2.5(+/−0.6)	65
Benign histology	93	2.4(+/−0.5)	60
Malignant histology	7	4.2(+/−0.7)	5
FNA unsatisfactory	7	2.6(+/−1.5)	6
Malignant histology	2	4.0(+/−1.0)	2
Benign histology	5	2.3(+/−1.4)	4

smear preparation and staining are important to avoid these errors. Proper smear and staining techniques have been well described.[39,104,131,152] Erroneous interpretation of adequately prepared smears is the most common reason for false-positive diagnoses and this frequently results from a failure to recognize the wide morphological spectrum many benign lesions possess. Familiarity with the cytological appearance of breast lesions and technical situations responsible for the majority of diagnostic errors should aid in improving the overall accuracy of breast FNA.

SOURCES OF FALSE-NEGATIVE DIAGNOSES

Technical difficulties are generally related to five variables: expertise, lesion size, circumscription, location, and cellular composition. Within our series, the size of the mass correlated with the presence of histologically documented cancer but not with the accuracy of the cytological examination. Breast masses associated with a false-negative diagnosis were generally 3 to 5 cm in diameter and did not vary significantly from the mean tumor diameter (3.1 cm) for carcinomas correctly diagnosed. In our material, large lesions (greater than 4 cm) were more likely to be the source of false-negative results than were smaller neoplasms (Table 3). Others who corroborated our experience, reported increased false-negative rates for tumors larger than 4 cm[7,150] due to large areas of necrosis, hemorrhage, or cystic degeneration. On the other hand, several series[5,24,27,33,44,51,73,77,79,80,98,106,112,113,145,150] reported that small malignant tumors were more likely to result in false-negative cytological diagnoses. Eisenberg et al[33] found that tumors less than 1 cm had a significantly higher rate of false-negative and unsatisfactory results than tumors between 2 and 3 cm. Other authors have reported similar results with neoplasms under 1 cm representing a large percentage of their false-negative reports.[5,24,27,33,44,73,79,81] Small tumors generally yielded fewer cells[53] with lesions 1 cm and less having false-negative rates within the range of 6[150] to 24 percent[106] while tumors between 2 and 3 cm were associated with false-negative rates of 3[150] to 6 percent.[106] From these data it may be concluded that lesions at the extreme ends of the size spectrum may be associated with increased false-negative rates. Finally, breast size is also an important factor since large breast size may prevent adequate palpation and sampling of underlying breast masses.[7,44,48,81] Grossly irregular or deep-seated masses may result in nonrepresentative aspirate specimens because the needle fails to enter the main bulk of the neoplasm.[27,44,51]

The cellular composition of the lesion is clearly a significant factor in sample acquisition. Several authorities have considered scirrhous tumors to be an important source of false-negative aspiration biopsies.[44,130,135] Marked desmoplasia in some breast adenocarcinomas may result in increased false-negative rates.[44,51,69,74,79,80,81,91,130,133] The tight fibrotic stroma is believed to inhibit the release of neoplastic cells.[46,135] At UCLA, smaller caliber needles (25 g) are used for all breast lesions suspected of having a markedly desmoplastic stroma. The smaller needle size may facilitate the removal of neoplastic cells due to enhanced cutting action of the needle. Predominately cystic lesions can cause false-negative FNA reports[114] because intracystic carcinomas may yield scanty partially degenerate material.[127]

Aspirator experience plays a significant role in achieving an acceptable frequency of false-negative breast FNA specimens. While the majority of the specimens in the present study were obtained by two cytopathologists performing over 500 aspirates per year, a small number of procedures were performed by less experienced aspirators (Table 4). Accuracy rates were lower for those who had performed fewer aspirates. Similar findings have been demonstrated for those performing thyroid needle aspirations.[55] A study of community clinicians, university hospital endocrinologists, and fine-needle aspiration cytopathologists demonstrated an inverse correlation between the number of aspirates performed (both total number and number performed per month) and the number of insufficient specimens. Community-based clinicians performing fewer aspirates had a significantly higher frequency of unsatisfactory specimens (32 percent than cytopathologists performing hundreds of aspirates per year (6.4 percent.) Dixon et al[27] compared unsatisfactory rates for breast aspirations in two different time periods. In the first period, the aspirates were performed by several individuals each doing only a few aspirates. In the second period, a single surgeon performed all aspirates. One quarter of all aspirates were unsatisfactory in the first period but only 3 of 280 aspirates performed by the single aspirator were unsatisfactory. Similarly, Lee et al[82] documented a technical failure rate of 9.8 percent for a single experienced aspirator and a 45.9 percent failure rate for a group of less experienced clinicians. Barrows et al[5] demonstrated that the physician performing the aspirate was the most important variable determining success in obtaining adequate material in their study of 689 women with primary breast carcinoma.

Interpretative errors appear to be less often responsible for false-negative results than are technical mistakes. In our material, there was only a single case reported to be cytologically benign, in which malignant cells were found on independent review. This patient had a well-differentiated adenocarcinoma with minimal cytological atypia and was studied relatively early in our series. Other authors have had similar experiences with most errors occurring early in their FNA experience.[7,77,128,142] Certain histological types of carcinoma appear to be associated with increased false-negative rates. Histologically well-differentiated

TABLE 4. CORRELATION OF ACCURACY WITH EXPERIENCE OF ASPIRATOR

	Cases (No.)	Total (%)	Overall Accuracy (%)
Cytopathologist #1	121	48	89
Cytopathologist #2	87	35	85
Cytopathologist #3	21	8	90
Total nonspecialists	21	8	67

adenocarcinomas lacking obvious malignant features appear to be more often associated with false-negative results than other histological types.[82,148,150] The bland nuclear cytology (Fig. 1) belies the malignant nature of the lesion. Consequently, tubular carcinoma has been associated with a disproportionate number of false-negative aspirates.[26,27,33,49,50,68,106] While the cytological appearance is frequently quite bland, the presence of angular microacini[33] and the lack of bipolar cells should suggest the diagnosis of adenocarcinoma (Table 5). Similar difficulties have been reported with lobular carcinoma, both in situ and invasive.[3,27,33,50,66,68,106,113,145] The small size and frequently bland appearance of cells (Fig. 2) obtained from these neoplasms often result in their underdiagnosis. The increased cellularity, absence of bipolar cells, "Indian file" clusters and magenta bodies should result in recognition of the malignant nature of these processes. Aspirates from intraductal carcinomas can result in false-negative diagnoses.[3,4,36,106] The small amount of tumor surrounded by relatively abundant stroma may cause sampling errors with few or no malignant cells being obtained. Comedocarcinomas with extensive necrosis may yield few recognizable tumor cells[7] obscured by necrotic debris. Several reports have noted a particularly high false-negative rate (42 percent) for colloid carcinomas[33,140] which may be due to dilution of the neoplastic cells by large volumes of mucin. Papillary carcinomas can result in false-negative dignoses.[106,130] Due to the difficulty in distinguishing

TABLE 5. DIFFERENTIAL DIAGNOSTIC FEATURES OF COMMON BREAST LESIONS

Lesion	Cellularity	Naked Nuclei	Necrosis	Dissociated Cells	Mitotic Rate	Nucleoli
Benign proliferative changes	Sparse to moderate	Numerous	Absent	Few	Rare	Rare Small
Fibroadenoma	Sparse to high	Numerous	Absent	Few	Absent	Rare Small
Radiation atypia	Sparse	Present	Rare	Moderate	Rare	Present Small
Fat necrosis	Moderate	Present	Prominent	Moderate	Rare	Present
Pregnancy	High	Abundant	Absent (except in infarct)	Moderate	Rare	Present
Lobular carcinoma	Low to moderate	Rare	Absent	Moderate	Rare	Absent
Tubular carcinoma	Low	Rare	Absent	Few	Rare	Absent
Ductal carcinoma[a]	High	Rare	Variable	Many	Present	Present
Colloid carcinoma	Moderate	Absent	Absent	Moderate Mucin present	Variable	Present

[a]Ductal carcinoma not otherwise specified both in situ and invasive.

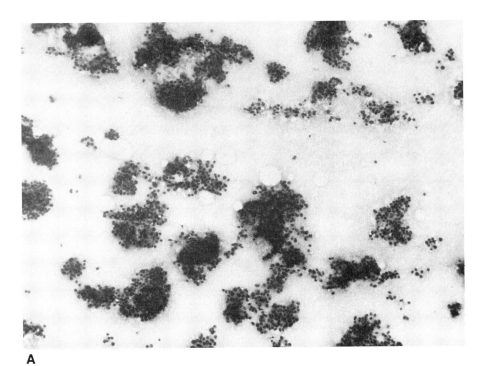

A

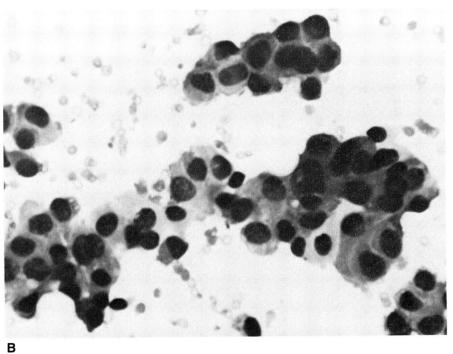

B

Figure 1. A. Well-differentiated adenocarcinoma demonstrating high cellularity. **B.** Note that single naked nuclei are infrequent. Within the epithelial sheets, the nuclei show mild variation in size and shape. (May-Grunwald-Giemsa ×40)

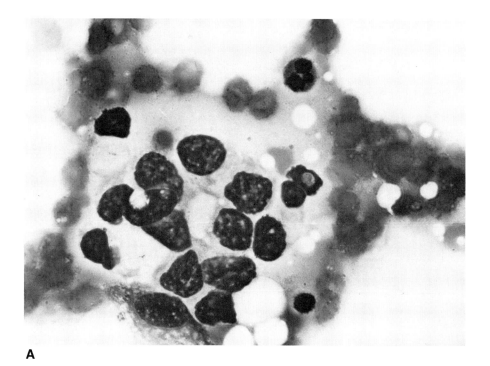

A

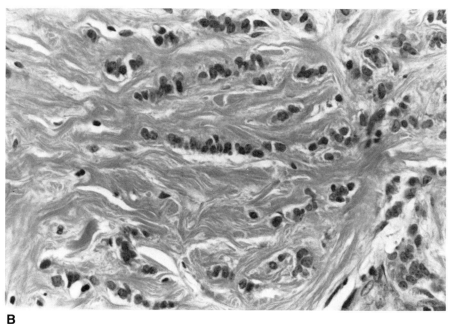

B

Figure 2.A. Fine-needle aspiration material from a lobular carcinoma of the breast. The specimen is composed of round epithelial cells with slightly enlarged nuclei surrounded by a small amount of cytoplasm. The cells are loosely cohesive with nuclei only slightly larger than the background erythrocytes. **B.** Histological section from a lobular carcinoma demonstrating single file strands of neoplastic cells invading the stroma. The individual cells are bland and of uniform appearance, (**A.** May-Grunwald-Giemsa ×630, **B.** H&E ×100)

these neoplasms from papillomas, it appears preferable to include these neoplasms in the diagnostic category of papillary neoplasm rather than attempt a definitive diagnosis in a needle aspiration specimen.

SOURCES OF FALSE-POSITIVE DIAGNOSIS

As with false-negative diagnoses, technical and interpretative errors are responsible for false-positive FNA results. Lesion size, shape, and composition are of less concern as causes of false-positive diagnoses than poor fixation and inadequate staining. Slow fixation with air drying of Papanicolau-stained specimens may result in ballooning of nuclei and incorrect interpretation of the nuclear enlargement as atypia (Fig. 3). Slow air drying of Giemsa-stained specimens may result in apparent nuclear enlargement and hyperchromasia creating suspicion of a malignant tumor for the unwary (Fig. 4). The smudged appearance of the nuclei and a background of red blood cells serve as markers for this artifact.

Within the literature, relatively few lesions were responsible for the majority of reported false-positive fine-needle aspirations (Table 6). In our material and that of others,[77,106] the majority of errors occurred early in the cytologists' experience.

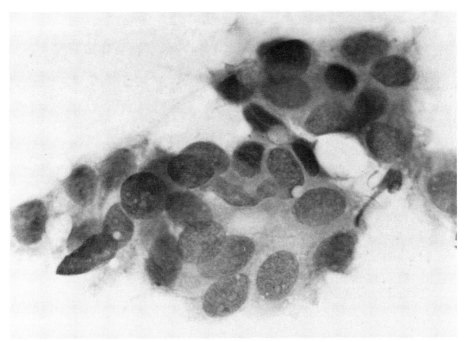

Figure 3. Ethanol-fixed and Papanicolau-stained smear of benign breast epithelium demonstrating nuclear enlargement and smudging due to inappropriate air drying. (Pap ×400)

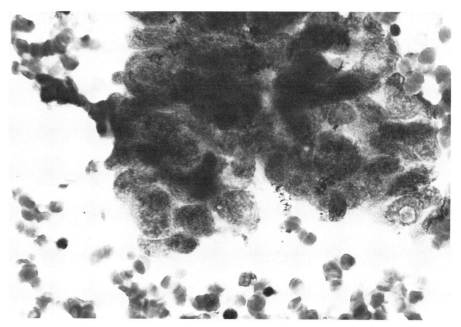

Figure 4. Ballooning degeneration and hyperchromasia secondary to slow drying of a May-Grunwald-Giemsa-stained smear. (MGG ×400)

Fibrocystic disease (mammary dysplasia) is responsible for the majority of false-positive diagnoses reported.[5,19,30,34,73,81,91,106,125,129,133,137,143,150,151] Our series confirms this because five of nine cytologically suspicious aspirates were shown on open biopsy to be benign proliferations within the spectrum of fibrocystic disease. Those who described the specific changes in fibrocystic disease responsible for false-positive diagnoses, most frequently reported apocrine metaplasia,[133] papillomatosis,[19,34] hyperplasia,[30,106] and atypical hyperplasia[5,73,129] as being associated with false-positive diagnoses. Increased cellularity, small but distinct nucleoli, and mild-to-moderate nuclear hyperchromasia (Fig. 5) can result in the interpretation of some of these proliferations as adenocarcinoma. The presence of bipolar cells scattered throughout the background along with interspersed small dark nuclei within the epithelial sheets should suggest the benign nature of the process (Fig. 6; Table 5).[76,92] Intraductal papillomatosis can be associated with large sheets of atypical epithelial cells and rare microacini-like structures but these smears generally contain bipolar cells and lack the high cellularity of most adenocarcinomas.

Fibroadenomas have also been a common cause of false-positive cytological reports[19,30,34,73,81,88,91,106,125,130,133,142,150] and they were responsible for two cytologically suspicious breast aspirates in our material. The high cellularity, large epithelial sheets with nuclear crowding, and occasional papillary structures can cause confusion with adenocarcinoma (Fig. 7). The distinction from adenocarci-

TABLE 6. LESIONS DESCRIBED IN THE LITERATURE ASSOCIATED WITH FALSE POSITIVE OR SUSPICIOUS DIAGNOSES

Lesion	References
Benign proliferations including atypical hyperplasia and papillomatosis	5,19,30,34,73,81,91,106,125,129,133,137, 143,150,151
Fibroadenoma	19,24,30,34,73,77,81,91,106,125,130,133, 142,150
Intraductal papilloma	72,73,77,91,92,94,95,137,143
Fat necrosis	7
Abscess and mastitis	7,51,88,133
Radiation change	9
Hematoma and granulation tissue	73,134
Tubular adenoma	73
Cystosarcoma	33,37
Gynecomastia	73
Galactocele	73
Pseudolymphoma	129

noma (Table 5) can be made by recognizing the uniformly bland nuclear cytology, "honeycomb" appearance, and blunt branching nature of the epithelial sheets in fibroadenomas (Fig. 8). Myoepithelial cells and naked nuclei are usually easily recognized in fibroadenomas[89,92] but are generally absent in adenocarcinomas. Fibroadenomas often contain many fragments of myxoid or loose fibrous tissue

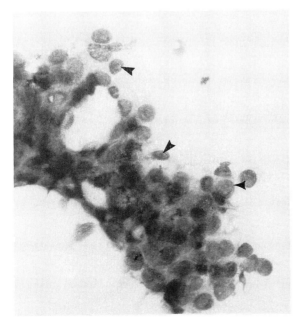

Figure 5. Aspirated material from an area of benign proliferative changes showing a cellular cluster. The individual cells have mild nuclear enlargement and hyperchromasia. Rare small but distinct nucleoli (*arrows*) are present. (Pap ×250)

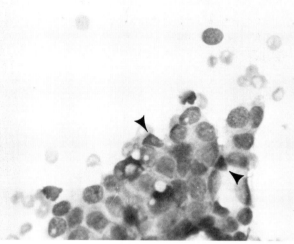

Figure 6. Cluster of cells aspirated from an area of benign proliferative changes. The cells contain oval nuclei with an open or fine chromatin pattern. Interspersed cells contain small dark nuclei (*arrows*). Naked nuclei are present within the background. (Pap ×250)

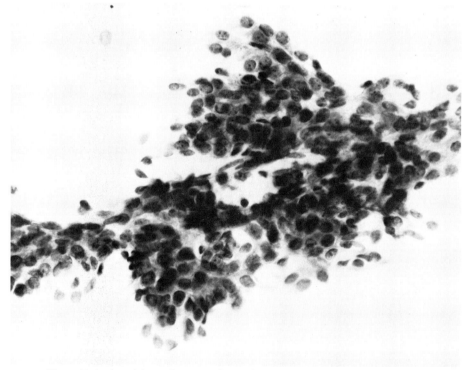

Figure 7. Aspirated tissue fragments from a fibroadenoma demonstrating nuclear crowding. The individual nuclei show mild nuclear enlargement and occasionally contain small but distinct nucleoli. (Pap ×250)

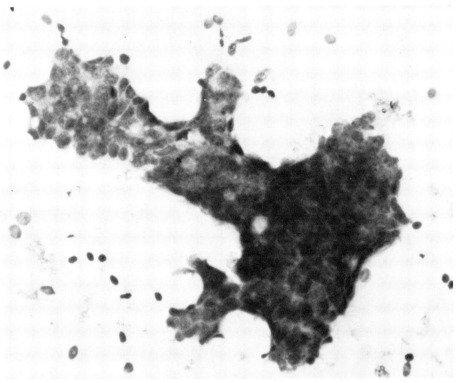

Figure 8. Epithelial cluster aspirated from a fibroadenoma. The cells form a tight aggregate with blunt branching "finger-like" protrusions. Note scattered bipolar cell nuclei in the background. (Pap ×250)

(Fig. 9) while adenocarcinomas contain only rare small fragments of fibrous stroma. Fibroadenomas in elderly patients may be clinically suspicious for carcinoma and cellular aspirates in postmenopausal patients are of concern but the bland nuclear features should alert the cytologist to the benign nature of these lesions. Fine-needle aspirates of edematous fibroadenomas may contain a prominent myxoid-watery background with scattered small clusters of epithelial cells mimicking the appearance of some colloid carcinomas (personal communication from P.P. Rosen, M.D.). The distinction between these two lesions can be achieved by recognizing the bipolar cells within the smears of fibroadenomas and the greater nuclear atypia generally present in the colloid carcinomas. Lactational changes can complicate the cytological appearance of fibroadenomas by increasing the cellularity of aspirates, producing moderate nuclear atypia, and increasing the prominence of nucleoli. The cellularity and vascularity of the stroma can be increased mimicking cystosarcoma phyllodes. Many fibroadenomas show focal epithelial atypia on histological section (Fig. 10) but the low power pattern renders their diagnosis straightforward. Cytological diagnosis of these same neoplasms may pose a significant hazard as the presence of cyto-

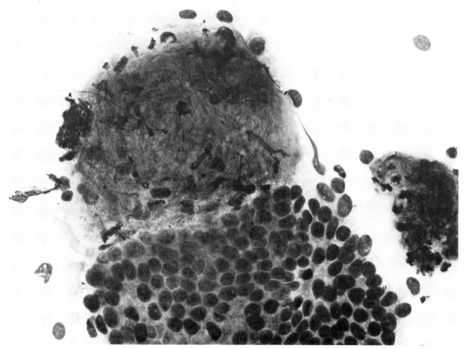

Figure 9. Aspirated tissue from a fibroadenoma demonstrating a core-like epithelial cluster composed of small nearly uniform cells. Immediately adjacent is a stromal fragment with bland oval nuclei. Occasional naked nuclei are present in the background. (May-Grunwald-Giemsa ×250)

logical atypia in the absence of the diagnostic architecture may result in their diagnosis as adenocarcinomas. Recognition of the tight cohesive "finger-like" clusters, regular rather uniform nuclei, scattered dark nuclei, and bipolar cells should suggest the benign nature of the process.

Inflammatory lesions of the breast have been reported as sources of false-positive diagnoses.[7,88,104] The single false-positive diagnosis within our series resulted from the overinterpretation of epithelial atypia and the misinterpretation of histiocytes in fat necrosis. Smears from fat necrosis are highly cellular with modest numbers of acute and chronic inflammatory cells. Occasional small sheets of epithelial cells are found which may show marked nuclear atypia, hyperchromasia, mitotic activity, and prominent nucleoli (Fig. 11). In addition, some histiocytes may contain enlarged vesicular nuclei with prominent nucleoli increasing the resemblance to adenocarcinoma (Fig. 12). The presence of inflammatory cells, free fat vacuoles, and few epithelial cells should distinguish this lesion from adenocarcinoma. Acute or granulomatous mastitis and breast abscesses have caused diagnostic difficulty.[7,88] These lesions may contain small cohesive sheets of epithelial cells with prominent reactive atypia and enlarged nucleoli (Fig. 13) resulting in the overdiagnosis of carcinoma. The presence of a heavy inflammatory cell infiltrate and the increased amount and spreading quality of the cytoplasm should alert the cytologist to the reactive nature of the atypia. Rarely, the presence of reactive fibroblasts and enlarged atypical histiocytes (Fig. 14) in organizing hematomas[134] and atypical granulation tissue[73] have resulted in erroneous diagnoses of malignancy. The paucity of epithelial cells may help avoid misdiagnosis in these aspirates.

Intraductal papilloma has been reported frequently as a cause of false-positive or suspicious diagnoses.[72,73,91,92,94,95,137,143] These neoplasms can be very cellular with large papillary clusters mimicking papillary carcinoma. As mentioned earlier, in the absence of marked nuclear atypia, papillary tumors should be designated as papillary neoplasms with a recommendation for open biopsy.

Less common lesions associated with false-positive or suspicious FNA diagnoses have included pseudolymphoma,[129] gynecomastia,[73] tubular adenoma,[73] galactocele,[73] granular cell tumor,[33,104] pregnancy,[72] and radiation change.[9] Radiation may induce marked atypia and cell dissociation within mammary epithelium (Fig. 15) resulting in its confusion with adenocarcinoma. The cells showing radiation atypia have a degenerative appearance with nuclear and cytoplasmic

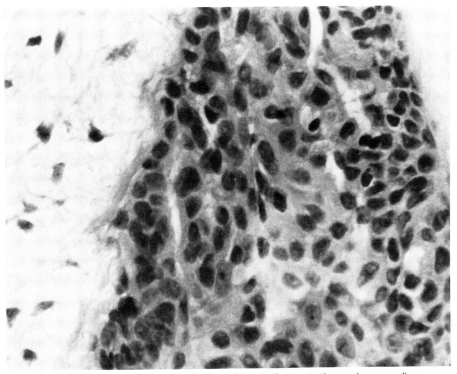

Figure 10. Histological section of a fibroadenoma demonstrating nuclear crowding, pleomorphism, and hyperchromasia of the epithelial component. (H&E ×400)

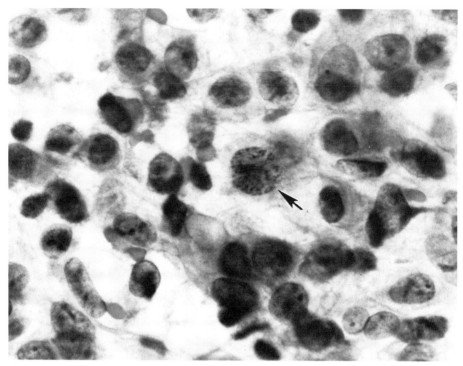

Figure 11. Aspirated tissue from an area of fat necrosis containing an epithelial sheet with marked nuclear enlargement, hyperchromasia, and crowding. Nucleoli are prominent. A single mitotic figure (*arrow*) is present. (Pap ×650)

enlargement. Cellularity is often scant with rare bipolar cells aiding in the differential diagnosis from adenocarcinoma. While tubular adenomas are highly cellular, their nuclear characteristics are bland and monotonous with scattered dark myoepithelial cells within the epithelial sheets and bipolar cells in the background.

Granular cell tumors may present with clinically and mammographically malignant features which when combined with this lesion's characteristic high cellularity on aspiration and prominent nucleoli can result in a misdiagnosis of carcinoma. The large number of cytoplasmic and dispersed background granules should alert one to the proper diagnosis.[90]

Gynecomastia may show mild nuclear enlargement and small nucleoli (Fig. 16) but lacks the cellularity and nuclear atypia of adenocarcinoma.

The pregnant patient with a breast infarct presents particular difficulties. Smears of these lesions show the abundant cellularity associated with pregnancy, the necrotic debris of an infarct, and the nuclear atypia and prominent nucleoli associated with both (Fig. 17). The reactive atypia is alarming but the clinical history of rapid onset and enlargement, pain, and pregnancy should suggest the correct interpretation.

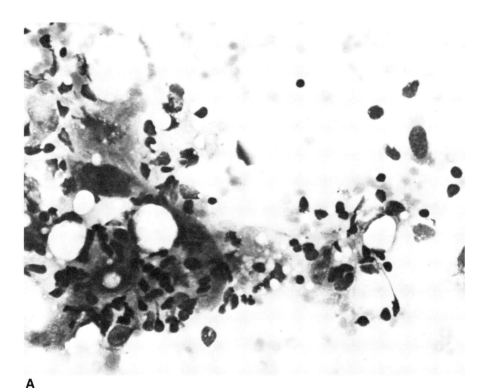

A

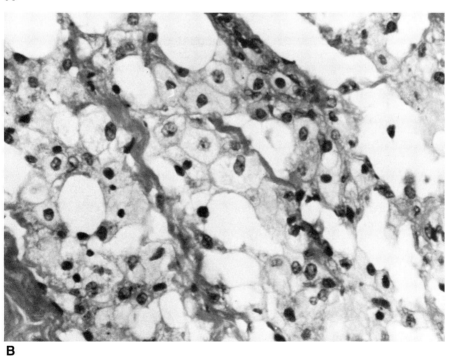

B

Figure 12.A. Atypical histiocytes with foamy cytoplasm associated with background lymphocytes and debris from an area of fat necrosis. **B.** Histological section from an area of fat necrosis demonstrates numerous histiocytes with abundant foamy cytoplasm and large vesicular nuclei with nucleoli. (**A.** May-Grunwald-Giemsa ×250, **B.** H&E ×250)

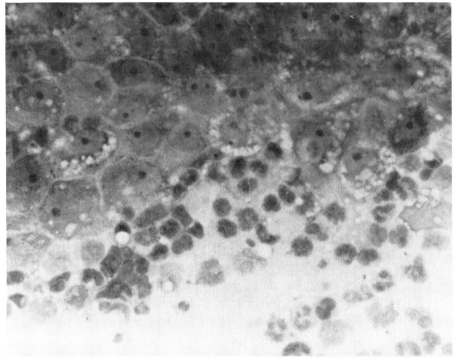

Figure 13. Aspirated tissue from a breast abscess containing a sheet of epithelial cells which show marked enlargement of the nuclei and prominent nucleoli. The epithelial cells lie in a syncitial pattern. Degenerating neutrophils are seen in the background. (May-Grunwald-Giemsa ×400)

Lymphomas of the breast are rare but their misinterpretation as high grade adenocarcinomas can result in inappropriate therapy. Atypical Reed–Sternberg cells and their variants can be prominent in lymphocyte-depleted Hodgkin's disease. These variant forms when associated with few background lymphocytes and no classic Reed–Sternberg cells can be confused with the cells of a poorly differentiated carcinoma. The young age of the patient in our case and the lack of cellular cohesion should have suggested the correct diagnosis. The distinction between large cell non-Hodgkin's lymphoma and high grade carcinoma can also be a problem. Specimens from such a lymphoma are generally very cellular and consist of a rather monomorphic population of neoplastic lymphoid cells.

DIAGNOSTIC ACCURACY AND THE "TRIPLE DIAGNOSIS" METHOD

Successful strategies for the preoperative management of breast masses require techniques with high diagnostic sensitivity and specificity. Diagnostic tests for breast lesions should detect nearly all carcinomas in an early phase of their

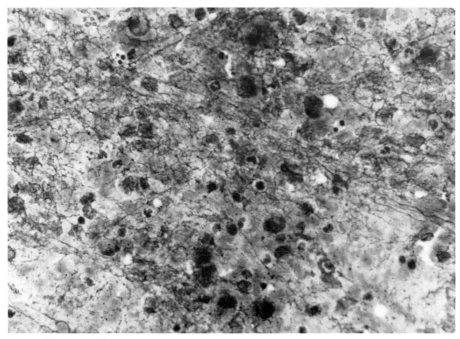

Figure 14. Cytological preparation from a hematoma containing degenerating histiocytes. The histiocytes show nuclear enlargement and atypia with smudging of the nuclear outline. (May-Grunwald-Giemsa ×100)

biologic evolution so that timely and appropriate therapy may be instituted. On the other hand, diagnostic methods with high false-positive rates may result in inappropriate therapy for benign breast lesions. Classic management of palpable noncystic breast masses dictates open biopsy but approximately 80 percent of these specimens will reveal benign changes.[144] While the high sensitivity of open biopsy is desirable, the low specificity of this procedure subjects some women to multiple operations. Alternate diagnostic techniques (palpation, mammography, and FNA) suffer from significant false-negative and false-positive rates but combinations of these methods may have sufficient diagnostic accuracy to substitute for open biopsy in many clinical situations (Table 7).

FALSE-NEGATIVE TEST RESULTS: RATES AND STRATEGIES FOR IMPROVED SENSITIVITY

Careful physical examination of all breast lesions is a mandatory part of a routine work-up but previous studies[20,52,80,83] indicate clinical diagnosis is inaccurate in as many as 20 to 40 percent of cases. Indeed, in our series, if palpation were the

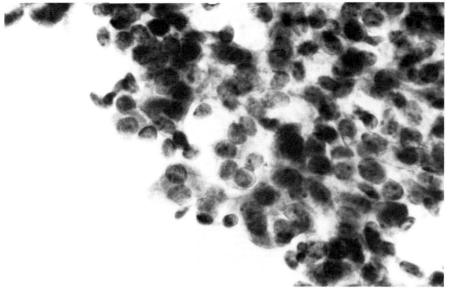

A

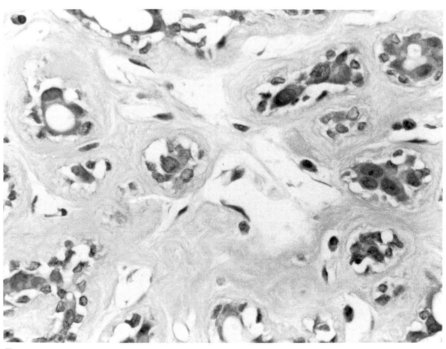

B

Figure 15.A. Epithelial cells demonstrating marked atypia secondary to radiation therapy. The cells have enlarged nuclei containing prominent nucleoli. The nuclei are hyperchromatic and often have indistinct margins. Differentiation from adeno-carcinoma can be extremely difficult. **B.** Histological section from an area of breast tissue showing radiation-induced atrophy and nuclear atypia. Some nuclei are enlarged, hyperchromatic, and have irregular borders. (**A.** Pap ×400, **B.** H&E ×250)

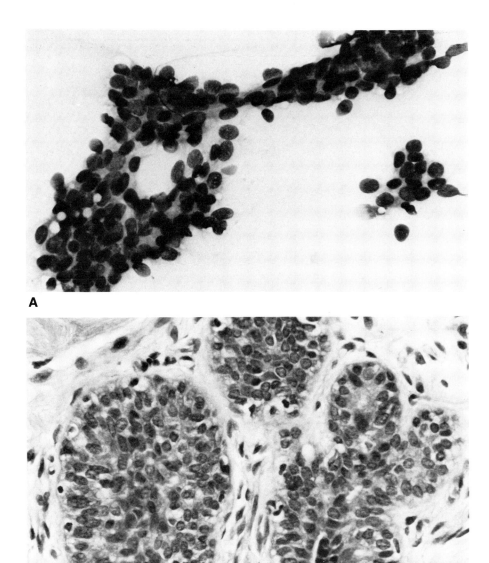

A

B

Figure 16.A. Bland but crowded epithelial cells from a patient with gynecomastia. The epithelial clusters are generally small and the total amount of material obtained at aspiration is usually scanty. Occasionally, nuclear enlargement and variation in size can be prominent but the presence of naked bipolar nuclei aids in the differentiation from adenocarcinoma. **B.** Microscopic section of a breast biopsy from a patient with gynecomastia. The epithelial cells are generally small with oval nuclei but some nuclear crowding is seen as is mild nuclear atypia. (**A.** May-Grunwald-Giemsa ×250, **B.** H&E ×250)

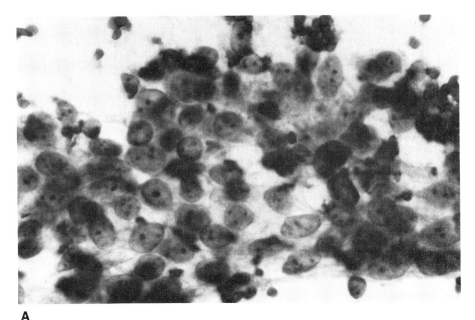

A

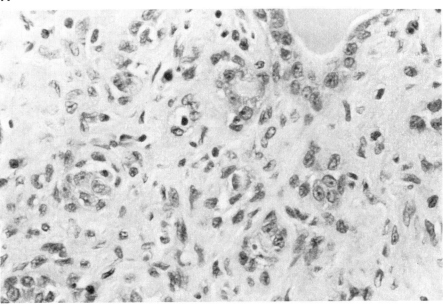

B

Figure 17.A. Aspirated tissue fragments from a pregnant patient with a breast infarct. The epithelial cells show marked nuclear enlargement with prominent nucleoli. The background contained a large amount of blood and cellular debris. In some areas of the smear (not shown) inflammatory cells were prominent. **B.** Histological section of tissue near an area of infarction in the breast of a pregnant patient. The tissue shows inflammatory cells surrounding glands composed of cells with enlarged hyperchromatic nuclei. (**A.** Pap ×400, **B.** H&E ×250)

sole criterion for open biopsy, 143 biopsies would have been performed but 25 cancers would not have been detected (false-negative rate of 17 percent). From these data, it is apparent that palpation failed to discover all patients with malignant tumors even though several open biopsies were performed on women not harboring carcinomas. This is in accord with prior studies reporting false-negative rates for clinical palpation of 3 to 38 percent.[13,28,43,80,109,132] In one series, one third of all carcinomas were nonpalpable.[86] If data from our material are pooled with three "triplet" studies[59,77,132] where complete figures are available (Tables 8 and 9), 9.4 percent of patients with benign physical findings harbored a carcinoma (Table 10). From these data, physical examination clearly has insufficient sensitivity to serve as the sole screening test for breast abnormalities.

Screening mammography has a sensitivity of 84 to 91 percent[29,103,119] but mammography performed on patients with palpable masses suspicious for carcinoma has been shown to be less sensitive, detecting only 78 percent of the cancers.[32] At UCLA, 191 of the 250 study patients had accompanying mammography. Only 9 of 20 carcinomas which were diagnosed as benign lesions by palpation were regarded as malignant by mammography. Twelve tumors correctly interpreted as malignant by palpation were considered benign by mammography. The false-negative rate for mammography in our material was 25.6 percent. Kreuzer and Boquoi[77] reported a false-negative rate of 3.3 percent for mammography but others have reported false-negative rates of up to 69 percent.[45,86,101,106] Indeed, Edeiken in his review of the literature found the sensitivity of mammography for palpable cancers to range from 42 to 87 percent.[32] Based on these data, he concluded that mammography was detrimental if used to avoid biopsy when a persistent mass was present and suggested that biopsy be performed on all undiagnosed persistent dominant masses.[32] The presently available data indicate that mammography alone is not sufficiently sensitive to negate the need for open biopsy of breast lesions which appear benign in mammograms.

Even though physical examination and mammography appear somewhat complementary with mammography being more accurate in women over 50 years of age and in those with large or fatty breasts while palpation is more accurate in younger women and in those with small or dense breasts,[35] the combination of physical examination and mammography failed to lead to the correct diagnosis of 19 carcinomas in 494 patients who had benign clinical and mammographic examinations (Table 9). In one series, the combination of mammography and palpation failed to correctly diagnose 33 percent of the carcinomas.[38] Even when used together, it appears that physical examination and mammography have insufficient sensitivity to replace open biopsy in the diagnosis of breast lesions.

While low cost screening mammography may improve the overall detection rate of breast carcinoma,[29,65,97,121] management of clinically and mammographically suspicious lesions requires a tissue diagnosis before definitive therapy can be undertaken. False-negative rates for FNA of breast lesions have varied widely within the literature ranging from 0 to 35 percent.[34,38,49,98,128,138] False-

TABLE 7. ACCURACY IN PREVIOUSLY PUBLISHED SERIES OF FNA OF THE BREAST

Author	# Cases	Cases with Histology		False (+) Cases		False (−) Cases		Unsatisfactory Cases	
		No.	(%)	No.	(%)a	No.	(%)a	No.	(%)b
Adye[2]	140	140		0	(7)c	5	(4)	NGd	
Aretz[3]	329	190	(58)	0	(9)c	14	(7)	35	(11)
Azzaselli[4]	1498	1138	(76)	3	(0.3)	65	(6)	375	(25)
Barrows[5]	1283	1283		2	(0.1)	48	(4)	273	(21)
Bell[6]	1680	584	(35)	0		27	(5)	230	(14)
Biedrzycki[7]	1438	593	(41)	1	(0.2)	44	(7)	22	(2)
Boquoi[10]	860	860		4	(0.5)	41	(5)	NG	
Coleman[16]	347	NG		4		9			(4)
Cornillot[17]	2267	1335	(59)	15	(1)	162	(12)	NG	
Davies[19]	131	131		5	(4)	46	(35)	41	
Degrell[21]	310	310		96% accuracy				NG	
Deschenes[22]	2050	405	(20)	0	(16)c	9	(2)	277	(68)
Devitt[24]	100	100		0	(1)c	11	(4)	2	(2)
DiPietro[25]	534	454	(85)	0	(14)c	34	(7)	98	(18)
Dixon[26]	1655	680	(41)	0	(16)c	24	(4)	110	(7)
Dua[30]	865	63	(7)	3	(12)c	15		NG	
Duguid[31]	294	NG		0	(18)c	2		37	
Eisenberg[33]	1942	1627	(84)	0		212	(13)	298	(15)
Elston[34]	163	163		5	(3)	51	(31)	NG	
Frable[37]	853	NG		1	(13)c	27		46	(5)

Frazier[38]	38	38		0		0		0	0
Furnival[42]	237	237		2	(1)	5	(3)	59	(25)
Gardecki[44]	444	242	(54)	0	(6)c	6	(2.5)	108	(24)
Geier[47]	974	NG		6		4		NG	
Glant[48]	523	244	(47)	8	(3)	6	(2.5)	15	(3)
Griffith[50]	335	236	(71)	0	(15)c	16	(7)	NG	
Gupta[51]	613	152	(25)	1	(0.6)(1)c	2	(1)	63	(10)
Hahn[53]	179	179		88% accuracy				NG	
Hajdu[54]	456	456		0		64 neg. or unsat.			
Hammond[56,57]	678	159	(23)	1	(0.6)	4	(3)	17	(11)
Hermansen[58]	292	222	(76)	0	(5)c	6	(3)	7	(2)
Hermansen[59]	650	465	(72)	0	(13)c	12	(3)	7	(1)
Hindle[60]	1196	206	(17)	0		11	(5)	NG	
Joffe[64]	30	30		0		0		0	
Kambouris[66]	38	35	(92)	0	(1)c	1	(3)	4	(10)
Kaufman[67]	480	163	(34)	1	(0.6)	1	(0.6)	87	(18)
Kern[68]	161	161		0	(8)c	19	(12)	NG	
Kher[69]	80	80		0		2	(3)	3	(4)
Kline[72]	4241	1286	(30)	61c		NG		NG	
Kline[73]	3545	1103	(31)	60c		35	(3)	NG	
Knox[74]	200	130	(65)	0		3	(2)	28	(14)
Koivuniemi[75]	503	503		0	(27)c	21	(4)	46	(9)
Kreuzer[77]	602	602		4	(0.6)	33	(5)	NG	
Lange[80]	714	367	(61)	11	(3)	27	(7)	NG	

(Continued)

TABLE 7. Continued

Author	# Cases	Cases with Histology		False (+) Cases		False (−) Cases		Unsatisfactory Cases	
		No.	(%)	No.	(%)[a]	No.	(%)[a]	No.	(%)[b]
Lange[81]	128	73	(57)	2	(3)	5	(7)	NG	
Lee[82]	503	169	(34)	0		13	(8)	54	(11)
Marasa[91]	328	328		4	(1)[16][c]	10	(3)	40	(12)
McSwain[94]	595 (cysts)	NG		1		1		NG	
Manheimer[95]	221	127	(57)	0	(2)[c]	11	(9)	NG	
Masukawa[96]	94	94		0		2	(2)	35	(37)
Murad[98]	292	96	(33)	0		3	(2)	98	(17)
Murrell[99]	31	NG		0		10		3	(10)
Norton[102]	49	49		0	(5)[c]	1	(2)	18	(37)
Padarha[105]	92	57	(62)	0		1	(2)	5	(5)
Pilotti[106]	4834	1173	(24)	2	(0.1)	63	(5)	362	(7)
Rajcic[108]	2890	1759	(61)	0	(20)[c]	0		91	(3)
Rimsten[109]	984	381	(39)	0		4	(1)	NG	
Rosen[112]	208	206	(99)	0		32	(16)	NG	
Russ[113]	257	143	(56)	0	(16)[c]	8	(6)	18	(7)
Schondorf[115]	1400	396	(28)	3	(0.8)	51	(13)	NG	
Shabot[117]	81	81		0		1	(1)	3	(4)
Shiller-Vokova[118]	263	165	(63)	4	(2)	44	(27)	NG	
Silver[122]	387	NG		NG	(2)[c]	6		9	(2)
Silverman[123]	219	93		0		4	(4)	15	(7)

Smallwood[124]	480	480		0		6	(1)	117	(24)
Smith[124]	100	100		3	(3)	8	(8)	NG	NG
Stavric[128]	250	250		2	(0.8)	5	(2)	NG	NG
Strawbridge[129]	3724	890	(24)	3	(0.3)	46	(5)	1205	(32)
Thomas[132]	196	196		4	(2)	0		37	(14)
Tribe[133]	311	311		2	(0.6)	16	(5)	NG	NG
Ulanow[134]	449	318	(71)	1	(0.3)	19	(6)	36	(8)
Van Bogaert[135]	164	34	(21)	0	(9)c	6	(18)	4	(2)
Vilaplana[137]	660	406	(62)	5	(1)	7	(2)	28	(4)
Wanebo[140]	398	247	(62)	0		1	(0.4)	38	(10)
Webb[142]	168	108	(64)	1	(0.9)	1	(0.9)	NG	NG
Wilson[143]	1792	322	(18)	2	(0.6)	15	(5)	734	(41)
Winchester[144]	158	158		9	(5.5)	8	(5)	NG	NG
Winship[145]	487	487		0		33	(7)	NG	NG
Wollenberg[147,148]	321	184	(57)	0		28	(15)	14	(4)
Zajdela[150]	2772	2772		3	(0.1)	63	(2)	155	(6)
Zajicek[151]	2111	2111		1	(0.05)	73	(4)	168	(8)
Zajicek[152]	2200	1220	(55)	0	(19)c	72	(6)	NG	NG

a % of cases with histology.

b % of total cases.

c Cases reported as cytologically suspicious for malignancy but histologically benign.

NG = Not Given

TABLE 8. TRIPLET RESULTS FROM THE UCLA SERIES

Physical Exam	Mammogram	FNA	# Cases	Histological Diagnosis Malignant	Benign
B[a]	B	B	47	1	46
M	M	M	36	36	0
S	M	M	15	15	0
M	S	M	10	9	1
M	S	B	8	6	2
S	S	M	8	8	0
B	M	M	8	8	0
M	B	M	7	7	0
B	B	M	7	7	0
M	B	S	6	6	0
M	S	S	3	3	0
S	M	B	3	1	2
S	B	M	3	3	0
M	M	B	2	0	2
S	M	S	2	1	1
M	M	S	1	1	0
B	M	B	1	0	1
B	S	M	1	1	0
M	B	B	0	0	0
S	S	S	0	0	0
S	S	B	0	0	0
S	B	S	0	0	0
S	B	B	0	0	0
B	M	S	0	0	0
B	S	S	0	0	0
B	S	B	0	0	0
B	B	S	0	0	0

[a]B = benign; S = suspicious; M = malignant.

negative rates at the higher end of the spectrum suggest that FNA is unacceptable as a substitute for open biopsy in the diagnosis of mammary carcinoma[87] and some authors continue to recommend open biopsy of all breast lesions with benign cytological reports. [2,64,80,92,106] Our false-negative rate was 3.6 percent indicating a significant potential for undiagnosed breast carcinoma if further diagnostic modalities are not used. More importantly, our data and that of Hermansen et al,[59] Kreuzer et al,[77] and Thomas et al[132] show that 2 percent of the 613 patients with benign physical and cytological examinations would have had undetected carcinoma if only palpation and FNA were used for diagnosis (Table 10).

The value of mammography as an adjunct to clinical palpation and FNA examination is not clear from the available literature. Thomas et al[132] stated that xeromammography was not a useful adjunct to the combination of aspiration cytology and physical examination for palpable breast lesions. In their material, xeromammography failed to diagnose any of four histologically confirmed carcinomas reported as benign by aspiration cytology. In contrast, Kreuzer et al[77] showed that mammography was positive in three and suspicious in four of eight carcinomas reported as benign by both cytology and physical examination. Similarly, Hermansen et al[59] demonstrated suspicious mammographic findings

TABLE 9. COMBINED TRIPLET RESULTS FROM THE UCLA EXPERIENCE AND THE LITERATURE[59,77,132]

Physical Exam	Mammography	FNA	# Cases	Histological Diagnosis	
				Malignant	*Benign*
B[a]	B	B	475	3	472
M	M	M	239	238	1
B	S	B	146	6	140
S	M	M	81	80	1
S	B	B	67	3	64
S	S	B	47	2	45
M	S	M	33	32	1
B	S	S	28	7	21
S	S	M	26	25	1
B	B	S	25	4	21
M	M	B	24	21	3
M	M	S	23	21	2
B	M	M	18	18	0
M	B	B	17	3	14
S	M	B	16	10	6
S	S	S	14	7	7
M	B	M	12	12	0
S	M	S	12	11	1
B	B	M	12	12	0
M	S	B	11	2	9
S	B	S	11	3	8
M	S	S	10	8	2
B	M	B	10	3	7
B	S	M	10	10	0
S	B	M	7	6	1
B	M	S	6	4	2
M	B	S	5	4	1
Totals			1385	1 false +	3 false −

[a]M = malignant; S = suspicious; B = benign.

TABLE 10. EXAMINATION OUTCOME IN PATIENTS WITH A BENIGN PHYSICAL EXAMINATION[59,77,132]

	Benign Physical Examination 712 (9.4%)[a]	
Benign Cytology 613 (2%)	**Suspicious Cytology** 59 (25%)	**Malignant Cytology** 40 (100%)
	Mammography	
Benign: 457 (0.7%) Suspicious: 146 (4%) Malignant: 10 (30%)	Benign: 25 (16%) Suspicious: 28 (25%) Malignant: 6 (67%)	Benign: 0 Suspicious: 0 Malignant: 40 (100%)

[a]Number in parentheses indicates percentage of patients in whom histological examination demonstrated adenocarcinoma.

in both carcinomas reported as benign by the combination of FNA and physical examination. Logistic regression analysis of our data combined with that of Hermansen et al,[59] Kreuzer et al,[77] and Thomas et al[132] demonstrated that FNA is the most predictive test for the nature of a breast mass (p > .001) but mammography significantly increases diagnostic sensitivity for breast carcinoma in the group of patients where both FNA and physical examination are falsely benign (Table 10). In the group of ten patients with benign physical examinations and FNAs but malignant mammograms, 30 percent proved to harbor carcinoma on open biopsy (Table 10). While the actual number of patients identified by mammography who require open biopsy is small, the percentage of these patients with carcinoma is significant indicating that mammography is an important component in the preoperative diagnosis of breast lesions.

The diagnostic triplet of palpation, mammography, and FNA was introduced to improve the overall accuracy of prebiopsy diagnosis of breast masses. While each technique has limitations and diagnostic biases, many authors have found the combination of the three methods to have high diagnostic sensitivity and specificity.[10,26,53,59,77,78,80,132,135] Some authors report no false-negative triplet results.[26,58,59] We encountered a single false-negative triplet (Table 8) and others have corroborated our findings of occasional false-negative triplets.[10,25,53,77,78] In fact, in the combined data (Tables 9 and 10), 3 of 457 (0.7 percent) patients with benign triplets demonstrated adenocarcinoma on open biopsy. Nonetheless, the "triple diagnosis" method appears to have a high diagnostic sensitivity and many authors conclude that when all three tests are benign open biopsy is unnecessary and the patient may be followed by simple observation.[59,77,78] Using this protocol, Hermansen et al[59] could have avoided open biopsy in 282 (43 percent) of their patients presenting with a breast mass. We believe, patients with discordant triplet results should undergo open biopsy. Careful palpation and FNA can be performed at the initial patient visit followed by mammography which should be at least 2 weeks later to avoid a false-positive mammogram secondary to FNA hematoma.[71,120] The management of patients with negative triplet results is less clear. The triplet protocol would leave undetected approximately 2 cancers in every 100 women with negative triplets. We believe that the majority of persistent dominant breast masses should be subjected to surgical biopsy regardless of triplet results.

FALSE-POSITIVE TEST RESULTS: RATES AND STRATEGIES FOR IMPROVED SPECIFICITY

Physical examination also has a false-positive rate with five patients within the UCLA study having malignant clinical findings but benign diagnoses on open biopsy. Similarly, 33 patients in the combined series (Table 9) had false-positive clinical examinations. In our data, mammography was responsible for 6 false-positive diagnoses occurring among the 191 patients studied with that method. The combination of palpation and mammography was more specific than either method alone since only two patients had clinical and mammographic studies interpreted as malignant but benign findings on open biopsy (Table 8). The 1 percent false-positive rate associated with the combined use of mammography and palpation appears too high for interpretations based on these techniques to substitute for open biopsy.

Since false-positive FNA diagnoses can lead to inappropriate radical surgery if cytology is used as the sole criterion for therapy, considerable discussion has appeared in the literature concerning the proper management of patients with positive FNA diagnoses. Some authorities[8,15,30,34,61,80,129,132] believe the FNA diagnosis of carcinoma must be comfirmed by open biopsy or intraoperative frozen section, while others suggest that mastectomy may be performed on the basis of a cytological diagnosis of carcinoma in the appropriate clinical setting.[25,33,37,44,67,68,82,106,116,151] False-positive rates reported in the literature have varied from 0 to 11 percent[6,90,106] with false-positive rates as high as 20 percent described for cystic lesions.[110] Our series included a single false-positive diagnosis (0.4 percent of total cases) which occurred early in our experience. An additional nine cases (3.6 percent) were considered cytologically suspicious for carcinoma prompting open biopsy which disclosed benign disease. Similarly, if our data were combined with those of Hermansen et al,[59] Kreuzer et al,[77] and Thomas et al[132] (Table 9), 5 of 438 cytological diagnoses of adenocarcinoma would have been falsely positive. This represents a 1 percent false-positive rate which could translate into unnecessary radical surgery in 1 percent of women referred for mastectomy if cytology were the sole basis for therapy. Clinical examination was benign or equivocal in all but two of these patients (Table 9) indicating the value of combining FNA and palpation in the decision algorithm.

The triple diagnosis protocol was developed to improve the overall specificity of the nonoperative management of breast masses. Each component of the triplet has a significant false-positive rate but it has been proposed that the combination of the three methods is sufficiently specific to allow definitive therapy to be based on a positive triplet.[59,77,78] Using the above protocol, mammography would be performed on all patients in whom the initial clinical and FNA examinations were positive for carcinoma and these patients could be referred for definitive therapy following a positive mammogram. When all three tests are in agreement, the "diagnostic triplet" has a high degree of accuracy with some authors reporting no false-positive results.[58,59,132] While our experience has been similar (Table 8), some authors have reported false-positive combinations.[25,77,78] In the combined data of UCLA, Hermansen,[59] Kreuzer,[77] and Thomas[132] (Table 9), only 1 false-positive triplet was encountered in 1367 patients (1 error in 239 positive triplet results). The combination of all three methods more accurately predicts the nature of a breast lesion than any one or two of the methods alone and some authors conclude that when all three tests are positive for carcinoma definitive therapy can be undertaken.[59,77,78] Due to the false-positive rate (0.07 percent in the combined data) of triplet diagnosis, we believe that a confirmatory intraoperative frozen section is desirable before mastectomy is performed. FNA diagnosis allows earlier and more definitive consultation before operative management is begun. FNA may also be of value in patients with clinically malignant breast lesions who wish a minimally invasive and inexpensive confirmatory test before submitting to open biopsy or intraoperative frozen section examination. In this context, FNA with a higher sensitivity and specificity appears to be superior to mammography.

FNA IN COMPARISON TO OTHER BIOPSY METHODS

Few comparative studies of FNA and Tru-Cut needle biopsies exist. Shabot et al[117] reported that aspiration cytology was superior to Tru-Cut needle biopsy with FNA being diagnostic in 96 percent and needle biopsy diagnostic in only 79 percent of cases. Elston et al[34] reported significantly different results with a correct positive diagnosis by Tru-Cut biopsy in 73.5 percent of cases but in only 52 percent of cases by FNA. Our experience has been limited, but we have found needle aspiration cytology to be a more sensitive test for the presence of carcinoma than Tru-Cut needle biopsy. In a group of eight patients undergoing FNA and needle biopsy, no false-positive diagnoses were obtained with either method. While FNA successfully identified all six carcinomas, Tru-Cut needle biopsy was associated with two false-negative diagnoses.

   The frozen section method is known to have a high diagnostic reliability with false-negative rates ranging from 0.3[11] to 1.66 percent[36] and reported false-positive rates between 0[12] and .09 percent[100] (Table 11). In our material, frozen sections were performed in 167 cases after FNA. One (0.6 percent) false-positive frozen section diagnosis was obtained, four frozen section diagnoses were deferred to permanent section evaluation, and one (0.6 percent) false-negative diagnosis was reported. In the same group of patients, a single false-positive FNA was obtained and five cases were cytologically suspicious for carcinoma but benign on frozen and permanent sections. In no case were the FNA and frozen section diagnoses both falsely positive.

TABLE 11. FROZEN SECTION RELIABILITY IN THE DIAGNOSIS OF BREAST LESIONS AS REPORTED IN SELECTED SERIES FROM THE LITERATURE

Author	No. of Cases	False Negatives		False Positives	
		No.	%	*No.*	%
Jennings[63]	212	2	0.95	0	
Pitts et al[107]	327	0		0	
Winship[146]	1004	8	0.8	0	
Ackerman[1]	440	4	0.9	0	
Sparkman[126]	571	0		0	
Desai[23]	1006	6	0.6	0	
Nakazawa[100]	1001	7	0.7	1	0.09
Lerman[84]	1085	10	0.9	0	
Holaday[62]	1616	8	0.5	1	0.06
Lessells[85]	2197	13	0.6	1	0.04
Rosen[111]	556	8	1.4	0	
Clemente[14]	1416	15	1.1	0	
Fessia[36]	4436	74	1.7	0	
Totals	15867	155	0.9	3	0.01

SUMMARY

The exact role of FNA in the diagnosis of palpable breast lesions is still uncertain. False-positive and false-negative cytological diagnoses occur and raise questions regarding the diagnostic utility of FNA as a replacement for open biopsy in many clinical situations. False-positive diagnoses may result from atypical epithelial proliferations, fibroadenomas, or inflammatory lesions. False-negative aspirates may occur because of technical errors, cystic lesions, and underdiagnosis of low grade neoplasms. The triple diagnosis protocol has been suggested as a replacement for open biopsy of palpable breast masses in many clinical situations. Following this algorithm, the results of palpation, mammography, and cytology are combined to guide management. Mammography should precede FNA or follow the cytologic procedure by 2 or more weeks.[71,120] Patients with a positive triple diagnosis should undergo open biopsy or confirmatory intraoperative frozen section. Positive FNA results would be useful for preoperative counselling as well as serving as a diagnostic procedure for clinically suspicious lesions in patients wishing a confirmatory test before open biopsy is performed. Patients with discordant triplet results should be referred for open biopsy. The management of patients with negative triplet results is less clear. From the available data, it appears that approximately 2 percent of patients with negative triplet results have carcinoma. Based on these results, we cannot recommend replacing open biopsy by the triple diagnosis method in most patients with a persistent dominant mass. In most cases, a biopsy is indicated. Surgeons, who plan to follow a breast mass with clinical examination, may be able to reduce their false-negative rate by performing FNA. Further study is necessary to establish the best way to use FNA in the diagnosis of breast carcinoma, to determine the cost effectiveness of the triple diagnosis method as a substitute for open biopsy, and to assess the utility of aspiration cytology in the mammographically directed diagnosis of nonpalpable breast lesions.

REFERENCES

1. Ackerman LV, Ramirez GA: The indications and limitations of frozen section diagnosis. Br J Surg 46:336, 1959
2. Adye B, Jolly PC, Bauermeister DE: The role of fine-needle aspiration in the management of solid breast masses. Arch Surg 123:37, 1988
3. Aretz HT, Silverman ML, Kolodziejski JL, Witherspoon BR: Fine-needle aspiration. Why it deserves another look. Postgrad Med 75:49, 1984
4. Azzaselli A, Guzzon A, Pilotti S, et al: Accuracy of breast cancer diagnosis by physical, radiologic and cytologic combined examinations. Tumori 69:137, 1983
5. Barrows GH, Anderson TJ, Lamb JL, Dixon JM: Fine-needle aspiration of breast cancer. Relationship of clinical factors to cytology results in 689 primary malignancies. Cancer 58:1493, 1986
6. Bell DA, Hajdu Sl, Urban JA, Gaston JP: Role of aspiration cytology in the diagnosis and management of mammary lesions in office practice. Cancer 51:1182, 1983
7. Biedrzycki T, Dabska M, Sikorowa L, Kubicki T: On cytologic vagaries in the diagnosis of breast tumors. Tumori 66:191, 1980
8. Blumgart LH, Hughes HE: Aspiration cytology in breast cancer. Lancet Nov 22:1033, 1975
9. Bondeson L: Aspiration cytology of radiation-induced changes of normal breast epithelium. Acta Cytol 31:309, 1987
10 Boquoi E, Kreuzer G: Die stellung der feinnadelbiopsie in rahmen der modernen mammadiagnostik. Arch Geschwulstforsch 47:616, 1977
11. Bredhal E, Simonsen J: Routine performance of intraoperative frozen section microscopy, with particular reference to diagnostic accuracy. Acta Pathol Microbiol Scand (suppl) 212:104, 1970
12. Breuer MJ: Frozen-section biopsy at operation. Am J Clin Pathol 8:153, 1938
13. Cardona G, Cataliotti L, Ciatto S, Del Turco MR: Reasons for failure of physical examination in breast cancer detection (analysis of 232 false-negative cases). Tumori 69:531, 1983
14. Clemente C, Pilotti S, Cattaneo M, Rilke F: Valutazione statistica della diagnosi istopatologica intraoperatoria su sezioni al microtomo criostato. Pathologica 73:561, 1981
15. Coleman DV: Aspiration cytology in preoperative management of breast cancer. Lancet 2:1083, 1980
16. Coleman DV: Cytologic screening for cancer of the breast. Proc Roy Soc med 69:494, 1976
17. Cornillot M, Verhaeghe M, Cappelaere P, Clay A: Place de la cytologie par ponction dans le diagnostic des tumeurs du sein. Presse Med 79:1813, 1971
18. Curling M: Part 2. Fine needle aspiration of breast lesions. The Practitioner 229:221, 1985

19. Davies CJ, Elston CW, Cotton RE, Blamey RW: Preoperative diagnosis in carcinoma of the breast. Br J Surg 64:326, 1977
20. Degrell I: Needle-biopsy cytology in the preoperative diagnosis of breast diseases. Acta Morphol Acad Sci Hung 28:297, 1980
21. Degrell I: Aspiration cytology of breast carcinoma. Acta Morphol Acad Sci Hung 30:277, 1982
22. Deschenes L, Fabia J, Meisels A, et al: Fine needle aspiration biopsy in the management of palpable breast lesions. Can J Surg 21:417, 1978
23. Desia SB: Uses and limitations of frozen section in diagnosis of lesions of the breast. Br J Surg 53:1038, 1966
24. Devitt JE, Curry RH: Role of aspiration breast biopsy. Can J Surg 20:450, 1977
25. Di Pietro S, Fariselli G, Bandieramonte G, et al: Systematic use of the clinical-mammographic-cytologic triplet for the early diagnosis of mammary carcinoma. Tumori 71:179, 1985
26. Dixon JM, Anderson TJ, Lamb J, et al: Fine needle aspiration cytology, its relationships to clinical examination and mammography in the diagnosis of a solid breast mass. Br J Surg 71:593, 1984
27. Dixon JM, Lamb J, Anderson TJ: Fine needle aspiration of the breast: Importance of the operator. Lancet 2:564, 1983
28. Dobreva PV, Kirov SM: Results from fine-needle biopsy in diagnosis of breast lesions. Acta Cytol 25:91, 1981
29. Dodd GD: The major issues in screening mammography. The history and present status of radiographic screening for breast carcinoma. Cancer 60(suppl):1671, 1987
30. Dua NK, Montana J, Sirkin B, Singh J: Aspiration cytology of the breast: An analysis of 865 cases. NY State J Med 83:867, 1983
31. Duguid HL, Wood RAB, Irving AD, et al: Needle aspiration of the breast with immediate reporting of material. Br Med J 2:185, 1979
32. Edeiken S: Mammography and palpable cancer of the breast. Cancer 61:263, 1988
33. Eisenberg AJ, Hajdu SI, Wilhelms J, et al: Preoperative aspiration cytology of breast tumors. Acta cytol 30:135, 1986
34. Elston CW, Cotton RE, Davies CJ, Blamey RW: A comparison of the use of the "Tru-Cut" needle and fine needle aspiration cytology in the pre-operative diagnosis of carcinoma of the breast. Histopathology 2:239, 1978
35. Feig SA, Shaber GS, Pathchefsky A, et al: Analysis of clinically occult and mammographically occult breast tumors. Am J Roentgenol 128:403, 1977
36. Fessia L, Ghiringhello B, Arisio R, et al: Accuracy of frozen section diagnosis in breast cancer detection. A review of 4436 biopsies and comparison with cytodiagnosis. Pathol Res Pract 179:61, 1984
37. Frable MJ: Needle aspiration of the breast. Cancer 53:671, 1984
38. Frazier TG, Rowland CH, Wollery CL: Comparative value of aspiration cytology in the diagnostic evaluation of breast masses. J Surg Oncol 12:353, 1979
39. Friedman M, Panahon AM, Fox S, et al: Needle aspiration cytology. Int Adv Surg Oncol 6:89, 1983
40. Forbes JF: Fine-needle aspiration cytology in the management of breast disease. Med J Aust 2:181, 1984
41. Furnival C: Aspiration cytology in breast disease. Med J Aust 11:548, 1979
42. Furnival C, Hocking MA, Hughes HE, et al: Aspiration cytology in breast cancer: Its relevance to diagnosis. Lancet 2:446, 1975

43. Furnival C, Stewart HJ, Weddell JM, et al: Accuracy of screening methods for the diagnosis of breast disease. Br Med J 4:461, 1970

44. Gardecki TIM, Melcher DH, Hogbin BM, Smith RS: Aspiration cytology in the preoperative management of breast cancer. Lancet 2:790, 1980

45. Gebhard PG, Feingold SG: Legal aspects of mammography screening. Cancer 60(suppl):1692, 1987

46. Geier GR, Korner BH, Schuhmann R: Differential cytology of breast cancer. Expl Cell Biol 45:167, 1977

47. Geier G, Schuhmann R, Kraus H: Mammapunktionszytologie. Beitr Pathol Bd 156:223, 1975

48. Glant MD: Aspiration biopsy cytology: Biopsy method of the eighties. India Med 8:595, 1984

49. Goodson WH, Mailman R, Miller TR: Three year follow-up of benign fine-needle aspiration biopsies of the breast. Am J Surg 154:58, 1987

50. Griffith CH, Kern WH, Mikkelsen WP: Needle aspiration cytologic examination in the management of suspicious lesions of the breast. Surg Gynecol Obstet 162:142, 1986

51. Gupta SK. Ghosh AK, Choudhary T, et al: Aspiration cytology in diagnosis of breast cancer. Indian J Cancer 16:1, 1979

52. Haagensen CD, Bodian C, Haagensen DE: Breast Carcinoma, Risk and Detection, 1st ed. Philadelphia, Saunders, 1981

53. Hahn P, Hallberg O, Schnurer LB: Combination of clinical examination, mammography and aspiration cytology in the diagnosis of carcinoma of the breast. Strahlentherapie 156:475, 1980

54. Hajdu SI, Melamed MR: The diagnostic value of aspiration smears. Am J Clin Pathol 59:350, 1973

55. Hall TL, Layfield LJ, Philippe A, Rosenthal DL: Sources of diagnostic error in fine needle aspiration of the thyroid. (in review)

56. Hammond S, Keyhani-Rofagha S, O'Toole RV: Statistical analysis of fine needle aspiration cytology of the breast. Acta Cytol 29:943, 1985

57. Hammond S, Keyhani-Rofagha S, O'Toole RV: Statistical analysis of the fine needle aspiration cytology of the breast. A review of 678 cases plus 4,265 cases from the literature. Acta Cytol 31:276, 1987

58. Hermansen C, Poulsen HS, Jensen J, et al: Palpable breast tumours: "Triple Diagnosis" and operative strategy. Results of a prospective study. Acta Chir Scand 150:625, 1984

59. Hermansen C, Poulsen HS, Jensen J, et al: Diagnostic reliability of combined physical examination, mammography and fine-needle puncture ("triple-test") in breast tumors. A prospective study. Cancer 60:1866, 1987

60. Hindle WH, Navin J: Breast aspiration cytology: A neglected gynecologic procedure. Am J Obstet Gynecol 146:482, 1983

61. Hirst E: Detection and diagnosis of early breast cancer. Med J Aust 4:566, 1977

62. Holaday WJ, Assor D: Ten thousand consecutive frozen sections. A retrospective study focusing on accuracy and quality control. Am J Clin Pathol 61:769, 1974

63. Jennings ER, Landers JW: The use of frozen section in cancer diagnosis. Surg Gynecol Obstet 104:60, 1957

64. Joffe SN, Hughes HE, Primrose JN, Williamson BWA: Aspiration cytology and outpatient excision of breast lumps. Lancet 8:294, 1979

65. Kalisher L, Schaffer DL: Xeromammography in early detection of breast cancer. JAMA 234:60, 1975
66. Kambouris AA: The role of fine needle aspiration cytology in the management of solid breast tumors. Am Surg 49:311, 1983
67. Kaufman M, Bider D, Weissberg D: Diagnosis of breast lesions by fine needle aspiration biopsy. Am Surg 49:558, 1983
68. Kern WH: The diagnosis of breast cancer by fine-needle aspiration smears. JAMA 241:1125, 1979
69. Kher AV, Marwar AW, Raichur BS: Evaluation of fine needle aspiration biopsy in the diagnosis of breast lesions. Indian J Pathol Microbiol 24:100, 1981
70. Kjellgren O: The cytologic diagnosis of cancer of the breast. Acta Cytol 8:216, 1964
71. Klein DL, Sickles EA: Effects of needle aspiration on the mammographic appearance of the breast: A guide to the proper timing of the mammography examination. Radiology 145:44, 1982
72. Kline TS: Masquerades of malignancy. A review of 4,241 aspirates from the breast. Acta Cytol 25:263, 1981
73. Kline TS, Joshi LP, Neal HS: Fine-needle aspiration of the breast: Diagnoses and pitfalls. A review of 3545 cases. Cancer 44:1458, 1979
74. Knox RA, Marshall T, Kingston RD: Fine needle aspiration breast cytology in district general hospital practice. Clin Oncol 10:369, 1984
75. Koivuniemi AP: Fine-needle aspiration biopsy of the breast. Ann Clin Res 8:272, 1976
76. Kreuzer G: Aspiration biopsy cytology in proliferating benign mammary dysplasia. Acta Cytol 22:128, 1978
77. Kreuzer G, Boquoi E: Aspiration biopsy cytology, mammography and clinical exploration: A modern set up in diagnosis of tumors of the breast. Acta Cytol 20:319, 1976
78. Kreuzer VG, Boquoi E: Die bedeutung der feinnadelbiopsie in der diagnostik des mammakarzinoms. Teil 2: Treffsicherheit und leistungsfahigkeit im rahmen der tripeldiagnostik. Fortschr Med 103:385, 1985
79. Kreuzer G, Zajicek J: Cytologic diagnosis of mammary tumors from aspiration biopsy smears. III. Studies on 200 carcinomas with false negative or doubtful cytologic reports. Acta Cytol 16:249, 1972
80. Lange M, Brebner D, Klempman S: Cytology and mammography in the diagnosis of breast cancer. SA Med J 14:2132, 1976
81. Lange M, Klempman S: Fine needle aspiration biopsy in the diagnosis of breast disease. SA Med J 10:143, 1972
82. Lee KR, Foster RS, Papillo JL: Fine needle aspiration of the breast. Importance of the aspirator. Acta Cytol 31:281, 1987
83. Leis HP: Diagnosis and treatment of breast lesions. New York, Medical Examination Publ, 1970
84. Lerman RI, Pitcock JA: Frozen section experience in 3249 specimens. Surg Gynecol Obstet 135:930, 1972
85. Lessells RI, Simpson JG: A retrospective analysis of the accuracy of immediate frozen section diagnosis in surgical pathology. Br J Surg 63:327, 1976
86. Letton AH: Breast cancer: Improved survival by routine screening. Int Adv Surg Oncol 6:127, 1983
87. Lever JV, Webb AJ: Aspiration cytology in breast cancer. Lancet 2:775, 1975
88. Lever JV, Trott PA, Webb AJ: Fine needle aspiration cytology. J Clin Pathol 38:1, 1985
89. Linsk J, Kreuzer G, Zajicek J: Cytologic diagnosis of mammary tumors from aspira-

tion biopsy smears. II. Studies on 210 fibroadenomas and 210 cases of benign dysplasia. Acta Cytol 16:130, 1972

90. Lowhagen, T, Rubio CA: The cytology of granular cell myoblasfoma of the breast. Report of a case. Acta Cytol 21:314, 1977

91. Marasa L, Tomasino RM: Aspiration cytology of the breast. I. Comparison of cytologic and histologic findings. Pathologica 74:183, 1982

92. Marasa L, Tomasino RM: Aspiration cytology of the breast. II. Significance of bipolar naked nuclei. Pathologica 74:193, 1982

93. Martin RE, Graham R: Office evaluation of breast tumors, with emphasis on needle aspiration therapy. MD State Med J 31:51, 1982

94. McSwain GR, Valicenti J, O'Brien PH: Cytologic evaluation of breast cysts. Surg Gynecol Obstet 146:921, 1978

95. Manheimer LH, Rywlin AM: Fine needle aspiration cytology. South Med J 70:923, 1977

96. Masukawa T: Breast cytology. Am J Med Tech 39:397, 1973

97. Moskowitz M: Cost-benefit determinations in screening mammography. Cancer 60 (suppl):1680, 1987

98. Murad TM, Snyder ME: The diagnosis of breast lesions from cytologic material. Acta Cytol 17:418, 1973

99. Murrell DS, Melcher DH: The role of aspiration cytology in a radiotherapy and oncology centre. Clin Radiol 34:337, 1982

100. Nakazawa H, Rosen P, Lane N, Lattes R: Frozen section experience in 3000 cases: Accuracy, limitations and value in residency training. Am J Clin Pathol 49:41, 1968

101. Niloff PH, Sheiner NM: False-negative mammograms in patients with breast cancer. Can J Surg 24:50, 1981

102. Norton LW, Davis JR, Wiens JL, et al: Accuracy of aspiration cytology in detecting breast cancer. Surgery 96:806, 1984

103. Ochsner A, Griffith WE: Critical evaluation of mammography in the management of breast disease. Am Surg 161:748, 1965

104. Oertel YC: Fine Needle Aspiration of the Breast, 1st ed. Boston, Butterworths, 1987, p 84

105. Padarha J, Gupta N, Gupta IC: Role of aspiration cytology in the early diagnosis of lumps in breast. J Indian Med Assoc 72:272, 1979

106. Pilotti S, Rilke F, Delpiano C, Di Pietro S: Problems in fine-needle aspiration biopsy cytology of clinically or mammographically uncertain breast tumors. Tumori 68:407, 1982

107. Pitts HH, Sturdy JH, Coady CJ: Frozen sections. II. Value in cases of suspected malignancy. Can Med Assoc J 79:110, 1958

108. Rajcic V: Cytologic studies of aspiration biopsy of the breast: Critical review of 2890 consecutive biopsies. Minerva Ginecol 23:417, 1971

109. Rimsten A, Stenkvist B, Johanson H, Lindgren A: The diagnostic accuracy of palpation and fine-needle biopsy and an evaluation of their combined use in the diagnosis of breast lesions. Report on a prospective study in 1244 women with symptoms. Ann Surg 182:1, 1975

110. Rosemond GP, Maier WP: Surgical pros and cons. Surg Gynecol Obstet 148:420, 1979

111. Rosen PP: Frozen section diagnosis of breast lesions. Recent experience with 556 consecutive biopsies. Ann Surg 187:17, 1978

112. Rosen P, Hajdu SI, Robbins G, Foote FW: Diagnosis of carcinoma of the breast by aspiration biopsy. Surg Gynocol Obstet 134:837, 1972

113. Russ JE, Winchester DP, Scanlon EF, Christ MA: Cytologic findings of aspiration of tumors of the breast. Surg Gynecol Obstet 146:407, 1978

114. Sartorius OW, Smith HS, Morris P, et al: Cytologic evaluation of breast fluid in the detection of breast disease. J Natl Cancer Inst 59:1073, 1977

115 Schoendorf NK: Possibilities and value of a differentiated cytology in the diagnosis of breast lesions. Acta Cytol 25:61, 1981

116. Schondorf H: Aspiration Cytology of the Breast, 1st ed. Philadelphia, Saunders, 1978

117. Shabot MM, Goldberg IM, Schick P, Nieberg R: Aspiration cytology is superior to Tru-Cut needle biopsy in establishing the diagnosis of clinically suspicious breast masses. Ann Surg 196:122, 1982

118. Shiller-Vokova NN, Agamova KA: Cytological study of punctates as a method of diagnosis of tumors of the breast. Vop Onkol 6:54, 1960

119. Sickles EA, Filly RA, Callen PW: Breast cancer detection with sonography and mammography: Comparison using state-of-the-art equipment. Am J Radiol 140:843, 1983

120. Sickles EA, Klein DL, Goodson WH, Hunt TK: Mammography after needle aspiration of palpable breast masses. Am J Surg 145:395, 1983

121. Sickles EA, Weber WN, Galvin HB, et al: Low cost mammography screening. Practical considerations with emphasis on mobile operation. Cancer 60(suppl):1688, 1987

122. Silver CE, Koss LG, Brauer RJ, et al: Needle aspiration cytology of tumors at various body sites. Curr Probl Surg 22:27, 1985

123. Silverman JF, Lannin DR, O'Brien K, Norris HT: The triage role of fine needle aspiration biopsy of breast masses: Diagnostic accuracy and cost effectiveness. Acta Cytol 30:588, 1986

124. Smallwood J, Herbert A, Guyer P, Taylor I: Accuracy of aspiration cytology in the diagnosis of breast disease. Br J Surg 72:841, 1985

125. Smith IH, Fisher JH, Lott JS, Thomson DH: The cytological diagnosis of solid tumors by small needle aspiration and its influence on cancer practice. Can Med Assoc J 80:855, 1959

126. Sparkman RS: Reliability of frozen sections in the diagnosis of breast lesions. Ann Surg 155:924, 1962

127. Squires JE, Betsill WL: Intracystic carcinoma of the breast. A correlation of cytomorphology, gross pathology, microscopic pathology and clinical diagnosis. Acta Cytol 25:267, 1981

128. Stavric GD, Tevcev DT, Kaftandjiev DR, Novak JJ: Aspiration biopsy cytologic method in diagnosis of breast lesions. A critical review of 250 cases. Acta Cytol 17:188, 1973

129. Strawbridge HTG, Bassett AA, Foldes I: Role of cytology in management of lesions of the breast. Surg Genecol Obstet 152:1, 1981

130. Takeda T, Takaso K, Isono S, et al: Studies on cytologic characteristics of mammary aspiration smears based on histologic types. Acta Cytol 21:424, 1977

131. Tallent DD, Halter SA: Cytologic examination of the breast. A safe, simple and accurate technique. Postgrad Med 69:91, 1981

132. Thomas JM, Fitzharris BM, Redding WH, et al: Clinical examination, xeromammo-

graphy and fine-needle aspiration cytology in diagnosis of breast tumours. Br Med J 2:1139, 1978

133. Tribe CR: Cytological diagnosis of breast tumours by the imprint method. J Clin Pathol 18:31, 1965

134. Ulanow RM, Galblum L, Canter JW: Fine needle aspiration in the diagnosis and management of solid breast lesions. Am J Surg 148:653, 1984

135. Van Bogaert LJ, Gilbert M: Reliability of the cyto-radio-clinical triplet in breast pathology diagnosis. Acta Cytol 21:60, 1977

136. Van Zyl JA, Van Zyl JJW, Street B, McCarthy E: Fine needle aspiration cytology in the management of patients with breast cancer. Int Adv Surg Oncol 4:241, 1981

137. Vilaplana D, Jimenez-Ayala M: The cytologic diagnosis of breast lesions. Acta Cytol 19:519, 1975

138. Vorherr H: Breast aspiration biopsy. Am J Obstet Gynecol 148:127, 1984

139. Walker-Brash RMT, Oatman SA, Randall KJ: Aspiration cytology in breast disease. Lancet Nov 8:1031, 1980

140. Wanebo HJ, Feldman PS, Wilhelm MC, et al: Fine needle aspiration cytology in lieu of open biopsy in management of primary breast cancer. Ann Surg 199:569, 1984

141. Webb AJ: The cytological diagnosis of breast lumps. Br J Surg 55:868, 1968

142. Webb AJ: The diagnostic cytology of breast carcinoma. Br J Surg 57:259, 1970

143. Wilson SL, Ehrmann RL: The cytologic diagnosis of breast aspirations. Acta Cytol 22:470, 1978

144. Winchester DP, Sener S, Immerman S, Blum M: A systematic approach to the evaluation and management of breast masses. Cancer 51:2535, 1983

145. Winship T: Aspiration biopsy of breast cancers by the pathologist. Am J Clin Pathol 52:438, 1969

146. Winship T, Rosvoll RV: Frozen sections: An evaluation of 1810 cases. Surgery 45:462, 1959

147. Wollenberg NJ, Caya JG, Clowry LJ: Fine needle aspiration biopsy of the breast: A ten-year correlation and statistical evaluation. Acta Cytol 27:562, 1983

148. Wollenberg NJ, Caya JG, Clowry LJ: Fine needle aspiration cytology of the breast. A review of 321 cases with statistical evaluation. Acta Cytol 29:425, 1985

149. Zagoren AJ, Waters DJ, Silverman D, Sonn RL: Aspiration biopsy for cytologic study of breast masses: An overview. J A O A 82:119, 1982

150. Zajdela A, Ghossein NA, Pilleron JP, Ennuyer A: The value of aspiration cytology in the diagnosis of breast cancer: Experience at the Foundation Curie. Cancer 35:499, 1975

151. Zajicek J, Caspersson T, Jakobsson P, et al: Cytologic diagnosis of mammary tumors from aspiration biopsy smears: Comparison of cytologic and histologic findings in 2111 lesions and diagnostic use of cytophotometry. Acta Cytol 14:370, 1970

152. Zajicek J, Franzen S, Jakobsson P, et al: Aspiration biopsy of mammary tumors in diagnosis and research: A critical review of 2,200 cases. Acta Cytol 11:169, 1967

Biopsy Interpretation in Bone Marrow Transplantation

Dale C. Snover

It has been 14 years since the last review of bone marrow transplantation (BMT) appeared in *Pathology Annual*.[1] In the intervening period, BMT has become a standard part of the treatment of a variety of neoplastic and non-neoplastic conditions affecting solid organs as well as the marrow itself. As the total number of transplants has increased, results have improved. There is a better understanding of the immunologic problems unique to BMT, in particular graft-versus-host disease (GVHD) with its many manifestations. This understanding includes the pathologic changes produced in a variety of organs that are frequently biopsied. The increased use of the biopsy in the assessment of the post-BMT patient has made the surgical pathologist an integral part of the transplant team. The major aim of this review is to provide a practical guide to biopsy interpretation. Bone marrow biopsy will not be included in this review, because it is in the realm of the hematopathologist rather than the surgical pathologist.

BONE MARROW TRANSPLANTATION: THE PROCEDURE

In order to understand the pathology of BMT, it is necessary to have a working knowledge of the procedures employed. These have been described in detail in previous reviews including the classic work by Thomas et al,[2] and will be described only briefly here.

This work is supported in part by Grant CA-P01-21737 from the National Institutes of Health.

There are three types of transplants performed in humans. The most common, the allogeneic transplant, involves transplantation of marrow from a genetically nonidentical member of the same species. The donor is usually a relative and frequently a sibling, since the goal in selecting a donor is to obtain the closest possible genetic match. In recent years, improvements in anti-GVHD prophylaxis have allowed attempts for the use of unrelated donors. In addition, donor banks are now being created to provide a source of better matched unrelated donors.

The second most common type of transplant, the autologous, involves removal and transplantation of the patient's own marrow. The obvious advantage of this type of transplant is that there is no problem with rejection since the marrow is genetically identical. In addition, GVHD is not generally a problem in this setting. The procedure, however, is limited by potential involvement of the marrow by malignancy, which makes recurrence of tumor more likely after this procedure. Attempts to purge the marrow of tumor cells by a variety of immunologic methods have met with some success.[3] Because of the risk for recurrence, however, allogeneic transplant is preferred for malignancies with marrow involvement. Obviously, the autologous transplant also cannot be used for aplastic anemia or other primary marrow diseases. The most common use for the autologous transplant is for the treatment of lymphoma or solid malignancies without marrow involvement, in which case, rescue of the patient with autologous marrow allows intensive chemotherapeutic and/or radiotherapeutic treatment of the tumor.

The least common transplant, the syngeneic, involves transplantation of marrow from a monozygotic twin. It can be used for all types of diseases except some genetic diseases.

The transplantation procedure involves ablation of the host immune system by chemo- or radiation therapy. This is necessary to prevent rejection of the graft in allogeneic transplantation and also to ablate tumor in the case of transplantation for malignancy. The extent and type of therapy will vary depending on the disease being treated and the idiosyncrasies of the transplant center. For diseases in which the immune system is already deficient, such as aplastic anemia or genetic immunodeficiency diseases, preparative treatment may be less intense. For malignancies, on the other hand, treatment usually consists of total body irradiation plus any of a variety of chemotherapeutic agents. Regardless of the particular preparative regimen used, the effects of the ablative agents must be taken into account when interpreting biopsies. While there are many similarities in the effects of various chemotherapeutic agents, some agents are more often associated with specific toxicities, such as the association of busulfan with venocclusive disease.[4,5] The effects of different agents will be discussed below.

Following ablation of the native marrow, the patient is infused with the donated marrow. In some cases, the marrow may be pretreated to remove residual malignant cells or to remove T cells in an effort to prevent GVHD. In other cases, immunosuppressive agents such as methotrexate and corticosteroids are used as prophylaxis against GVHD. The patient remains pancytopenic for a variable period following transplantation, during which time the patient is at risk for a variety of infections. Because of this, prophylactic antibiotics are administered. Since many of these agents are potentially toxic, they must be considered as possible causes of damage to biopsied organs.

In addition to the pancytopenia induced by the cytoreductive therapy, the patient often suffers from mucositis which may make eating difficult or impossible. This frequently results in the use of total parenteral nutrition, another factor to be taken into account in the assessment of biopsies, especially of the liver.

WHY BIOPSY THE TRANSPLANT PATIENT?

Biopsies are taken for several reasons such as diagnosing GVHD, ruling out potential infectious or toxic processes, and assessing the status of the primary disease. These processes are not mutually exclusive.

A biopsy taken to assess GVHD may serve two purposes. First is the diagnosis of GVHD itself. The second purpose is to provide a grade for the GVHD process. Although, as will be discussed below, the grading of acute GVHD seems to be of little prognostic significance, grading of the liver in chronic GVHD does play a role in the determination of prognosis and treatment. Other potential uses of the biopsy in regard to GVHD will be discussed in the appropriate section.

In regard to infectious diseases, the absence of an infectious disease diagnosis is often as important as the definitive positive diagnosis of GVHD. For example, the liver is commonly biopsied because liver function abnormalities fail to respond to anti-GVHD therapy given for GVHD diagnosed in other organs. The liver most often has been assumed clinically to be involved with the GVHD process so no prior biopsy was taken. The major purpose of a biopsy under these circumstances is not to absolutely confirm the diagnosis of GVHD. Instead, it is to be certain that the patient does not have some other cause of liver dysfunction, especially an infectious one that may be aggravated by immunosuppressive therapy. A similar situation often occurs regarding the lung.

Biopsies are often taken prior to transplantation to act as a baseline for future biopsies. The most common organ for such a biopsy is the liver, since many patients come into transplantation with liver dysfunction due to viral hepatitis or drug reactions. Since some diseases such as non-A non-B hepatitis may have histological features that can be confused with GVHD, it is important to document the status of the liver prior to transplantation.

One final reason to biopsy a patient is to assess progress of the transplant in correcting a metabolic disease for which the patient was transplanted. We have used biopsies of the liver and cartilage to follow the removal of mucopolysaccharide from patients transplanted for mucopolysaccharidosis.[6] Use of this technique in addition to enzyme measurements can detect successful engraftment as well as rejection of the graft, and it can provide visual evidence of the success of donated cells in removing storage products from non-donated cells such as hepatocytes.

GRAFT-VERSUS-HOST DISEASE: THE PROCESS

Graft-versus-host disease (GVHD) is a process that results from an attack by donated cells (or cells derived from donated cells) against tissue of the host. While originally defined for experimental purposes as requiring immunohisto-incompatibility for its occurrence, there are reported cases of acute GVHD occuring with syngeneic or autologous transplant.[7,8] There is also experimental evidence that GVHD may be produced under certain circumstances after autologous transplant.[9] This would imply that GVHD is not simply the result of T-cell attack on immunologically disparate tissue, but suggests that other mechanisms such as alteration in immune regulation may play a role in GVHD.[10] Support for this hypothesis comes from the fact that acute GVHD rarely occurs after a patient is fully reconstituted. Despite the suggestion that acute GVHD may occur in the autologous or syngeneic setting, as a practical clinical problem, GVHD occurs in the setting of the allogeneic transplant. It should be noted that chronic GVHD has not been described in autologous or syngeneic transplant patients.

As implied above, GVHD is categorized as acute or chronic. Originally the distinction was defined arbitrarily by occurrence before or after 100 days post-transplant.[2] Although this arbitrary distinction is still useful, it is now clear that the two processes can be better defined by clinicopathologic criteria including the pattern of organ involvement and histopathology of the process as well as the time of onset. Although it is rare in our experience to see what appears to be acute GVHD present after day 100, it is not so uncommon to see the onset of chronic GVHD before this time.

Acute GVHD involves predominantly three organ systems, the skin, liver and gastrointestinal (GI) tract.[2] Other organs such as the lung and bone marrow occasionally seem to be involved, although documentation of involvement of these latter organs has been difficult. The disease most often presents with a maculopapular skin rash, which is graded clinically based on extent of involvement and presence of bullae or desquamation. The second most commonly involved system is the GI tract. Patients with GI involvement present with diarrhea or upper abdominal pain, nausea, and vomiting depending on the portion of the tract involved. If diarrhea is present, the disease is graded by volume of stool; no quantitation exists for upper GI involvement. Somewhat less common is liver involvement. Patients with liver disease will manifest abnormalities in bilirubin, alkaline phosphatase, 5'-nucleotidase, or the amino-transferases. The process has been graded in the past by degree of bilirubin elevation, although it has been our impression that alkaline phosphatase and 5'-nucleotidase are more sensitive markers of disease.

Chronic GVHD involves a much larger range of organs than acute disease and the onset is frequently more insidious.[10,11] The skin, liver, and, to a lesser extent, gastrointestinal tract, are still targets, but salivary and lacrimal glands, mucosal surfaces, lung, and a host of other organs may be involved. The salivary or lacrimal glandular involvement commonly leads to a sicca syndrome, and the lung disease may lead to restrictive or obstructive lung disease.

Specifics of the grading and clinical features of GVHD as they relate to pathologic findings will be discussed below. For convenience sake, acute GVHD and other changes usually seen in the first 100 days post-transplant will be discussed first, followed by a discussion of chronic GVHD and related pathology.

ACUTE GVHD: THE BIOPSY

As described above, three organs are commonly biopsied to diagnose acute GVHD: the skin, gastrointestinal tract, and liver. Acute GVHD is an epithelial destructive lesion that, in the skin and GI tract, involves primarily the regenerative compartment, i.e., the basal layer of the skin, the crypt of the intestine, and the neck region of the gastric mucosa.[12–15] In these organs, the basic lesion is the single necrotic cell (Fig. 1). In the liver, a more varied picture is seen with damage primarily to biliary structures as well as a lesser degree of damage to hepatocytes and endothelial cells.[4,15–18] It is important to keep in mind that, although the tissue destruction in acute GVHD appears to be mediated by some type of lymphoid cell, the actual degree of lymphoid infiltration seen in routine sections is often minimal in large part due to the extreme lymphopenia that the patient may be experiencing early in the transplant course.

In the skin, the earliest sign of damage appears at the tip of the rete ridge, the location of the largest concentration of "stem" cells in the skin (Fig. 2).[19] The basal cells in these areas show evidence of hydropic degeneration characterized by vacuolation of their cytoplasm, usually in association with a mild lymphocytic dermal and epidermal infiltrate (Fig. 2). These changes, although characteristic of GVHD, are not diagnostic and are in fact quite nonspecific. They have been designated as grade 1 GVHD, despite the non-specificity.[12] At the next stage (grade 2), dyskeratotic epidermal cells appear near the base of the epidermis, occasionally with attached lymphocytes ("satel-litosis") (Fig. 1). The finding of such cells is considered "diagnostic" of GVHD if certain other conditions described below can be excluded. With increasing severity of disease, subepidermal clefting appears (grade 3) (Fig. 3), followed by total sloughing of the epidermis or by a toxic epidermal necrolysis-like picture (grade 4). Grade 4 lesions are, not surprisingly, associated with a poor prognosis. There is very little documented prognostic significance to histological grades 1 to 3 disease.

A variety of other nonspecific features may be seen with cutaneous GVHD, including intra- and perivascular lymphocytic inflammation with or without purpura (Fig. 4), cytological atypia of the epidermis, pigment incontinence, and

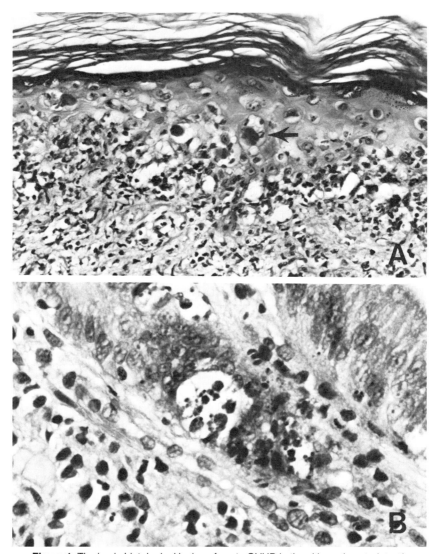

Figure 1. The basic histological lesion of acute GVHD in the skin and gastrointestinal tract is necrosis of individual cells in the regenerating compartment. **A.** Typical acute GVHD grade 2 with a junctional lymphocytic infiltrate, hydropic degeneration of the basal layer, and numerous single necrotic epithelial cells sometimes referred to as dyskeratotic cells or apoptotic bodies. Some of these have lymphocytes attached, a phenomenon known as satellitosis (*arrow*). **B.** Crypt of rectal mucosa with acute GVHD showing the typical single necrotic cell, also known as the "exploding crypt cell" because of its characteristic appearance with abundant karyorrhexic debris in an open space, presumably previously occupied by the dead cell. Scattered isolated karyorrhexic debris may also be seen in the lamina propria in these cases but in itself is insufficient for the diagnosis of GVHD. (H&E: **A.** =192, **B.** =480)

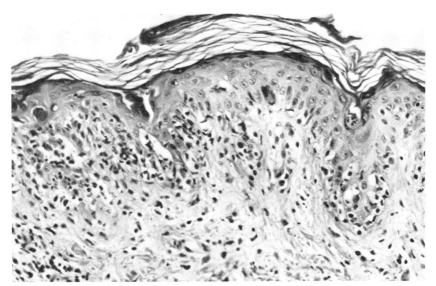

Figure 2. Acute GVHD of the skin showing a characteristic predilection for the tips of the rete ridges with relative sparing of the dermal plates. (H&E ×192)

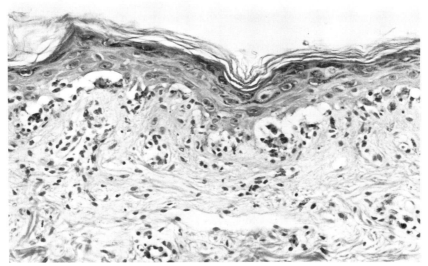

Figure 3. Grade 3 acute GVHD with confluence of basal hydropic degeneration leading to separation of the epidermis from the dermis. (H&E ×192)

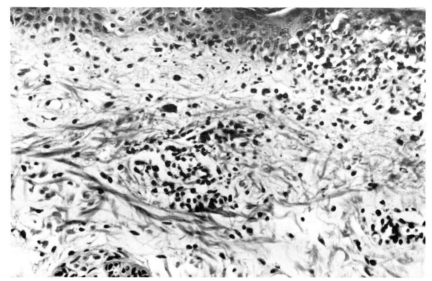

Figure 4. Acute GVHD of the skin showing a nonspecific perivascular infiltrate. (H&E ×192)

involvement of adnexal structures. This latter finding is considered to be suggestive of the possible progression of acute-to-chronic disease (see below).[15]

It is clear that the cytoreductive preparation of the patient can result in toxic changes in the epidermis that can precisely mimic those of GVHD, including dyskeratotic cells with satellitosis.[12] In general, these effects resolve by day 20 post-transplant, so that any biopsy taken before that time can result in an unreliable interpretation. It should be noted, however, that the 20-day figure is not an absolute one and that mild changes shortly after that time may also need to be interpreted with caution. In addition, under some circumstances, the effect of irradiation may be prolonged, particularly in the case of higher than usual doses.

Having set a cautionary stage, there are some features that will help the pathologist *favor* a diagnosis of GVHD or cytotoxic effect, even in an early biopsy. First, the process of chemotherapy or radiation damage is generally more diffuse than that of GVHD. Secondly, since there is always some time elapsed since the point of cytotoxic injury, dyskeratosis and cytological atypia will often be more prominent than basal hydropic degeneration in cytotoxic injury. If one views the changes of GVHD as a progression, then hydropic degeneration is the active process, while dyskeratosis and atypia are the end stage. In disease produced by a cytoreductive agent, the later stages predominate without evidence of active damage in the form of basal degeneration (Fig. 5).

The problem of drug reaction may be more difficult to deal with than cytoreductive damage. We have seen trimethoprim–sulfamethoxazole result in a skin rash bearing all of the histological findings of a grade 2 GVHD. Under such circumstances, failure to respond to immunosuppressive therapy may be the only clue to the diagnosis, although this is a weak clue since not all GVHD responds either. The presence of eosinophils, if present, favors a hypersensitivity diagnosis. The only way to prove the diagnosis, of course, is to withdraw and readminister the potential offending drug.

The role of viruses in the production of a GVHD-like rash is not well documented. We have had several cases of a grade 2 GVHD-like rash occurring in patients whose other organ biopsies (liver, rectum) showed evidence of cytomegalovirus (CMV) infection, and indeed these patients died of the CMV without ever having responded to GVHD therapy.[14] In one case, CMV inclusions were identified in the skin at autopsy.

The gastrointestinal tract is the second most often biopsied site for GVHD. In most institutions, the rectum is the segment of choice to biopsy, although in our experience, this depends somewhat on the symptomatology.[14] In patients with diarrhea, the rectum would be the logical first choice, but in patients presenting with upper GI symptoms of pain, nausea, or emesis, biopsy of duodenum and stomach are more likely to be rewarding.[14] Even with diarrhea, the rectum is sometimes negative in the face of a positive duodenal biopsy. This is not too surprising since it is probable that the diarrhea is due to small intestinal, not rectal, disease.

The sine qua non of GI GVHD is single cell necrosis (SCN) or the so-

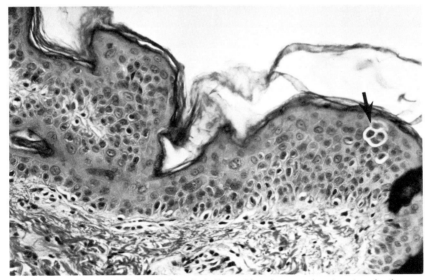

Figure 5. Scattered dyskeratotic cells in the epidermis secondary to cytoreductive therapy (*arrow*). Despite these cells, the absence of active damage to the basal layer indicates that whatever caused this cell death is no longer an active process. (H&E ×192)

called "exploding crypt cell" which is the diagnostic equivalent of the dysker-atotic cell in the skin (Figs. 1 and 6).[13] This structure is characterized by a vacuole in the regenerative compartment of the biopsied organ (the crypt of the small or large intestine and neck of gastric glands). The vacuole contains frag-ments of cytoplasm and karyorrhexic nuclear debris. Several caveats must be placed on the use of this as a diagnostic feature, however. First, it is of signifi-cance only if seen in the regenerating compartment rather than on the surface of the mucosa being examined. Fragments of cells similar to SCN are common on the surface and may represent either normal cell death, residual dead cells from cytoreductive preparation, or possibly the effects of preparative hypnotic enemas (Fig. 7).[20] Second, SCN can be produced by cytoreductive therapy, so interpretation of biopsies in the first 20 days post-transplant must be done with caution.[13] Criteria similar to those of the skin can be applied to the GI tract in that evidence of old rather than ongoing damage (e.g., cytological atypia out of proportion to SCN) favors a diagnosis of cytotoxic effect (Fig. 8). Finally, other factors, in particular viral infections, can produce histological findings identical to GVHD. Foremost among these is CMV, which has been shown in non-BMT patients to be associated with SCN (Fig. 9).[21] For this reason, if CMV inclusions are present in a GI biopsy, the presence of GVHD can neither be diagnosed nor excluded. The tissue must be considered inadequate for the diagnosis of GVHD. Whether other viruses can mimic GI GVHD remains to be proven.

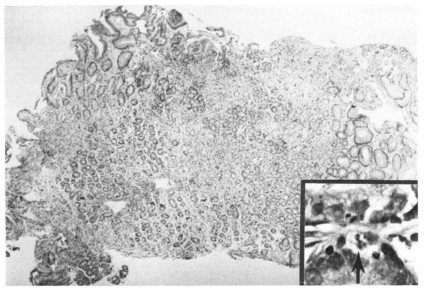

Figure 6. Acute GVHD of the stomach. At low power the mucosa looks altered with areas in which the crypts are missing alternating with retained crypts. *Inset:* Typical single necrotic cell of GVHD (*arrow*). In the stomach and duodenum these dead cells often lack the "explosive" character of acute GVHD of the rectum as seen in Figure 1B. (H&E: **A.** ×30, **B.** ×480)

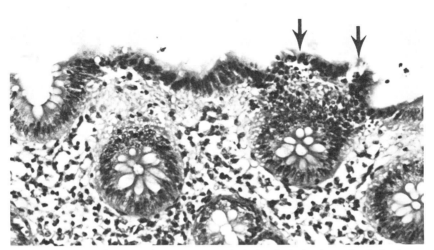

Figure 7. Rectal mucosa from a nontransplanted patient showing cells similar to the exploding crypt cells of GVHD located in the surface absorptive layer (*arrow*). These changes are a very common finding in rectal biopsies and are not indicative of damage to the mucosa. (H&E ×192)

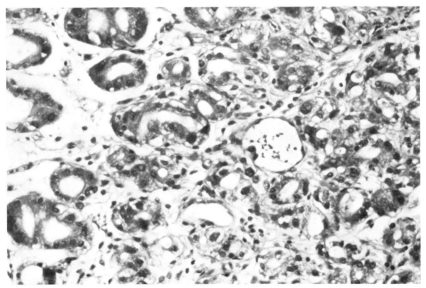

Figure 8. Gastric biopsy showing cytoreductive damage. There is nuclear atypia and occasional loss of crypts. There is no active single cell necrosis, which presumably was present at the time of administration of the cytoreductive agents. (H&E ×192)

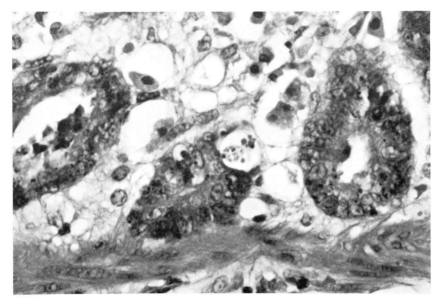

Figure 9. Single cell necrosis in the crypt of a renal transplant patient with cyto-megalovirus colitis. This infection can simulate GVHD and therefore the diagnosis of GVHD cannot be made or excluded in the presence of CMV inclusions. (H&E ×480). *(Reproduced from Snover DC, 1985, with permission.[21])*

Interestingly, GVHD-like changes are also commonly seen in ulcerative colitis and in neoplastic epithelium.

Other features seen in GI biopsies with GVHD are nonspecific and include crypt abscesses, fibrosis of the lamina propria, relative preservation of the neuroendocrine cells, and necrosis and loss of crypts. The latter feature is the basis for current grading systems as detailed below. Crypt abscesses are, in our experience, relatively uncommon and entirely nonspecific.

The preservation of neuroendocrine cells is an interesting phenomenon of uncertain significance.[22] In badly damaged biopsies, these cells may be the only cells remaining in some crypts. The neuroendocrine cells are recognized by their pink granular cytoplasm, which may lead to confusion with Paneth cell metaplasia induced by persistent inflammation. They are distinguishable because of the fine character and abluminal location of the granules compared to the coarse luminal granules of Paneth cells. In case of doubt, argyrophil or immunoperoxidase staining for neuropeptides or chromogranin will allow definitive distinction. Why neuroendocrine cells are spared in GVHD is unclear, but it may be due to destruction of undifferentiated stem cells rather than differentiated cells in acute GVHD.[10,19]

A common problem in the diagnosis of GVHD by GI biopsy is the question of minimal criteria. If one carefully searches a biopsy at high power, one will inevitably find a cell which may fit the description of SCN. However, is one cell adequate to make the diagnosis? In our opinion, the answer is clearly no. As a general rule, we scan the biopsy at medium power to look for evidence of SCN which is then confirmed by high power. The biopsy with GVHD will also frequently look disorganized and reactive at low power (Fig. 6). If there is only a rare SCN, the biopsy may be interpreted as "suggestive, but not diagnostic of GVHD." If the SCN is easily found, however, then the diagnosis of GVHD can be made.

Another problem in the interpretation of biopsies for GVHD is caused by the fact that the changes are likely to be found only in the regenerating compartment. This means that if the regenerating compartment is not seen, as in a rectal biopsy cut tangentially, then GVHD cannot be ruled out (Fig. 10). Under such circumstances, deeper levels of the tissue must be obtained to examine the deep crypts.

GVHD of the rectum is graded on the basis of destruction of crypts following the suggestion of the Seattle group[13] (Fig. 11). We have slightly modified the Seattle criteria because most cases seem to fall into grade 1 or 3 in their system, while very few are grade 2. Our system is shown in Table 1. In addition to expanding grade 2, we have added the "consistent with" category. There is no published grading system for the upper GI tract, although one can adapt the rectal system to stomach or duodenum without too much difficulty. As in the skin, there is little documented prognostic information contained in the grading of GI biopsies with the exception that patients with total sloughing (grade 4) do poorly. Several traps should be noted in the grading of rectal GVHD. Most important is to not diagnose all biopsies with loss of crypts as being GVHD. Crypts can be displaced (squeezed out, if you will) by the biopsy forceps leaving empty crypt sheaths at the edge of the biopsy (Fig. 12). These can be recognized by their peripheral location as well as by the fact that the epithelium can often be found lying beside the specimen in the block. Another common cause of "pseudoloss" of crypts is the depleted lymphoid aggregate. In this situation, the normal lymphoid aggregates of the large intestine are depleted of lymphocytes by cytoreductive therapy (Fig. 13). In their absence, one sees a space in the mucosa which is generally rounded and located near the base of the mucosa. In addition, the muscularis mucosae is frequently disrupted in the area of a

TABLE 1. GRADING OF ACUTE RECTAL GVHD

Grade	Definition
Consistent with but nondiagnostic	Rare exploding crypt cells, no loss of crypts
Grade 1	Exploding crypt cells easily found with medium power scan, no loss of crypts
Grade 2	Grade 1 plus loss of up to two contiguous crypts
Grade 3	Grade 1 plus loss of three or more contiguous crypts
Grade 4	Total loss of epithelial cells

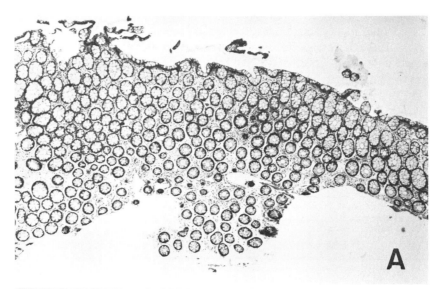

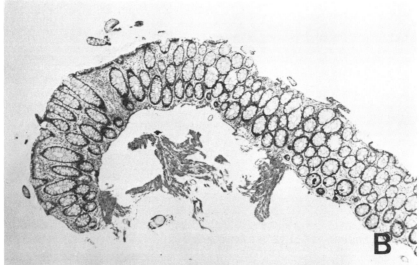

Figure 10. A. Since the primary lesion of acute GVHD occurs in the deep crypt, tangential sections such as this one are insufficient to make a diagnosis. In such a case deeper levels should be obtained, as in **B**, until the crypts are adequately visualized. (H&E ×30)

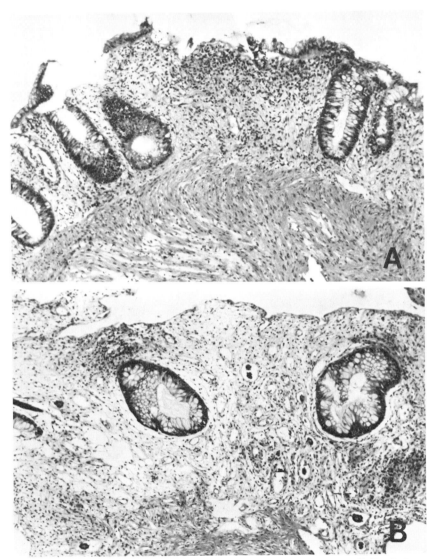

Figure 11. A. Grade 2 rectal GVHD with two adjacent missing crypts. **B.** Grade 3 rectal GVHD with loss of more than three adjacent crypts but without complete loss of epithelium. Careful examination revealed ongoing damage to other crypts in the area of the missing ones. (H&E ×75).

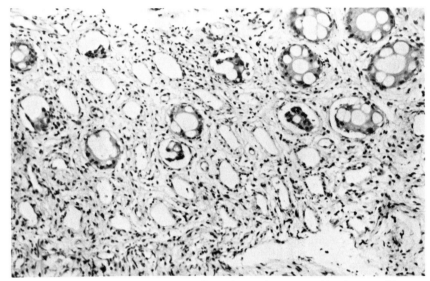

Figure 12. Rectal biopsy showing artifactual loss of crypts resulting from crushing of the specimen. Note that the epithelium in the remaining crypts is intact without necrosis or regenerative changes. (H&E ×120)

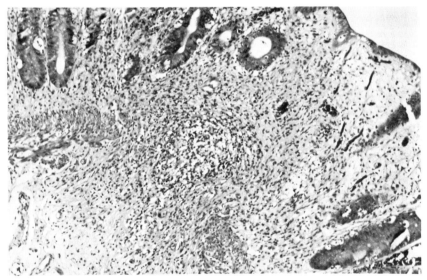

Figure 13. Depleted lymphoid aggregate simulating loss of crypts in rectal mucosa. Note the rounded character of the area as well as the disruption of the muscularis mucosae in the same area. (H&E ×75)

lymphoid aggregate. An important clue to the fact that GVHD may not have caused these spaces, as well as the empty crypt sheaths described above, is the fact that the diagnostic exploding crypt cell is not seen in crypts adjacent to the missing crypts. As a rule of thumb, crypts destroyed by GVHD are usually accompanied by degenerating crypts in the same area of the specimen.

Acute GVHD of the liver is characterized clinically by abnormalities of liver function tests (LFTs), particularly alkaline phosphatase and bilirubin. However, LFTs are quite nonspecific. In our institution, if a patient develops liver function abnormalities concurrently with biopsy-proven GVHD of other organs, the liver disease is assumed to be GVHD. This is in large part a decision of necessity since the platelet count often does not allow biopsy in the early period following transplant. The liver is biopsied in one of several circumstances including (1) failure of abnormal LFTs to improve following treatment for GVHD, (2) development of LFT abnormalities during treatment of GVHD of other organs, and (3) development of LFT abnormalities not accompanied by evidence of GVHD elsewhere. In the first two of these circumstances, the patient has already received immunosuppressive therapy, and therefore the histology of GVHD, if present, will be modified. In all cases, a major reason for biopsy is to rule out an infectious cause for the liver abnormalities which may be treatable in itself or may lead to caution in the use of immunosuppression. In the case of isolated LFT abnormalities without GVHD elsewhere, the biopsy may obviously be the only way of explaining the dysfunction. Other disorders to be included in the differential diagnosis (in addition to GVHD and infections) are drug reactions, diseases related to cytoreductive therapy, recurrent primary disease, and other primary liver diseases such as extrahepatic obstruction due to stones.

Acute GVHD in the liver is manifest by damage to interlobular bile ducts, usually associated with mild portal lymphocytic infiltration (Fig. 14).[4,16,17] Hepatocellular inflammation and necrosis may be present as well. Endothelialitis, i.e., lymphocytic infiltrate and damage to venous endothelium, is probably the most specific feature of GVHD (Fig. 15).[16] It is not commonly identified in GVHD, however, in distinction to the case of liver allograft rejection, where it is almost invariably present.[23] This difference is in part due to the fact that most cases of hepatic GVHD are treated aggressively with immunosuppressive agents prior to biopsy. It has been the experience in liver transplantation in which one has the luxury of repeated serial biopsies, that endothelialitis is the first feature to disappear after such therapy.[23] In addition, even in those cases of GVHD with endothelialitis, it is not nearly as florid as in allograft rejection, probably due to the leukopenic nature of most BMT patients.

More consistent, although less specific, is the bile duct damage, usually in association with intraepithelial lymphocytes. This finding is the sine qua non of the diagnosis of hepatic GVHD. The bile ducts can show a variety of features including vacuolation of the epithelial cytoplasm, nuclear pleomorphism, pseudostratification, nuclear vesiculation with prominent nucleoli, loss of nuclei, loss of the ductal lumen, and eventually total loss of ducts (Fig. 14). At

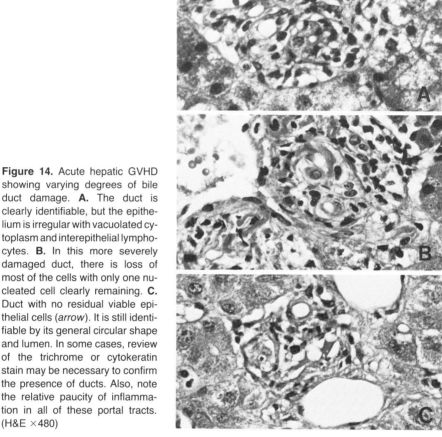

Figure 14. Acute hepatic GVHD showing varying degrees of bile duct damage. **A.** The duct is clearly identifiable, but the epithelium is irregular with vacuolated cytoplasm and interepithelial lymphocytes. **B.** In this more severely damaged duct, there is loss of most of the cells with only one nucleated cell clearly remaining. **C.** Duct with no residual viable epithelial cells (*arrow*). It is still identifiable by its general circular shape and lumen. In some cases, review of the trichrome or cytokeratin stain may be necessary to confirm the presence of ducts. Also, note the relative paucity of inflammation in all of these portal tracts. (H&E ×480)

times, especially in the presence of a prominent lymphocytic infiltrate, the ducts may be difficult to identify. In this circumstance, use of the trichrome or cytokeratin stain will often allow better definition of the ductal structure. It should be noted that the ducts of interest are the interlobular ducts that are accompanied by arterioles. Smaller, proliferating ductules of any cause often have many features of atypia described above, and therefore they are unreliable indicators of damage.

Although bile duct damage is characteristic of GVHD, it is certainly not specific. Certain immune diseases such as allograft rejection and primary biliary cirrhosis show identical changes.[16] Obviously, these diseases are not primary considerations for liver dysfunction in this setting. Of more interest is the fact that bile duct damage is not uncommonly seen in viral hepatitis, particularly of

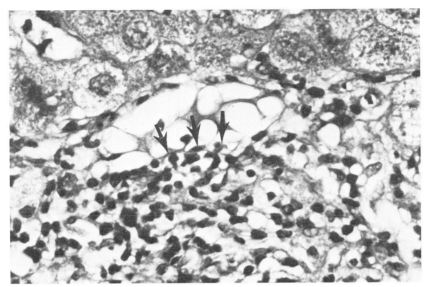

Figure 15. Portal vein in acute GVHD showing lymphocytes raising and damaging the endothelium (*arrows*), a process known as "endothelialitis," which is an uncommon but specific finding for GVHD. (H&E ×480)

the non-A non-B type.[24] In addition, a number of drug reactions have been associated with bile duct damage. Most worrisome in this regard are several cases of possible sulfonamide reactions that we have seen. Although bile duct damage can occur in these circumstances, it usually involves only a small percentage of ducts, and therefore a differential can usually be made on the basis of degree of damage.

The final and least specific features of GVHD are the mild portal infiltrate and hepatocellular damage. The infiltrate is usually almost entirely composed of small lymphocytes without eosinophils or polymorphonuclear cells; features useful in the distinction of GVHD from drug reactions. The hepatocellular damage can consist of ballooning degeneration or acidophil bodies, and it is thus very similar to changes seen in viral infection of the liver. The degree of hepatocellular damage is usually less than the degree of portal inflammation and bile duct damage.

When confronted with the differential of viral infection versus GVHD, we rely on the ratio of hepatocellular to bile duct damage as a major aid to diagnosis. If more than 50 percent of the bile ducts are damaged, with minimal hepatocellular damage, the process is probably GVHD. The converse, marked hepatocellular damage with less than 50 percent bile duct damage, favors a diagnosis of hepatitis. Endothelialitis assures the diagnosis of GVHD, regardless of degree of bile duct damage (as long as there is some). When degree of hepatocellular and bile duct damage appear relatively equal, either diagnosis may be correct and other clinical or biopsy findings must be used to make the diagnosis.

The grading of hepatic GVHD proposed by Lerner[25] is based on degree of bile duct damage. Grades 1 to 4 correspond to increasing quartiles of bile duct damage, i.e., grade 1 is up to 25 percent, grade 2 is 25 to 50 percent, etc. Although this grading system is of some value in giving an assessment of the degree of certainty of a diagnosis of GVHD as described above, there is no documented prognostic value to the grading.

Acute GVHD of organs other than skin, stomach, duodenum, rectum, and liver has not been well documented. The esophagus seems resistent to involvement. Although there were a few early reports of renal involvement, this has not been documented in the more recent experience.[26] Similarly, one early report on cardiac involvement has not been confirmed, and post-transplant cardiac problems are minimal.[27] In point of fact, the only other organ which seems a likely candidate for acute GVHD is the lung, although clearcut documentation is not available. An early report of the specificity of "lymphocytic bronchitis" for pulmonary GVHD has not been confirmed in a repeat study.[28,29] However, the possibility that lymphocytic bronchitis is characteristic, if not diagnostic, cannot be totally excluded. In addition, there are many anecdotal cases of pulmonary interstitial pneumonitis occurring concomitantly with GVHD of other organs, and responding to appropriate immunosuppressive therapy. Although certainly not specific, it would appear that interstitial pneumonitis can be caused by acute GVHD. The major value of lung biopsy, however, is to rule out other specific, usually infective, causes for lung disease.

THE ACUTE PERIOD: OTHER PATHOLOGY

Although GVHD is of primary interest in the acute period following transplantation, numerous other processes may occur. First and foremost are the infectious diseases. Although briefly discussed in the context of differential diagnosis of GVHD, it should be reiterated that any and all sorts of unusual bacterial, protozoal, viral, and fungal infections may occur and must always be sought. Although these are too numerous to detail, the most common include CMV, *Aspergillus*, and *Candida* plus unusual systemic infections by *Fusarium* and *Scopulariopsis*, and *Toxoplasma* hepatitis.[30–33]

Occasionally noninfectious processes will mimic infections. We have encountered this most often in the esophagus where glycogenic acanthosis simulates *Candida* esophagitis as seen by the endoscopist. Both processes appear as white plaques, although *Candida* infections generally have a hyperemic border with areas of ulceration.[34] Microscopically, *Candida* infection has ulceration with fungal elements, whearas glycogenic acanthosis is characterized by thickening of the mucosa by clear, glycogen-filled squamous cells (Fig. 16).

There are two liver diseases that are found more commonly in BMT pa-

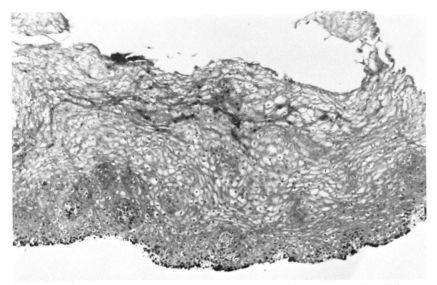

Figure 16. Esophageal biopsy from a white plaque in the esophagus thought by the endoscopist to possibly represent candidal esophagitis. Microscopically, the mucosa is thickened and the individual squamous cells have abundant clear cytoplasm due to glycogen accumulation, features characteristic of glycogenic acanthosis. (H&E ×75)

tients than in the general population, and they deserve special mention. One is venocclusive disease (VOD), an obstruction of hepatic outflow at the level of the terminal hepatic vein. First described in Jamaican children secondary to consumption of "bush tea" containing toxic alkaloids, the disease has now been associated with a variety of chemotherapeutic agents as well as irradiation.[4,5,35] In post-transplant patients, it clinically presents with symptoms of portal hypertension including weight gain, ascites, hepatomegaly, or jaundice, usually in the first 30 days. Histologically, there is a marked centrilobular congestion, atrophy of central hepatocytes, and eventually occlusion of the central veins by a delicate network of reticulin fibers (Fig. 17). These features are often best appreciated with the trichrome or reticulin stain. The changes are not absolutely diagnostic since they are similar to those seen in any outflow obstruction including heart failure or Budd–Chiari syndrome. Therefore clinical correlation is imperative.[5]

The group in Seattle has recently reported an incidence of 21 percent of VOD among patients treated for malignancy based on clinical criteria (not confirmed by biopsy, since biopsy of these lesions may be hazardous).[35] Because the symptoms of VOD are not specific, the possibility exists that some of these cases, particularly those that do not succumb to the disease, are actually something other than GVHD. In our experience, nodular regenerative hyperplasia (NRH) may produce similar symptoms and may be responsible for some

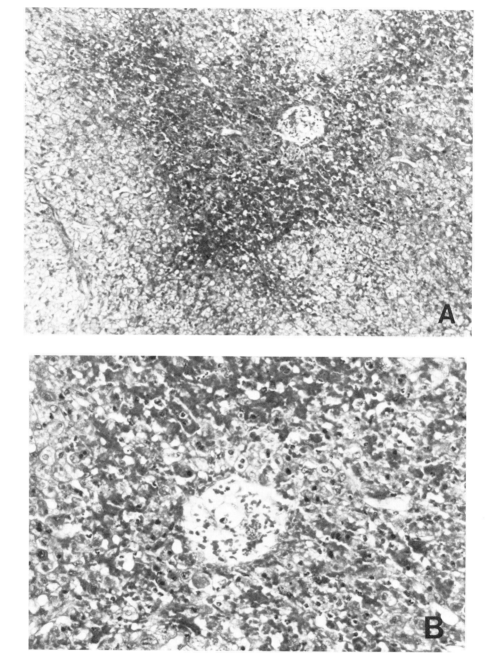

Figure 17. A Venocclusive disease of the liver is characterized by marked centri-lobular congestion and sinusoidal dilatation with occlusion of the central veins. **B.** The central veins, if identifiable, may be occluded by mature fibrous tissue or by loose fibrinoid material. Note the residual diminished lumen. (H&E: **A.** ×75, **B.** ×192)

cases of VOD-like disease.[36,37] NRH consists of diffuse regenerative nodulation of the liver without fibrosis (Fig. 18). Although sometimes noted as an incidental finding, it most commonly occurs in the setting of collagen vascular diseases and especially in patients receiving corticosteroids or other immunosuppressive drugs. In our retrospective study, we found NRH to be approximately three times more common than VOD in biopsy or autopsy material. The diagnosis on needle biopsy is difficult because the regenerative nodules are frequently wider than the needle width and hence not readily apparent. On reticulin stain, however, one sees alternating areas of hepatocellular atrophy and regeneration with the regeneration in the periportal areas (Fig. 19). In addition, the central veins are frequently compressed and not visible on routine hematoxylin and eosin stain. It seems likely that NRH accounts for some cases of nonfatal "VOD."

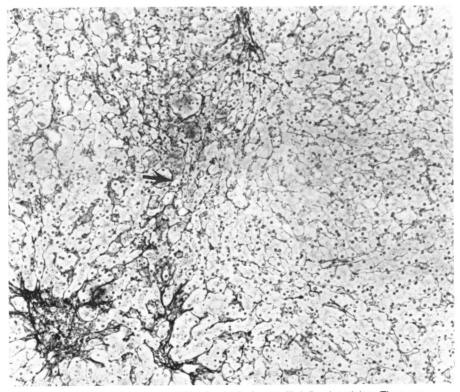

Figure 18. Nodular regenerative hyperplasia was ill-defined nodules. They are composed of regenerating hepatocytes with thickened cell plates in the periportal area separated by areas of hepatocellular atrophy. The atrophy is characterized by collapse of the reticulin framework usually in a more central location (*arrow*). (Reticulin ×75)

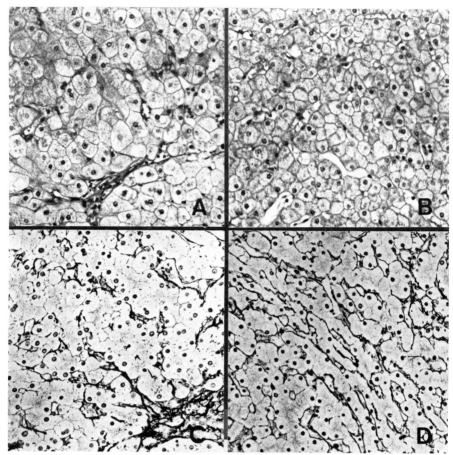

Figure 19. A. The regenerating cells of nodular regenerative hyperplasia are generally larger with clearing of the cytoplasm in comparison to cells in the atrophic areas (**B**). **C.** This hematoxylin and eosin impression is confirmed by the reticulin stain which identifies thickened cell plates characteristic of regeneration in areas similar to panel **A. D.** A reticulin stain of atrophic single cell layers in areas corresponding to panel **B.** (**A, B,** H&E ×192, **C, D,** reticulin ×192)

CHRONIC GVHD: THE BIOPSY

A larger number of organs may be involved with chronic GVHD than acute GVHD. Traditionally, chronic GVHD is thought of as a fibrosing process characterized clinically by insidious onset and irreversibility.[11] This latter feature may not necessarily be so if the process is detected early while still in a "cellular" phase. The existence of such a reversible phase has not been clearly demonstrated, although it is well known that in the minor salivary glands the pathology can range from intact glands with a mild lymphoplasmacytic infiltrate to complete destruction and fibrosis.[38] It is our current working hypothesis that chronic GVHD can be detected at a reversible cellular phase. The role of protocol biopsies as a corollary to this hypothesis will be discussed in the section on lip biopsy.

We consider acute and chronic GVHD to be two different processes rather than different expressions of the same process, which appears to be true for acute and chronic rejection of a solid organ.[10] For this reason, chronic GVHD is not, by definition, an irreversible process such as chronic rejection in solid organs. An important corollary to this statement lies in the fact that all chronic GVHD cases do not need to be preceded by acute GVHD (in fact only two thirds of cases are).[11] It appears that chronic GVHD has more in common with autoimmune diseases than acute GVHD, and indeed it has been suggested that chronic GVHD may be initiated by some "irrelevant" process such as a viral infection or radiation therapy. In reality, acute GVHD may be one of the nonspecific initiators of chronic GVHD. If this hypothesis is true, the proposed cellular and end stage fibrotic types of "chronic" GVHD, suggested in the preceding paragraph, may be the functional equivalents of acute and chronic rejection of solid organs in the "traditional" sense.

Chronic GVHD is graded as limited if there is localized involvement of skin and/or liver alone. This assumes the liver does not show certain features to be described below. If skin disease is generalized, or if other organs are involved, the process is designated as extensive and carries a somewhat worse prognosis.[11] The skin is the first organ biopsied in chronic as well as in acute GVHD because of its relative safety. However, in order to determine extent of disease a second organ is usually biopsied. The lip is a common choice since it is easy to biopsy and frequently is involved.[38] The liver is also commonly biopsied because its histological features alone may be enough to thrust a patient into the extensive category. Biopsy of other organs, particularly the lung and GI tract, are usually performed to rule out other disease, particularly infectious diseases. Unfortunately, chronic GVHD has an adverse effect on the immune system so that patients with chronic GVHD commonly are secondarily infected.

Biopsy of the skin can have several changes in chronic disease. The distribution may be localized or generalized, and these different clinical manifestations may have somewhat different histopathologic features.[15]

Localized chronic GVHD, which is the pattern found in approximately 20 percent of chronic cutaneous GVHD, clinically resembles lichen sclerosus et atrophicus with areas of depressed depigmentation of various sizes. The lesions will sometimes be confined to skin under tight clothing. Histologically, it is characterized by gradual collagenization of the reticular dermis with little involvement of the epidermis or other epithelial structures. Eventually the entire reticular dermis will become thickened and sclerotic. The epidermis may become atrophic at this time. At this stage, the lesion will resemble late generalized chronic GVHD (see below), although clinically it will appear quite different and may eventually undergo resolution. Because the early changes are in a deep location, a punch or even small incisional biopsy may not detect diagnostic histological abnormalities despite the clearcut clinical appearance.

Generalized chronic GVHD, as the name implies, involves a greater proportion of the skin than the localized form, and it has a different clinical as well as histopathologic appearance. The early lesions may be erythematous or papular, and they have a predilection for the palms and soles. There may be an accompanying brawny edema with eventual sloughing of the epidermis. Areas of depigmentation may develop. In many cases, the changes are found predominantly in areas of sun exposure or previous intense irradiation. In one case, the lesions developed in areas involved with a measles rash.[39] These changes are often accompanied by alterations of the mucous membranes including dryness and lichen planus-like papules.

As the disease progresses, the skin may take on a tight hidebound appearance typical of scleroderma. There may also be areas of telangiectasia and alternating hypo- and hyperpigmentation. Severe contractures of large joints may develop, as well as cutaneous ulceration.

From a histopathologic perspective, the process of generalized chronic GVHD often begins as a lichen planus-like eruption with irregular acanthosis, a band-like lymphoplasmacellular infiltrate at the dermal–epidermal junction, and hydropic degeneration of the basal layer with resultant dyskeratotic cells (Fig. 20). There is often hyperkeratosis as well. These features combine to produce papules and foci of hypopigmentation. Because of the epidermal involvement, punch biopsy will usually produce a positive result. Since the

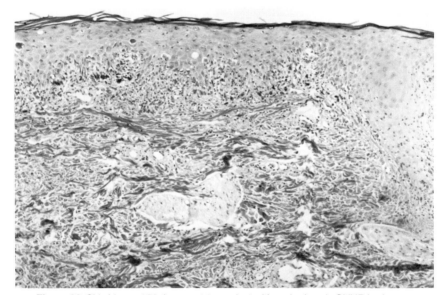

Figure 20. Skin biopsy 120 days post-transplant with early chronic GVHD is characterized by a band-like lymphocytic infiltrate and degeneration of the basal layer with some dyskeratotic cells. Note that the entire epidermis is involved with no apparent predilection for the rete ridges. There is inflammation and epithelial degeneration in the hair follicle at the right. (H&E ×75)

changes are not strikingly different from those of acute GVHD, distinction based on histology at this stage may not always be possible. However, a clue to the presence of GVHD appears to be the fact that acute GVHD tends to involve predominantly the tips of the rete ridges with sparing of the dermal plates, whereas chronic GVHD tends to be less localized in its damage (Fig. 20).

In addition to the above changes, early chronic GVHD may show lymphocytic infiltration of adnexal structures such as sweat glands and hair follicles plus nerves (Figs. 20 and 21). These structures, with the exception of hair follicles, are not commonly involved in acute disease. A true leukocytoblastic vasculitis has also been described. Eventually the inflammatory infiltrate may extend to the subcutaneous fat, leading to the deep fibrosis that is characteristic of the late stages of the disease. Obviously, a deep biopsy is necessary to see any of these adnexal, nerve, and fatty changes.

As the disease progresses to the later stages, the deep inflammatory and fibrotic picture predominates and the epidermal changes diminish. In the transition period from early-to-late generalized disease, the papillary dermis shows progressive fibrosis (Fig. 21). This characteristic fibrotic pattern is said to distinguish GVHD from scleroderma, which shows its earliest fibrosis in the reticular dermis. Eventually, the fibrosis of GVHD extends to involve the entire reticular dermis as well as underlying adipose tissue with entrapment of adnexal structures. At this stage, the process resembles both late localized GVHD and scleroderma (Fig. 22). The epidermis in the late stage becomes atrophic with loss of rete ridges although there may still be hyperkeratosis. Signs of active epithelial destruction such as dyskeratotic cells are generally scant or absent. Pigment incontinence may be prominent. As with localized disease, late generalized GVHD may be difficult to diagnose on a superficial punch biopsy. Generally a deep incisional biopsy is necessary.

The liver in chronic GVHD most commonly shows a mixed lymphoplasmacellular portal infiltrate with bile duct damage not unlike that of acute GVHD (Fig. 23). The infiltrate is in general more intense than in acute disease, reflecting the more complete immune reconstitution of the patient.[11,16] If the bile ducts have been destroyed as part of the "vanishing bile duct syndrome," the inflammation will diminish (Fig. 24). There is generally little hepatocellular involvement with the exception of piecemeal necrosis. In point of fact, if there is much hepatocellular damage in a biopsy taken in the chronic period, another diagnosis such as viral or drug-induced hepatitis should be strongly considered. Because of this lack of hepatocellular involvement, chronic GVHD actually looks more like acute liver transplant rejection than like acute GVHD. It should be noted that venous endothelialitis is only rarely seen in chronic GVHD.

Other features sometimes seen in association with chronic hepatic GVHD include cholestasis, piecemeal necrosis, fibrosis, cirrhosis, and paucity of bile ducts (the vanishing bile duct syndrome).[15,40] The presence of cholestasis is not surprising in a bile duct destructive lesion and is more commonly seen in the vanishing bile duct syndrome. The presence of piecemeal necrosis, fibrosis, or cirrhosis places a patient in the extensive disease category mentioned above

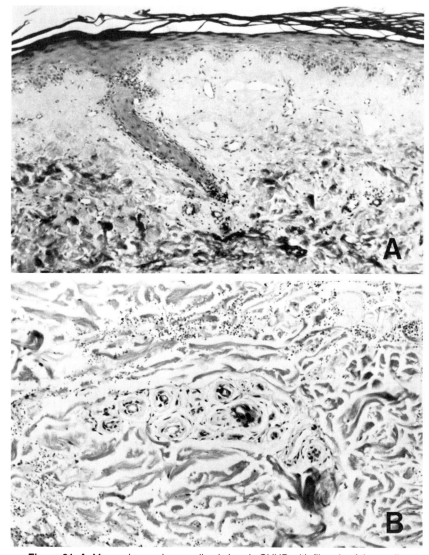

Figure 21. A. More advanced generalized chronic GVHD with fibrosis of the papillary dermis including degeneration of the hair follicle. **B.** There was also degeneration and atrophy of sweat glands in the specimen. (H&E: **A.** ×75, **B.** ×120)

(Fig. 23). Although not proposed in the original publications, it would seem that the vanishing bile duct syndrome falls in the extensive disease category.

The differential diagnosis of liver disease in the chronic phase usually includes viral infections, cholestasis of sepsis, and drug reaction in addition to GVHD. Acute viral infections, as mentioned above, present little diagnostic difficulty. Neither does cholestasis of sepsis since it is characterized by bland

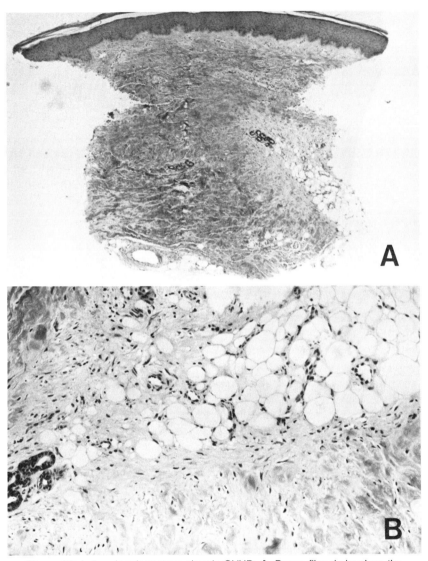

Figure 22. Late sclerodermatous chronic GVHD. **A.** Dense fibrosis involves the entire dermis with extension into subcutaneous fat. **B.** There is entrapment of sweat glands by the fibrosis which infiltrates the fat. (H&E: **A.** ×30, **B.** ×75)

canalicular cholestasis without the bile duct damage or infiltrate of GVHD. It should be noted that cholestasis of sepsis can have ductular bile plugs. Differentiation from drug reactions and chronic viral infections (hepatitis B or non-A non-B) can be impossible. However, many drug reactions manifest hepatocellular damage and/or an eosinophilia, thus allowing the differential diagnosis. Chronic active or persistent hepatitis of any cause may be impossible to distin-

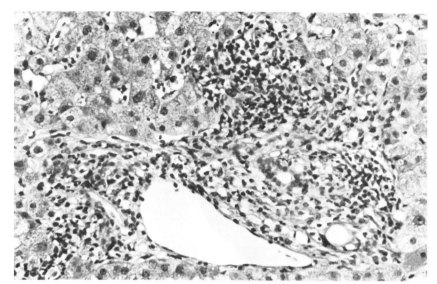

Figure 23. Chronic hepatic GVHD with a dense patchy lymphoplasmacellular portal infiltrate, piecemeal necrosis, and mild bile duct damage. This pattern may be histologically indistinguishable from chronic active viral hepatitis. (H&E ×192)

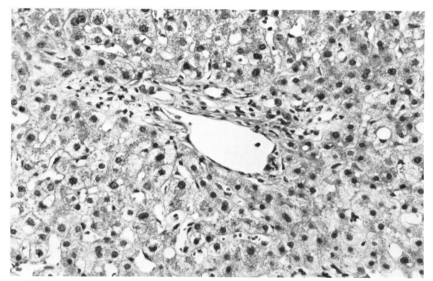

Figure 24. Portal tract from liver with chronic GVHD manifest as the "vanishing bile duct syndrome." Note the absence of an interlobular bile duct, even in the presence of an arteriole, as well as the paucity of inflammation. (H&E ×192)

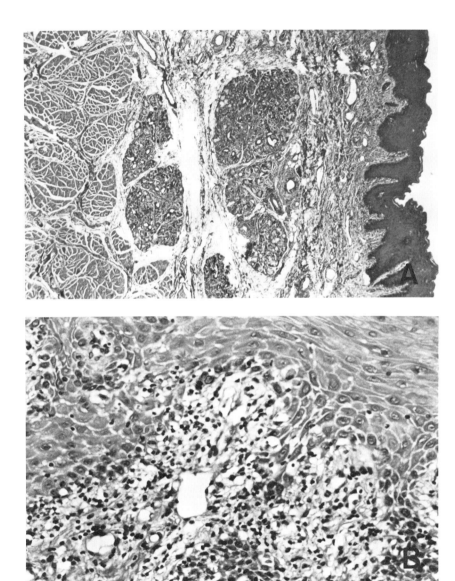

Figure 25. A. Deep full thickness lip biopsy showing abundant salivary gland tissue as well as mucosa for evaluation. **B.** The mucosa shows a lichenoid lympho-plasmacellular infiltrate with basal degeneration and dyskeratotic cells similar to those seen in acute GVHD of the skin. (*continued*)

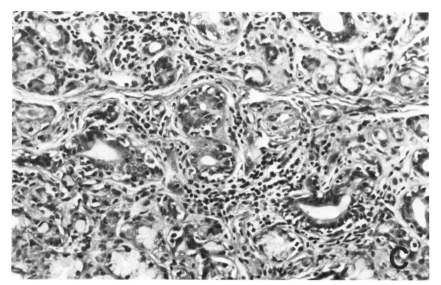

Figure 25 (cont.) C. Salivary gland shows a lymphoplasmacellular infiltrate with inflammation and degeneration of the ducts and acinar tissue. (H&E: **B., C.** ×192)

guish although the degree of bile duct damage may be helpful. As a rule of thumb, more than 50 percent damaged ducts favors GVHD. It should be remembered that viral hepatitis, particularly that due to non-A non-B may also show significant bile duct damage.[24,41]

Evaluation of the lip biopsy in chronic GVHD involves two separate pathologic processes: a lichen planus-like mucosal involvement and a Sjögren-like involvement of minor salivary glands.[38] Ideally both tissues should be available for examination although occasionally minor salivary glands are not present in the tissue obtained. As a technical point, however, deeper sections should always be obtained if salivary tissue is not present in the initial cuts.

The mucosa of the lip has features similar to the skin in acute GVHD with a band-like lymphoplasmacellular infiltrate, disruption and hydropic degeneration of the basal layer and dyskeratotic cells (civotte bodies) with satellitosis.[38] In general, the features are those of lichen planus (Fig. 25).

The salivary gland involvement resembles that of Sjögren syndrome. In early stages, there is a mild lymphocytic or plasma cellular infiltrate centered on the ducts with extension into the acini (Fig. 25). There may be infiltration of lymphocytes into the ductular or acinar epithelium associated with necrosis. As the disease progresses, the acinar portion of the gland becomes atrophic and eventually fibrotic. The patient may develop xerostomia (Fig. 26). Xerophthalmia results from similar changes in the lacrimal glands.[42] Of all of the organs biopsied, the lip may have the greatest potential as a predictor of development of chronic GVHD prior to development of symptoms. This is in large part due to the ease of biopsy plus the relative specificity of the pathology.

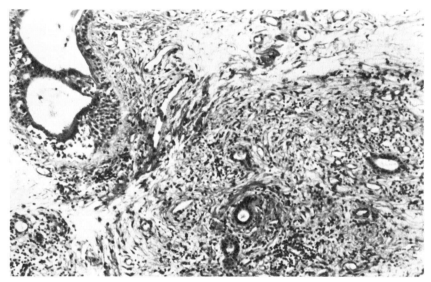

Figure 26. Severe chronic GVHD with almost total destruction of minor salivary gland. (H&E ×75)

Involvement of the GI tract in chronic GVHD has been reported to result in stenosis of the esophagus with resultant dysphagia. This was attributed to submucosal and subserosal fibrosis rather than fibrosis of the muscularis propria, thus distinguishing the process from scleroderma.[11,15] It appears, however, that esophageal involvement is much less common than early reports suggest. Stenosis of the small intestine and colon has also been reported.[14,43] Histologically, these lesions have shown denudation of the mucosa and fibrosis of the submucosa and subserosa. We have recently seen a case with active lymphocytic infiltration of the lamina propria, submucosa, and Auerbach's plexus. In addition to stenosis of the jejunum, the patient had delayed emptying of the stomach suggesting a motility problem. It is of some interest in this regard that similar changes have been reported in dog models of small intestinal allograft rejection.[44] Unfortunately, since the bowel changes reported in chronic GVHD are mild and nonspecific in the mucosa, endoscopic biopsy is rarely helpful in the diagnosis. Nonetheless, the biopsy is of value if infectious diseases must be ruled out.

The only other organ commonly biopsied to assess chronic GVHD in our institution is the lung. As with acute GVHD, considerable controversy exists over the existence, not to mention the histopathology, of pulmonary chronic GVHD. It is clear that many cases will have nonspecific interstitial pneumonitis. Most viral diseases also manifest that pattern, so the necessity to rule out infectious diseases is paramount. We have recently become aware of a subset of patients with reversible lung disease found in association with chronic GVHD of other organs who have lung biopsies characterized by, in addition to variable interstitial pneumonitis, endothelialitis as seen in the liver in GVHD or in most

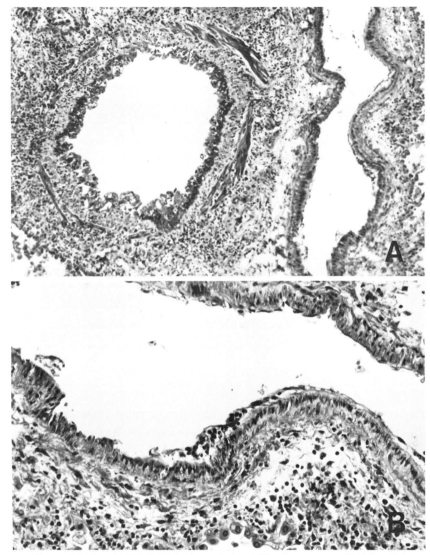

Figure 27. Chronic GVHD of the lung. **A.** In addition to a nonspecific interstitial infiltrate, there is a dense lyphocellular infiltrate of the bronchioles and veins which has resulted in subepithelial fibrosis in the bronchiole. **B.** The vein shows damage to the endothelium by a lymphocytic infiltrate identical to endothelialitis as seen in the liver. (H&E: **A.** ×75, **B.** ×192)

other organs in allograft rejection (Fig. 27). This endothelialitis is usually accompanied by lymphocytic infiltration of the respiratory bronchioles, often with destruction of the epithelium. It seems likely that this latter lesion may lead to cases of obstructive bronchitis that have been reported from a number of centers in association with chronic GVHD (Fig. 28).[45] Although the obstructive

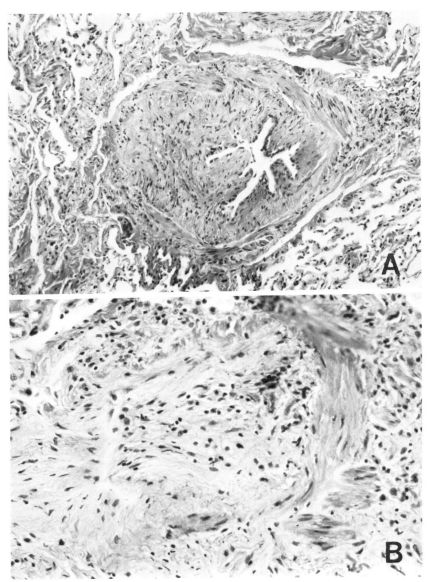

Figure 28. If not successfully treated, the bronchial lesion of chronic GVHD may eventually lead to partial (**A**) or total (**B**) fibrous occlusion. (H&E ×100). *(Reprinted from Rosenberg et al, Bronchiolitis obliterans after bone marrow transplantation. Am J Hematol 18:325, 1985, with permission.)*

bronchitis is irreversible if total, the lesion with endothelialitis and non-occlusive lymphocytic bronchitis appears to respond to steroid therapy.

A large number of other organs have been reported to be targets for chronic GVHD although the histopathology and diagnostic usefulness of biopsy are not well documented. Included among these are the heart, kidney, musculoskeletal system, and lymphoid system.[11,46,47] In theory, any organ should be a potential target for chronic GVHD. The specific reason for the particular distribution seen is unclear. However, if previous injury is necessary to initiate chronic GVHD, then organs commonly injured by GVHD post bone marrow transplant such as skin, GI tract and liver, as well as lung by infectious agents are rational targets.

THE CHRONIC PERIOD: OTHER PATHOLOGY

As in the acute phase, infectious diseases top the list of "other" pathology in the chronic period. There is some decrease in overall incidence of infection because the patients have generally undergone relatively complete marrow recovery. Nevertheless, chronic GVHD may diminish the immune response, leading to infections. It appears that viral agents, in particular CMV, are most common.

The only other problem unique to transplant patients is that of post-transplant lymphomas that begin to arise in the chronic phase.[48] These may be related to uncontrolled infections with the Epstein–Barr virus and are difficult to distinguish from atypical immunoproliferative processes by light microscopy alone. In all suspected cases, analysis for lymphocyte subsets, gene rearrangement, and cytogenetic abnormalities should be undertaken.

REFERENCES

1. Slavin RE, Woodruff JM: The pathology of bone marrow transplantation. Pathol Annu 9:291, 1974
2. Thomas ED, Storb R, Clift RA, et al: Bone marrow transplantation. N Engl J Med 292:832, 1975
3. Ramsay NKC, LeBien T, Nesbit M, et al: Autologous bone marrow transplantation for patients with acute lymphoblastic leukemia in second or subsequent remission: Results of bone marrow treated with monoclonal antibodies BA-1, BA-2, and BA-3 plus complement. Blood 66:508, 1985
4. Beschorner WE, Pino J, Boitnott JK, et al: Pathology of the liver with bone marrow transplantation. Effects of busulfan, carmustine, acute graft-vs-host disease and cytomegalovirus. Am J Pathol 99:369, 1980
5. Shulman HM, McDonald GB, Matthews D, et al: An analysis of hepatic venocclusive disease and centrilobular helpatocellular degeneration following bone marrow transplantation. Gastroenterology 79:1178, 1980
6. Krivit W, Pierpont ME, Ayaz K, et al: Bone marrow transplantation in Maroteaux-Lamy syndrome (mucopolysaccharidosis type VI): Biochemical and clinical status 24 months post-transplantation. N Engl J Med 311:1606, 1984

7. Thein SL, Goldman JM, Galton DAG: Acute "graft-versus-host disease" after autografting for chronic granulocytic leukemia in transformation. Ann Int Med 94:210, 1981

8. Hood AF, Vogelsang GB, Black LP, et al: Acute graft-vs-host disease: Development following autologous and syngeneic bone marrow transplantation. Arch Dermatol 123:745, 1987

9. Glazier A, Tutschka PJ, Farmer ER, Santos GW: Graft-versus-host disease in cyclosporin A-treated rats after syngeneic and autologous bone marrow reconstitution. J Exp Med 158:1, 1983

10. Snover DC: Acute and chronic graft versus host disease: Histopathological evidence for two pathogenetic mechanisms. Hum Pathol 15:202, 1984

11. Shulman HM, Sullivan KM, Weiden PL, et al: Chronic graft-versus-host syndrome in man: A long term clinicopathologic study of 20 Seattle patients. Am J Med 69:204, 1980

12. Sale GE, Lerner KG, Barker EA, et al: The skin biopsy in the diagnosis of acute graft-versus-host disease in man. Am J Pathol 89:621, 1977

13. Sale GE, Shulman HM, McDonald GB, Thomas ED: Gastrointestinal graft-versus-host disease in man. A clinicopathological study of the rectal biopsy. Am J Surg Pathol 3:291, 1979

14. Snover DC, Weisdorf SA, Vercellotti GM, et al: The histopathology of gastric and small intestinal graft-versus-host disease following allogeneic bone marrow transplantation. Hum Pathol 16:387, 1985

15. Sale GE, Shulman HM (eds): The Pathology of Bone Marrow Transplantation. New York, Masson, 1984

16. Snover DC, Weisdorf SA, Ramsay NKC, et al: Hepatic graft versus host disease: A study of the predictive value of liver biopsy in diagnosis. Hepatology 4:123, 1984

17. Sloane JP, Farthing MJ, Powles RL: Histopathological changes in the liver after allogeneic bone marrow transplantation. J Clin Pathol 33:344, 1980

18. Gale GE, Storb R, Kolb H: Histopathology of hepatic acute graft-versus-host disease in the dog. A double blind study confirms the specificity of small bile duct lesions. Transplantation 26:103, 1978

19. Sale GE, Shulman HM, Gallucci BB, Thomas ED: Young rete ridge keratinocytes are preferred targets in cutaneous graft-versus-host disease. Am J Pathol 118:278, 1985

20. Meisel JL, Bergman D, Graney D, et al: Human rectal mucosa. Proctoscopic and morphological changes caused by laxatives. Gastroenterology 72:1274, 1977

21. Snover DC: Mucosal damage simulating acute graft-versus-host reaction in cytomegalovirus colitis. Transplantation 39:669, 1985

22. Lampert IA, Thorpe P, Noorden SV, et al: Selective sparing of enterochromaffin cells in graft versus host disease affecting the colonic mucosa. Histopathology 9:875, 1985

23. Snover DC, Freese DK, Sharp HL, et al: Liver allograft rejection: An analysis of the use of biopsy in determining outcome of rejection. Am J Surg Pathol 11:1, 1987

24. Kryger P, Christoffersen P, Copenhagen Hepatitis Acuta Programme: Light microscopic morphology of acute hepatitis non-A, non-B. A comparison with hepatitis type A and B. Liver 2:200, 1982

25. Lerner KG, Kao GF, Storb R, et al: Histopathology of graft-vs.-host reaction (GvHR) in human recipients of marrow from HL-A matched sibling donors. Transplant Proc 6:367, 1974

26. Woodruff JM, Hansen JA, Good RA, et al: The pathology of the graft-versus-host reaction (GVHR) in adults receiving bone marrow transplants. Transplant Proc 8:675, 1976

27. Buja LM, Ferrans VJ, Graw RG: Cardiac pathologic findings in patients treated with bone marrow transplantation. Hum Pathol 7:17, 1976

28. Beschorner WE, Saral R, Hutchins GM, et al: Lymphocytic bronchitis associated with graft-vs-host disease in recipients of bone marrow transplants. N Engl J Med 299:1030, 1978

29. Hackman RC, Sale GE: Large airway inflammation as a possible manifestation of a pulmonary graft-versus-host reaction. Lab Invest 44:26A, 1981

30. Winston DJ, Gale RP, Meyer DV, et al: Infectious complications of human bone marrow transplantation. Medicine 58:1, 1979

31. Blazar B, Hurd DD, Snover DC, et al: Invasive *Fusarium* infection in bone marrow transplant recipients: A report of three cases and a review of the literature. Am J Med 77:546, 1984

32. Neglia JP, Hurd DD, Ferrieri P, Snover DC: Invasive *Scopulariopsis* in the immunosuppressed host. Am J Med 83:1163, 1987

33. Hirsch R, Burke BA, Kersey JH: Toxoplasmosis in bone marrow transplant recipients. J Pediatr 105:426, 1984

34. Rywlin AM, Ortega A: Glycogenic acanthosis of the esophagus. Arch Pathol 90:439, 1970

35. McDonald GB, Sharma P, Matthews DE, et al: Venocclusive disease of the liver after bone marrow transplantation: Diagnosis, incidence and predisposing factors. Hepatology 4:116, 1984

36. Snover DC, Weisdorf SA, Bloomer J, McGlave P: Nodular regenerative hyperplasia: A possible cause of liver disease following bone marrow transplantation. Lab Invest 54:60A, 1986

37. Stromeyer FW, Ishak KG: Nodular transformation (nodular "regenerative" hyperplasia) of the liver: A clinicopathologic study of 30 cases. Hum Pathol 12:60, 1981

38. Sale GE, Shulman HM, Schubert MM, et al: Oral and ophthalmic pathology of graft-versus-host disease in man. Predictive value of the lip biopsy. Hum Pathol 12:1022, 1981

39. Fenyk JR Jr, Smith CM, Warkentin PI, et al: Sclerodermatous graft-versus-host disease limited to an area of measles exanthem. Lancet 1:472, 1978

40. Shulman HM: Graft-versus-host-induced cirrhosis: Possible mechanisms. Hepatology 7:1385, 1987

41. Christoffersen P, Poulsen H, Scheuer PJ: Abnormal bile duct epithelium in chronic aggressive hepatitis and primary biliary cirrhosis. Hum Pathol 3:227, 1972

42. Jabs DA, Hirst LW, Green R, et al: The eye in bone marrow transplantation. II. Histopathology. Arch Ophthalmol 101:585, 1983

43. Fisk JD, Shulman HM, Greening RR, et al: Gastrointestinal radiographic features of human graft-vs-host disease. AJR 136:329, 1981

44. Banner BF, Dean P, Williams JW: Morphology of rejection in long-surviving canine small bowel transplants. Lab Invest 56:4A, 1987

45. Urbanski SJ, Kossakowska AE, Curtis J, et al: Idiopathic small airways pathology in patients with graft-versus-host disease following allogeneic bone marrow transplantation. Am J Surg Pathol 11:965, 1987

46. Graze PR, Gale RP: Chronic graft versus host disease: A syndrome of disordered immunity. Am J Med 66:611, 1979
47. Furst DE, Clements PJ, Graze P, et al: A syndrome resembling progressive systemic sclerosis after bone marrow transplantation: A model for scleroderma? Arthritis Rheum 22:904, 1979
48. Frizzera G, Hanto DW, Gajl-Peczalska K, et al: Polymorphic diffuse B-cell hyperplasias and lymphomas in renal transplant recipients. Cancer Res 41:4262, 1981

Histopathologic Parameters and DNA Analysis in Colorectal Adenocarcinomas

John D. Crissman, Richard J. Zarbo, Chan K. Ma, and
Daniel W. Visscher

Cancer of the colon and rectum is a common malignant neoplasm in Western countries. In the United States, it is second as a cause of mortality to cancer of the lung in men and third to cancer of the lung and breast in women.[1] In 1987, approximately 145,000 new cases of colorectal cancer were diagnosed in the United States.[1] The 5-year survival rates of colon cancer of whites for the period 1960 to 1963 was 43 percent and for the period of 1977 to 1983 was 53 percent.[1] These rates suggest some improvement in survival between these periods. Diagnosis at an earlier stage of the disease remains the best hope for continuing improvement in patient survival. There is increasing evidence that adjuvant radiation therapy of rectal carcinomas is helpful in improving patient outcome.[2] To provide optimal therapy, it has become important to identify groups of patients at higher risk for local recurrence and distant metastasis.

STAGING AND HISTOLOGICAL PROGNOSTIC PARAMETERS

Many clinicopathologic factors have been reported to have prognostic significance in colon carcinoma. The clinical factors which may influence prognosis, i.e., bowel obstruction, rectal bleeding, and anemia,[3-5] are beyond the scope of this discussion and are usually related to the stage and growth pattern (e.g., ulceration, circumferential involvement) of the neoplasm. The literature contains many studies of the relationship between a variety of pathologic parameters and survival for patients with colorectal cancer. The more widely accepted and time-honored prognostic factors are extent or depth of tumor invasion, presence of regional lymph node metastasis, degree of tumor differentiation, presence of vascular invasion, lymphocytic infiltrates, and pattern of tumor invasion. The relationship of tumor size to stage and ultimate survival is controversial. Cohen and associates found that 42 percent of ulcerative carcinomas greater than 4 cm penetrated through the rectal wall, compared to 12 percent of tumors less than 4 cm.[6] More recently, however Wolmark et al failed to find a significant correlation between tumor size and the presence of lymph node metastases.[7]

Pathologic Staging

The extent of tumor infiltration (depth of invasion) and lymph node metastasis are the two most important prognostic factors and they determine pathologic stage. The depth of tumor infiltration correlates well with the frequency of venous invasion, the presence of lymph node metastases, and survival at 5 years. Lockhart-Mummery was the first to stage rectal carcinoma, correlating stage with survival.[8] Based on the extent of the tumor, he classified rectal cancer into stage A, B, or C. Cuthbert Dukes refined this staging system in 1929 and further modified the staging system in 1932.[9,10] This latter staging system, originally described for rectal cancers but later extended to include all colon sites, represents "Dukes' Staging" defined as follows:

- Stage A: Carcinoma confined to the rectal wall defined as muscularis propria without lymph node metastases
- Stage B: Carcinoma penetrating through the muscularis propria into the perirectal (colonic) soft tissue without lymph node metastases
- Stage C: Lymph node metasases present regardless of the depth of tumor invasion

This staging system is simple, easy to reproduce and widely accepted. Dukes in 1935 divided his stage C into C1 (only perirectal lymph nodes involved) and C2 (involvement of apical mesenteric lymph nodes).[11] Unfortunately, subsequent authors (Simpson and Mayo in 1939[12]; Kirklin et al in 1949[13]; and Astler and Coller in 1954[14]) modified Dukes' classification but they retained the A, B, C system, redefined the depth of invasion for each stage and divided B into B1 and B2 and C into C1 and C2, but with different definitions. These alternate staging systems provided little additional useful information and greatly confused the staging terminology.[15] In 1967, Turnbull added stage D to Dukes' system to describe patients with either distant spread or invasion into adjacent organs.[16] Pihl et al, in reporting 1061 cases of carcinoma of the rectum and rectosigmoid, also added a stage D, similar to Turnbull's classification.[17] However, they further divided D into D1 (invading adjacent organs) and D2 (distant metastasis). Confusion arises when subsequent authors refer to these different systems merely as Dukes' classification or a modified Dukes' classification.[15] Table 1 compares various staging systems proposed by different authors.

TABLE 1. COMPARISON OF VARIOUS STAGING SYSTEMS USED BY DIFFERENT AUTHORS

Maximal Depth of Invasion	Lockhart-Mummery[8] 1926	Dukes 1932[10a]	Dukes 1935[11]	Simpson et al[12] 1939	Kirklin et al[13] 1949	Astler–Coller[14] 1954	Turnbull[16] 1967	Pihl et al[17] 1980
				Stage (% 5-Year Survival)				
Mucosa					A (100)	A (100)		
Submucosa	A (73.7)			A (100)				A1 (90)
Muscularis propria	B (44.1)	A (80)	A (91)	B (61.9)	B1 (75)	B1 (66.6)	A (98.9)	A2 (89)
Pericolic or rectal adipose tissue		B (73)	B (64)	C (49.4)	B2 (70)	B2 (53.9)	B (84.9)	B (76)
Positive nodes	C (44.4)	C (7)	C (16)		C (36.4)		C (67.3)	
Regional			C1			C1 (43)[b]		C1 (43)
Apical			C2			C2 (22.4)[c]		C2 (12)
Invades adjacent tissue or distant spread							D (14.3)	D1 (11) D2 (0)

[a] The "classic" Dukes' classification.
[b] C1 is stage B1 tumor with lymph node metastasis.
[c] C2 is stage B2 tumor with lymph node metastasis.

The subdivision of stage C tumors into C1 and C2 is even more confusing. Dukes defined C1 and C2 as follows:

- C1: Metastasis to proximal (perirectal lymph nodes only)
- C2: Involvement of distal (apical) nodes

whereas, Astler-Coller defined C1 and C2 as follows:

- C1: B1 lesions with positive lymph nodes
- C2: B2 lesions with positive lymph nodes

However, the Gastrointestinal Tumor Study Group (GISG) defined them as follows[18]:

- C1: 1 to 4 positive lymph nodes
- C2: More than 4 positive lymph nodes

Studies have indicated that each of these three staging classifications have independent prognostic value. Table 2 lists the 5-year survival rates of major series of colorectal carcinomas by Dukes' classification and the three modified C staging systems. Wolmark investigated the interrelationships between these three stage C systems based on data collected from 844 Dukes' C colorectal carcinomas.[19] He confirmed that each system had a highly significant predictive capacity as independent variables. When adjusting for the contribution of other variables, however, the effect attributable to the level of positive nodes (proximal or apical) was markedly attenuated. Of these three factors, the number of positive nodes appeared to be the strongest predictor of recurrence. Using depth of tumor penetration and the number of positive nodes, 98 patients with tumor limited to the muscularis propria (Astler–Coller's B1) and 1 to 4 positive nodes had 5-year survival rates similar to 593 Dukes' B cases (78 versus 70 percent). Phillips et al, in their study of 2518 cases of colorectal carcinoma, made similar observations[20] (Table 2). This indicates that not all Dukes' C cases fare poorly, depending on the depth of tumor penetration and the number of positive nodes.

Newland et al, who studied 1117 cases of colorectal carcinoma, observed the importance of serosal (free mesothelial surface) involvement by the tumor.[21] They subdivided stage A lesions into A2 with invasion into submucosa, and A3 with invasion into muscularis propria. Stage B lesions were subdivided into B1 with invasion beyond muscularis propria but not to the serosa and B2 with the serosa involved; stage C was divided into C1 with only proximal nodes involved and C2 with apical nodes involved. The corrected 5-year survival rates were A2: 97 percent, A3: 83 percent, B1: 77 percent, B2: 64 percent, C1: 54 percent, and C2: 26 percent. There was not a statistically significant difference in the 5-year survival rate between A3 lesions and B1 lesions. However, B2 lesions fared much worse than B1 lesions, having survival patterns similar to C1 lesions.

Prognosis tended to be much worse when the serosa was involved than when it was not (B2 versus B1). In most major series (Table 2), tumors that penetrated through the muscularis propria would be classified as Dukes' B

TABLE 2. 5-YEAR SURVIVAL RATE BY STAGE[a]

| Author | Total Cases | Sites | % Survival | | | | | | | | | |
| | | | Dukes | | | | | Astler–Coller[b] | | GITSG | |
			A	B	C	C1	C2	C1	C2	C1	C2
Astler–Coller[14]	352	Colon and rectum						42.8	22.4		
Dukes and Bussy[31]	2447	Rectum	99.7	77.6	32	40.9	13.6				
Freedman[8]	769	Rectum	72	57	35						
Phillips[20]	2518	Colon and rectum	82	65		46	22	68	40	60	21
Chapuis[3]	709	Colon and rectum	62	55	29						
Newland[21]	1117	Colon and rectum	89	75	49	54	26				
Jass[36]	710	Rectum	97	81		51	23			44	13

[a]Some authors used crude 5-year survival rate, whereas others used corrected 5-year survival rates.
[b]Astler–Coller's stages A and B differ from Dukes' A and B.

regardless of invasion of the serosal surface. Overall, Dukes' B lesions did not fare much worse than stage A tumors, although these differences in 5-year survival were statistically significant. If patients with serosal invasion were separated from the rest of Dukes' B cases, the difference in 5-year survival rates between A and B lesions would be even smaller. Because the number of Dukes' B cases with serosal involvement was small (in Newland's series, only 27 of 380 Dukes' B cases), the effect on the 5-year survival rate of Dukes' B lesions was minimal. Nevertheless, it is important to identify tumor invasion of the serosa since this significantly reduces the 5-year survival.

On the other hand, the division of "B" lesions into B1 (into but not beyond muscularis propria) and B2 (through the muscularis propria) by Astler–Coller does not have much prognostic significance as shown in the study of Newland et al.[21] The staging system of Astler–Coller, one of the more commonly used systems, has created most of the confusion regarding staging terminology. Astler–Coller "A" and "B1" correspond to Dukes' A and their "B2" corresponds to Dukes' B. The use of a subgroup of stage A with tumor limited to the mucosa is not practical since few such cases exist and metastases seldom occur.[22] Astler–Coller's original report only had one example of an "A" tumor among their 352 cases and Newland et al had none in their 1117 cases. Because of the lack of a generally accepted classification and confusion regarding Dukes' staging, the American Joint Committee on Cancer and the Union Internationale Contre Cancer developed a TNM (tumor staging) system for colorectal carcinoma.[23] However, this system is more complex and difficult to apply.[24] It would appear that the major contribution of the TNM system is to avoid confusion created by the various A, B, C staging systems. The classification of lymph node stage by number of lymph nodes with metastases appears to be statistically significant and it represents an improvement in the substaging of regional disease.[25]

Vascular Invasion
Vascular invasion, although closely related to the depth of invasion, is an independent prognostic factor in most studies.[20] The significance of extramural vascular invasion as a poor prognostic parameter is generally accepted; the importance of intramural vascular invasion remains controversial. In general, intramural vascular involvement includes both blood and lymphatic capillary spaces since these small vessels are impossible to differentiate. Extramural vascular invasion invariably involves tumor extension into draining veins, often with identifiable mural elastic tissue and smooth muscle (Fig. 1). Khankhanian et al studied 143 Dukes' B colorectal carcinomas and they found no statistically significant difference in tumor-free interval and overall survival time between patients with and without intramural vascular invasion.[26] Talbot and associates performed one of the most comprehensive studies of venous invasion of 703 cases of rectal carcinoma.[27] The corrected 5-year survival rate of 108 cases with intramural venous invasion (65.7 percent) did not differ significantly from that of 328 cases in which venous invasion was not demonstrated (73 percent). However, survival was reduced to 40.9 percent when extramural thin-walled

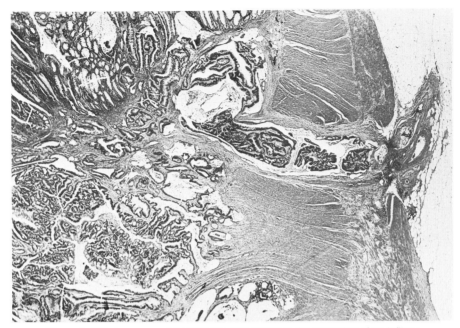

Figure 1. This low-power magnification demonstrates the extension of an infiltrating carcinoma into a large draining vein. The intravascular tumor extends beyond the bowel wall as extramural extension.

veins were involved. An additional reduction in survival to 19.4 percent was noted when extramural thick-walled veins contained intraluminal tumor. A recent report by Minsky et al further supports Talbot's observation.[28] In their study of 168 cases of rectosigmoid and rectal carcinomas, the 5-year survival rate for patients with extramural venous involvement was 33 percent, compared to 72 percent for patients without venous invasion or with only intramural venous invasion. Most large recent series confirmed the prognostic value of venous invasion, particularly when extramural veins are involved (Table 3).

Histological Grading

Studies have shown that a number of histopathologic parameters (degree of tumor differentiation, pattern of tumor growth, lymphocytic infiltrates, desmoplastic response) have prognostic significance.[29] The grading of colorectal carcinomas by most pathologists is usually based on the degree of tumor differentiation, reflected by structural and cytological features. It is widely accepted that the degree of tumor differentiation is an important prognostic factor independent of stage (Table 4). However, the assessment of differentiation remains a subjective exercise with substantial interobserver variability.[30] The problem is further complicated by a lack of strict guidelines for separating histological grades. A review of the literature indicated that most authors applied the

TABLE 3. 5-YEAR SURVIVAL RATE RELATED TO VENOUS INVASION

Author	Total Cases	Site	% Survival by Distribution of Venous Invasion						
			Absent	None or Submucosal	Not Specified	Intra-mural	Extra-mural	Thin-walled	Thick-walled
Talbot[27]	703	Rectum	73			65.7		40.9	19.4
Freedman[87]	769	Rectum	58			42	31		
Phillips[20]	2518	Colon and rectum	71		48				
Chapuis[3]	709	Colon and rectum	40		15				
Jass[29]	447	Rectum		67			41		

TABLE 4. 5-YEAR SURVIVAL RATE RELATED TO DEGREE OF DIFFERENTIATION

Author	Total Cases	Site	% Survival by Degree of Differentiation		
			Well	*Moderate*	*Poor*
Phillips[20]	2518	Colon and rectum	62	60	42
Freedman[87]	769	Rectum	62	54	35
Chapuis[3]	709	Colon and rectum	63	43	11
Jass[29]	447	Rectum	83	63	22

criteria of Dukes and Bussey.[31] Well-differentiated adenocarcinoma was composed of complex or simple tubules lined by epithelium closely resembling adenomatous epithelium (Fig. 2). Nuclear polarity was maintained. Poorly differentiated carcinoma showed little or no gland formation and a loss of nuclear polarity (Fig. 3). Tumors with morphology between those extremes were classified as moderately differentiated (Fig. 4).

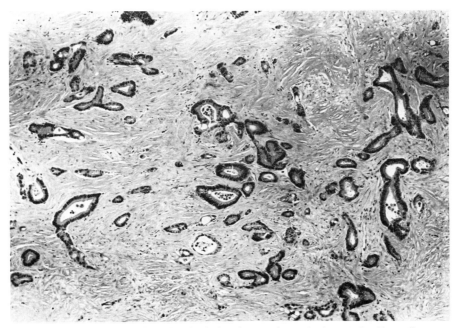

Figure 2. This well-differentiated colonic adenocarcinoma is characterized by well-formed ducts or tubules. The cells have organized basilar placed nuclei. The growth pattern and cytological features define this neoplasm as well differentiated.

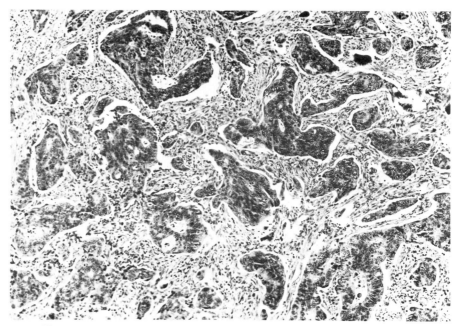

Figure 3. This poorly differentiated colonic adenocarcinoma grows in a disorganized manner. There are only rare abortive lumens and much of the neoplasm grows as sheets. The cells display little evidence of differentiation.

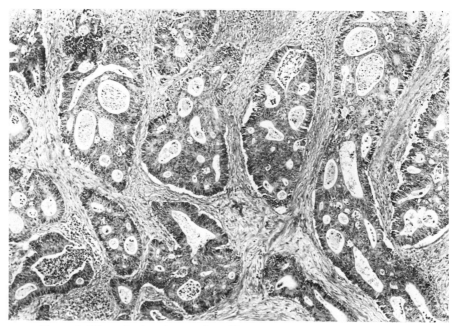

Figure 4. This moderate or intermediate differentiated tumor infiltrates as sheets of cribriform-appearing tumor with numerous irregular lumens. The cells attempt to form differentiated structures but are only partially successful.

Lymphocytic Infiltrate

The inflammatory response to a tumor has traditionally been regarded as an indication of host resistance to neoplastic spread (Fig. 5A). MacCarty, in 1922, reported a favorable association between lymphocytic infiltration in the primary tumor and survival.[32] Spratt and Spjut found that the 5-year survival rate was doubled when there was intense inflammatory response around the carcinoma of the colon and rectum.[33] These observations were confirmed by Murray et al.[34] Jass, in his comprehensive studies of 447 specimens of rectal carcinoma, semiquantitated the degree of lymphocytic infiltration around the tumor into pronounced, moderate, and little. The corresponding corrected 5-year survival rates were 92, 65, and 36 percent, respectively[35] (Table 5). He subsequently developed a prognostic classification based on the evaluation of multiple histological parameters, and lymphocytic infiltration was one of the four variables selected as statistically significant for predicting patient outcome.[36]

"Infiltrative" versus "Pushing" Invasion Pattern

The pattern of tumor growth (infiltrative peripheral border versus well defined or pushing) is also an important prognostic factor. Spratt and Spjut showed that tumors with expanding or pushing borders (Fig. 6) were less aggressive than tumors with infiltrative margins (Fig. 7).[33] Carlon and associates, in a study of 124 cases of rectal carcinoma, found pattern of tumor growth, staging, and lymphocytic response to be the most important histological parameters for defining prognosis.[37] The 5-year survival rates for expanding and infiltrative tumors were 75 and 40 percent, respectively.[37] In a series of 447 rectal carcinomas reported by Jass, the corrected 5-year survival rates for expanding and infiltrative tumors were 73 and 26 percent, respectively.[29] The pattern of tumor growth was also one of four variables selected by Jass in his prognostic classification for rectal carcinoma.[36]

TABLE 5. 5-YEAR SURVIVAL RATE RELATED TO AMOUNT OF LYMPHOCYTE INFILTRATE

Author	Total Cases	Site	Peri-tumoral	Intra-tumoral	Pro-nounced	Mod. to Marked	Moderate	Little or None
Murray[34]	148	Colon	+			78.2		40
Zhou[88]	1226	Colon and rectum	+	+	100		68.4	32.4
Carlon[89]	124	Rectum	+	+	92		59	51
Jass[35]	447	Rectum	+		92		65	36

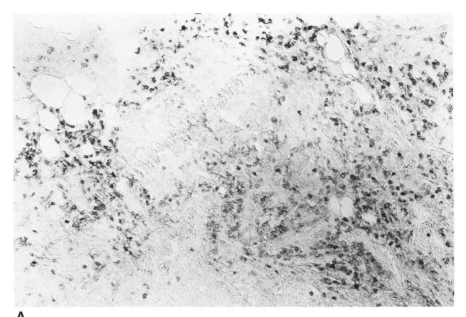

A

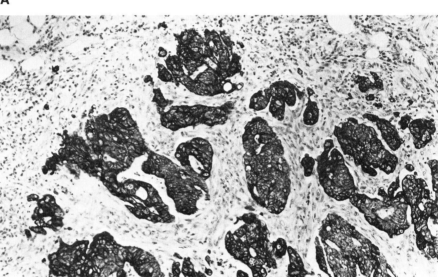

B

Figure 5. A. This microscopic section is stained with the antibody to leukocyte common antigen (LCA) and reveals numerous leukocytes in this invasive colonic adenocarcinoma. **B.** This microscopic section is from an area adjacent to that demonstrated in **A** stained with antikeratin antibody. This stains only epithelial cells which with careful selection are invariably neoplastic. The tumor is rimmed by leukocytes and separated by reacting stromal desmoplasia.

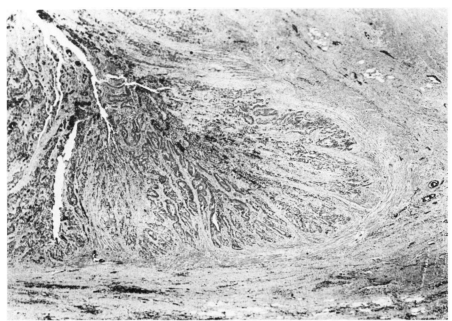

Figure 6. This low power magnification of adenocarcinoma shows the well-defined tumor–stromal interface characteristic of a pushing margin of invasion. This appears to be a tumor of moderate differentiation.

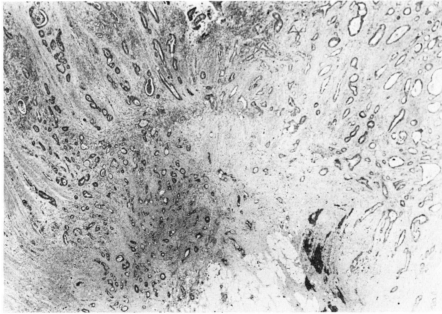

Figure 7. This photomicrograph documents a well-differentiated adenocarcinoma with infiltrative margins. The tumor dissects through normal structures with penetration into pericolonic adipose tissue.

DNA ANALYSIS BY FLOW CYTOMETRY

Initial clinical application of flow cytometry was directed at determining the subset distribution of cell surface markers of circulating leukocytes and leukemic cells. Subsequently, non-Hodgkin's lymphomas, neoplasms that are readily disaggregated into single cell suspensions, were also evaluated for cell surface markers indicative of lineage and clonality. Additional applications of flow cytometry have included DNA analysis using a number of fluorescent dyes that bind in a stoichiometric manner with nuclear DNA.

Subsequently, quantitation of DNA in solid tumors, including lymphomas, has become a common procedure in many laboratories. While it was initially applied only as a research tool, it has been gaining popularity because of its perceived importance as a prognostic parameter and its potential value in planning therapy. The essence of DNA analysis is the measurement of the DNA content in numerous single cells (10^4–10^5 cells) and the construction of a histogram representing the DNA distribution within the study cell population (Fig. 8). The largest proportion of any cell population is in the resting (G_0) or cycling (G_1) component of the cell cycle which contains similar quantities of DNA. In normal cells, the G_0/G_1 component has 46 chromosomes or a normal DNA (diploid) content. Replicating cells synthesize DNA prior to cell division and this intermediate population with an increasing quantity of DNA represents the synthesis phase fraction (SPF) located between the G_0/G_1 and G_2/M peaks (Fig. 8). The latter cell population has double the chromosomal DNA content of the G_0/G_1 cell population and represents synthetic cells preceding mitosis (G_2) and cells which have entered into mitosis (M) prior to completion of cell division.

The two major observations which result from flow cytometric DNA analy-

Figure 8. This idealized DNA histogram of a propidium iodide-stained test cell population also includes a reference peak of chick red blood cells. Increasing fluorescence intensity corresponds to increased DNA content of the individual cells. The distribution of the cell cycle compartments is also represented. The major peak contains G_0/G_1 cells with a 2N DNA content. The G_2/M peak contains double the normal amount of DNA and the dotted line represents the fraction of cells in the process of synthesizing DNA (SPF).

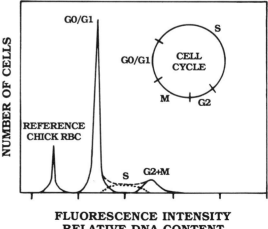

**FLUORESCENCE INTENSITY
RELATIVE DNA CONTENT**

sis are the presence (or absence) of G_0/G_1 populations containing an abnormal DNA content and the quantitation of the SPF (or rarely the SPF and G_2/M populations). The former is a measurement of cells in G_0/G_1 containing abnormal amounts of DNA (aneuploidy). The latter is an index of tumor replication or proliferation and is expressed as a percent of the total cell population.

Abnormal DNA-containing tumor cell populations are classified by comparing them to diploid control cells. This is the DNA index (DI), calculated as the ratio of the mean channel of the abnormal G_0/G_1 peak divided by the mean channel of the control normal (diploid) G_0/G_1 peak. The denominator is determined by the use of appropriate control cells which are known to have a diploid DNA content.[38,39] Cells which have established but lower DNA contents, such as chicken- and trout-nucleated erythrocytes, are also commonly used to establish the location of diploid DNA channels (Fig. 9). When the latter are used, the system must be carefully calibrated since slight shifts in DNA staining occur with different methods of solid tumor disaggregation. We have found that diploid cells in the tumor provide the most reliable basis on which to establish the diploid channel. Minor chromosomal abnormalities involving either arms of single chromosomes such as deletions, translocations, point mutations, and other marker changes associated with neoplastic transformation, may not appreciably change the total DNA content. In tumors with minor chromosomal abnormalities, identification of DNA content changes is dependent on the sensitivity and resolution of the histogram. Optimum sample preparation to provide a narrow peak width (low coefficient of variation or CV) for diploid control and tumor cells allows better resolution of peridiploid tumor populations. Instrument resolution and alignment are also critical for achieving maximum sensitivity in resolving diploid from peridiploid tumor cell populations.

We define abnormal or aneuploid DNA peaks as second peaks that can be resolved from the known diploid DNA peak. The limits of resolution are dependent on the quality of the sample preparation as reflected by the CVs of the normal and abnormal peaks. In most instances, we can resolve smaller differences than the 10 percent or two standard deviation differences in channels arbitrarily required by many investigators. Dissociation and fixation artifacts may alter DNA staining which mandates control cell (diploid human or nucleated erythrocyte calibrators) populations prepared by the same procedure as the tumor cell population. In many studies, human lymphocytes prepared and stored differently from the cells dissociated from solid tumors are used as controls and they may or may not correspond with diploid non-neoplastic cells from the tumor. The process of dissociation of human tumors has the potential to alter DNA staining characteristics, especially if enzymes are used.[40] We strongly recommend that if exogenous diploid control cells are used, they should be handled in a similar fashion as the dissociated tumor cells. In addition, we have found that sufficient diploid cells are present in human colon cancer to accurately determine the diploid standard channel. Ideally, normal diploid non-neoplastic cells within the dissociated tumor serve as the optimum internal diploid standard. When there is a question as to which peak represents

GREEN FLUORESCENCE   RED FLUORESCENCE

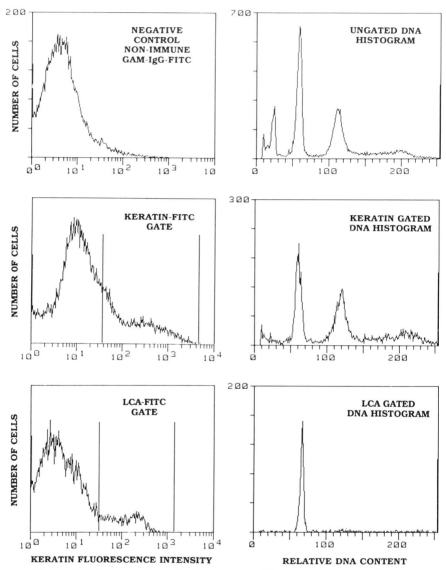

KERATIN FLUORESCENCE INTENSITY   RELATIVE DNA CONTENT

Figure 9. This figure shows the fluorescein isothiocyanate (green) conjugated nonimmune IgG (control), keratin and leukocyte common antigen (LCA) in the left column. The corresponding DNA histogram of propidium iodide fluorescence (red) in the dual labeled colon carcinoma cells is represented in the right column. These include ungated (*top panel*) cells, keratin positive cells (*middle panel*) and LCA-positive cells (*lower panel*). The ungated histogram reveals two populations, diploid and aneuploid. Both contain keratin-positive cells, indicating a biclonal tumor. The LCA-positive inflammatory cells are found only in the diploid range channels.

the non-neoplastic cells, we can document their location by dual labeling for keratin or LCA antigens (Fig. 9).

PREPARATION OF SINGLE CELL SUSPENSIONS

The major impediment to flow cytometric (FCM) analysis of solid tumors is the ability to produce single cell suspensions representative of the neoplastic cell population. Carcinomas and some sarcomas are characterized by intercellular desmosomes, attachment to extracellular matrix (basement membrane), and other complex interactions with stromal components which contribute to the cohesive nature of the tissue. Carcinomas with squamous differentiation have complex desmosomal attachments and are difficult to dissociate.[41,42] Adenocarcinomas have less well-developed desmosomes but are commonly surrounded by host stroma and extracellular matrix.

Two general approaches have evolved to produce single cell samples suitable for FCM DNA analysis. The most common method is the use of bare nuclei extracted from solid tumors by a combination of detergents and enzymes.[43] This approach was pioneered by Vindelov and is employed in many laboratories.[43] Similar techniques have been suggested for extracting nuclei from paraffin tissue blocks for DNA analysis and include the use of different proteases with varying digestion times.[44-48] At present, the most popular protocol is one proposed by Hedley.[48] A second method for preparation of samples for FCM analysis is to produce suspensions of intact cells by either enzymatic digestion or mechanical dissociation.[49] This approach is much more difficult because the disruption of desmosomes or attachments requires great care. In many instances, only portions of the cytoplasm remain and the injured cells are not viable. One critical issue in any dissociation technique is whether the resulting nuclear or cellular suspension is truly representative of the tumor population. As obvious as this statement appears, very few investigators have performed appropriate studies to define the efficiency of extraction and to determine if the recovered cells are representative of the cell components comprising the tumor.

Nuclear suspensions are technically less difficult and time consuming to prepare, but discrimination of diploid tumor from contaminating inflammatory and stromal nuclei is difficult or impossible to achieve. In addition, the possibility of applying multiparameter analyses using cytoplasmic or cell membrane markers is lost. The preparation of suspensions of intact cells is more difficult in squamous cell carcinomas which have well-developed desmosomes.[41,42] Mechanical disaggregation of most adenocarcinomas, including colonic adenocarcinomas, to produce intact cells is a relatively simple procedure which represents an attractive alternative to enucleation procedures.[40] However, we recommend quality control procedures for this method in each laboratory to assure that the dissociated cells are representative of the tumor.[41]

The ability of the flow cytometer to quantitate multiple markers has prompted the use of secondary tissue-specific markers for solid tumors to allow electronic gating to select defined cell populations. In suspensions of intact cells it is possible to use a variety of dual labeling techniques for cytoplasmic antigens which serve to better define tumor cell populations and by electronic gating, restrict the DNA analysis to tumor cells (Fig. 9).[50] The ultimate goal of observing multiple parameters is to identify tumor cell subsets, to restrict the DNA analysis to tumor cells, and to exclude contaminating host cell components. This results in "clean" nonoverlapping histogram peaks of defined cell populations with better resolution of tumor DNA content and more accurate SPF

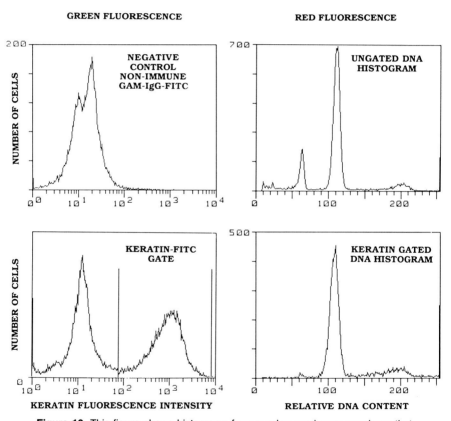

Figure 10. This figure shows histograms from a colon carcinoma specimen that was dual labeled for keratin and DNA. The first peak in the ungated DNA histogram represents non-neoplastic inflammatory and stromal cell components and the second peak aneuploid tumor cells. The keratin-gated DNA histogram (*lower right*) represents only the aneuploid tumor population. Dual labeling and selective gating enables more sensitive detection of aneuploid events and more specific calculation of the S-phase fraction, avoiding overlap of G_2/M from the contaminating diploid component.

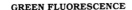
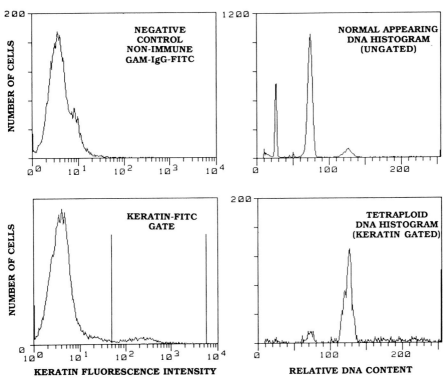

Figure 11. This figure is a histogram of a dual keratin-DNA-labeled colon carcinoma, the ungated histogram (*upper right*) with external chick RBC standard simulates a diploid DNA population. However, in the keratin-gated DNA histogram (*lower right*), it is obvious that the majority of diploid cells were non-keratin-containing stromal and inflammatory cells while the tumor cell population contained a tetraploid (4N) DNA content that coincided with the G_2/M of the normal diploid component.

calculations by excluding the dilutional effect of non-neoplastic cells and the overlap of diploid and aneuploid DNA histograms (Figs. 10 and 11).

At present, no true tumor-specific markers for epithelial-derived neoplasms are available. In our laboratory, we use antibodies directed to keratin intermediate filaments to discriminate epithelial cells (Fig. 5B). Keratin fluorescein isothiocyanate (green) labeling in conjunction with DNA staining by propidium iodide (red) enables one to restrict DNA analysis to epithelial cells. Although discrimination cannot be made on this basis between normal and neoplastic epithelial cells, normal host stroma and inflammatory cells can be excluded from the DNA analysis (Fig. 9). In colon carcinomas, the nonepithelial component can be significant, serving to dilute the malignant population of interest (Fig. 10). Even when the tissue is selected by a pathologist, the disag-

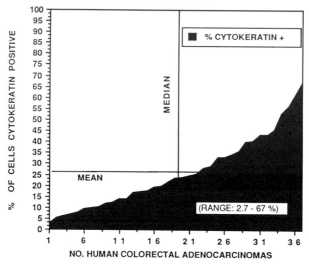

Figure 12. Graph demonstrating the distribution of keratin positive cells in a series of colon adenocarcinomas. The mean number of keratin-positive cells is 27 percent.

gregated cells represent a combination of normal and neoplastic epithelial cells and substantial numbers of host stromal and inflammatory cells (Fig. 12). The latter do not stain with antibodies to keratin but can be identified by antibodies directed to the leukocyte common antigen epitope.

A comparison of the disaggregation of fresh surgical specimens and formalin-fixed, paraffin-embedded colon carcinomas has been recently completed in our laboratory.[40] We compared mechanical versus enzymatic disaggregation methods, cell fixation parameters, nuclear extraction from paraffin blocks, and keratin gating of intact epithelial cells to exclude the abundant inflammatory and stromal cells associated with colon adenocarcinomas. These parameters were initially evaluated using established diploid and aneuploid murine colon adenocarcinoma lines grown in syngeneic mice. This permitted the comparison of results in sequential studies, including comparing cell yields and efficiency of dissociation techniques. Once optimum conditions were identified for the animal models, we studied a series of 30 human colon carcinomas for comparison of fresh and formalin-fixed, paraffin-embedded disaggregation techniques.

The aneuploid murine colon adenocarcinoma line (#36-A) was best dissociated by mechanical means with approximately 40 percent of the recovered cells being aneuploid. The remaining cells presumably represented stromal and inflammatory (diploid) populations. Enzyme (collagenase, class III) dissociation resulted in tumor cell yields approximately half those achieved by mechanical methods. No significant differences in G_0/G_1 peak resolution (CV) for cell suspensions were noted between the mechanical and enzymatic disaggregation techniques. This is an important observation because mechanical disaggregation is much simpler and requires less time to prepare.

Comparison of alcohol- and formalin-fixed cell suspensions has shown that the only histogram parameter adversely affected by formalin fixation is DNA PI staining intensity. The formalin-fixed cells have much lower staining intensity when compared to chick erythrocyte standards (CRBC).[44] The latter contain less DNA than human diploid cells and provide a convenient non-overlapping standard. Comparison of 30 fresh, mechanically disaggregated human colon adenocarcinomas with the same tumors that were formalin fixed and paraffin embedded revealed a decreased detection of aneuploid cells in the latter group. Twenty-two aneuploid human colonic adenocarcinomas were detected by analysis of fresh intact cells but only 17 were reportedly aneuploid by the standard Hedley analysis of corresponding paraffin-embedded tumor. The analysis of nuclei retrieved from paraffin often resulted in poor quality histograms (wide CVs) with less sensitivity in the detection of peridiploid DNA peaks. Small populations of aneuploid cells can also be masked by debris, especially when the efficiency of extraction of aneuploid cells is poor.

Modifications of the "standard Hedley" technique using additional pepsin digestion of the initial nuclear suspension and residual tissue resulted in better identification of aneuploid cell populations.[40] This was due to improved CVs and the release of additional aneuploid tumor cells. The modified procedure made it possible to detect aneuploidy in the five human tumors classified as diploid with the standard Hedley procedure. Despite the enhanced sensitivity for detecting aneuploid cell populations with the modified nuclear technique, we were able to measure SPF in only 15 of 22 (68 percent) of the aneuploid human colon adenocarcinomas. In contrast, we were able to analyze SPF in 21 of 22 (95 percent) aneuploid adenocarcinomas from the fresh disaggregated tumors with the dual cytokeratin/DNA labeling technique.

Part of the increased sensitivity of analyzing fresh intact tumor cells resulted from the use of keratin gating to measure only keratin-containing epithelial cells. Using the dual labeling technique, the aneuploid cell recovery rates could be improved by excluding contaminating inflammatory and stromal cells from the analysis. Our own prospective dual cytokeratin-labeled FCM analyses of human colon carcinomas have shown a wide range of cytokeratin-positive events (2.7 to 67 percent cytokeratin positive) in mechanically dissociated fresh specimens (Fig. 12).[51] This confirms the observation that in some human colon cancers inflammatory cells comprise the majority of the cells analyzed. Keratin labeling also avoids overlapping histograms in which the diploid component is composed of non-epithelial cells. In addition, the cleaner DNA histograms generated from intact cell suspensions result in a higher proportion of histograms with analyzable SPF. The application of enzyme enucleation procedures to paraffin-embedded tissue blocks is popular, but the pitfalls, including decreased sensitivity in detecting aneuploid cell population and the inability to measure SPF inherent with this procedure, must be recognized.

ASSESSMENT AND INTERPRETATION OF DNA HISTOGRAMS

Before addressing the clinicopathologic association of DNA and cell cycle measurements derived from flow cytometry, one must recognize what constitutes acceptable data and interpretable DNA histograms. The pitfalls of interpretation lie in the five following areas:

1. The quality of the prepared cellular/nuclear suspensions with degree of resolution attained measured by standard deviation divided by the mean channel and described as the coefficient of variation (CV)
2. The definition of histogram peak abnormalities; inability to discriminate tumor from nontumor cell populations, especially diploid and peridiploid tumor cell fractions
3. The discrimination of G_2/M cell populations from tetraploid cells and cell doublets
4. The biologic meaning of an aneuploid population
5. Mathematical calculations of cell cycle compartments, especially S-phase fraction

1. Sample Preparation

The quality of cellular/nuclear suspensions is dependent on the technique for producing the suspensions and the tumor system investigated. Mechanical dissociation of intact cells obviously requires viable, recently resected tumor tissue. Increased proportions of non-viable tumor, necrosis, or sclerotic stroma contribute to increased debris, bare nuclei, and nuclear fragments, resulting in background noise in the DNA histogram. In some tumors, such as colon carcinoma, substantial numbers of inflammatory and stromal cells are present and tumor necrosis is common. Enzymatic dissociation of intact cells and extraction of fixed nuclei from paraffin blocks can also result in poor quality histograms. Variable amounts of nuclear debris, reflected in increased CV values and background are noted with different protease digestion times and concentrations.[41] Our modifications of the standard Hedley procedure for retrieval of nuclei from paraffin blocks has resulted in the detection of additional instances of aneuploidy due to a combination of better defined histograms with tighter CVs and enhanced release of aneuploid tumor nuclei. The CV attained with nuclei from paraffin blocks is also greatly influenced by the following: (1) trimming blocks of necrotic tumor and host stroma to minimize debris; (2) obtaining sections at least 50 λm thick to avoid additional fragmentation of nuclei during sectioning[45]; and (3) the avoidance of suboptimally fixed tissue, improperly stored blocks, inadequately dehydrated or paraffin-infiltrated tissue which can contribute to poor quality histograms.[52] The DNA histogram CV is additionally affected by the specificity of the DNA stain and optimal and electronic measurement capabilities of the instrument.[53]

2. Resolution of Diploid and Peridiploid Cell Populations

Discrimination of small aberrations in DNA content is dependent on the CV of the G_0/G_1 peak. For example, discrimination of two G_1/G_0 peaks as separate peak means of DI 1.00 and 1.05 is not possible with a CV of 6 percent. Wide or abnormally skewed G_1/G_0 peaks, especially with a right-sided shoulder, are designated abnormal by some investigators, while others have assumed that all cell populations within 10 percent of the mean G_0/G_1 peak of the control cells cannot be reliably regarded as abnormal and define them as "diploid." This may be correct in some instances, but it is quite clear that the best method to achieve maximum sensitivity for detecting abnormal peridiploid tumor populations is with the "cleanest" narrow G_0/G_1 peaks and the use of appropriate controls which allow optimum resolution from adjacent abnormal cell populations. Some investigators have required that the adjacent G_0/G_1 peaks be separated by two or three standard deviations to be considered separate. Obviously, with this definition, the sensitivity of resolution of cell populations also improves with better histogram CVs.

Differences in cell size and cytoplasmic granularity can be detected by light scatter analysis. Some investigators have used these observations to gate on large nuclei, assuming the larger nuclei originate from tumor cells. Our own studies (unpublished), however, have found that tumor cells and nuclei can vary greatly in size within the same tumor. Gating on larger nuclei also tends to bias the SPF and G_2/M compartments. In addition, nuclear and cellular debris, commonly thought to produce light scatter signals lower than lymphocytes, actually displays a broad range of scatter characteristics and fluorescent intensity. The debris is presumed to represent nuclear fragments and, although the majority contain less DNA than intact cells, there is appreciable overlap with all components of a DNA histogram.

As previously mentioned, numerous definitions of DNA abnormality and/or aneuploidy have been suggested for FCM-generated DNA histograms. The strictest criterion for aneuploidy is the demonstration of two distinct G_0/G_1 populations. This requires an abnormal peak clearly separated from the internal normal/diploid cells. Some investigators have classified tumors with a single G_0/G_1 peak having a CV greater than 5 as a separate peridiploid group in their clinicopathologic analyses. They defend this approach by assuming that poor resolution could mask a separate peridiploid peak.[54] Still others accept non-Gaussian (skewed) distributions or peaks with shoulders as representing abnormal peridiploid cell populations.[55] These latter investigators assume that unresolved overlapping populations contribute to the wide CV and asymmetry of DNA distribution. As we have seen, however, numerous other technical parameters can significantly contribute to the large CVs and irregular histogram contours of individual samples. We have concluded that the identification of diploid internal standards composed of non-epithelial or inflammatory cells serve as the most reliable control cell population. Any peak that can be resolved as different from this internal standard (i.e., when both ascending and descending sides of the histogram peak are present allowing identification of a peak mean and not shoulders or wide CVs) is sufficient to conclude that there is an abnormal DNA-containing cell population present. Positive confirmation of the inflammatory cells in the diploid peak by LCA dual labeling or decrease of the diploid peak by keratin labeling confirm the presence of a non-neoplastic diploid channel in the histogram.

3. Resolution of G$_2$/M and Tetraploid Cell Population

The separation of G$_2$/M cells from tetraploid neoplastic cells can also be a problem. Some investigators have set an upper limit for G$_2$/M cell proportion of 15 to 20 percent of total cells. Cell populations greater than this are considered to represent tetraploid cells.[56] Binucleate cells in intact cell preparations may appear as an increased number of events in the G$_2$/M range and thereby simulate a tetraploid (4n) DNA-containing neoplasm.[57] Cell doublets may also cause an apparent increase in G$_2$/M peaks but can be distinguished by electronic doublet discrimination. When a significant tetraploid cell population is present, a discrete G$_2$/M peak in the octoploid range will usually allow identification of the second abnormal (tetraploid) cell population. In addition, gated analysis based on tissue-specific markers such as keratin will often enhance the detection of tetraploid tumors by reducing the G$_0$/G$_1$ peak contributed by non-neoplastic diploid host cells (Fig. 11).

4. Interpretation of Abnormal DNA Content (Aneuploidy)

Initially, it was thought that any cell population with abnormal DNA content (aneuploidy) represented a malignant neoplasm.[58] However, it has become evident that there are numerous exceptions to this observation. Major exceptions are a number of benign neoplasms, particularly of the endocrine system, and intraepithelial dysplasias that have also been documented to have an aneuploid DNA content. In endocrine neoplasms, the presence of an aneuploid cell population does not appear to predict for a clinically malignant course.[59] And, the presence of an abnormal DNA content in dysplasia does not indicate that the epithelium is irreversibly programmed to progress to invasive carcinoma.[60]

Recently, the sensitivity of flow cytometric DNA analysis has been studied and more fully defined. It is becoming clear that DNA analysis using DNA-specific dyes often fails to detect cells with minor aberrations in DNA content due to abnormal chromosomes.[61] In cell samples prepared from fresh tumors with optimum CVs, DNA alterations of 2 to 4 percent can be resolved. The degree of sensitivity decreases to 5 percent or greater in DNA quantitation of tumor nuclei removed from paraffin.[62,63] Unfortunately, many of the minor marker chromosome aberrations associated with neoplastic transformation, such as translocations, minor deletions, and other focal mutations, cause such small differences in total DNA content they cannot be detected by FCM means. We have documented this in a retrospective analysis from paraffin tissue blocks and in fresh tumors of the urinary bladder.[61–63]

However insensitive flow cytometric DNA analysis may be in comparison to chromosomal analysis, flow cytometry's measurement of DNA content has still been demonstrated to have prognostic significance. Studies of tumors from several organ systems, notably large cell lymphomas and breast carcinomas, have suggested that tumors with aneuploid DNA distributions have a more aggressive biologic course and appear to be more responsive to cytotoxic chemotherapy and possibly radiation therapy.[64,65] Conversely, neoplasms which have diploid DNA distributions are generally thought to be less aggressive as defined by growth rates and also less responsive to cytotoxic chemotherapy and possibly radiation therapy. The proliferative index (S + G_2M) or SPF identified in the DNA histogram appears to correlate with DNA content. Aneuploid neoplasms tend to have a higher proportion of cells actively synthesizing DNA, indicating an increased level of proliferation.[64-66]

5. SPF Calculation

SPF calculations are an important component in DNA histogram interpretation. Ideally, with optimum cell disaggregation and staining methods, the three cell cycle phases (G_0/G_1, SPF, and G_2/M) would be easily separated (Fig. 8). However, measurement errors can result because of overlap of cell cycle compartments in DNA histograms. Separation of the components is optimum on histograms with well-defined G_0/G_1 and G_2/M peaks. Measurement of SPF is based on mathematical modeling which is best applied to optimum histograms with little background debris. Non-optimal histograms (wide CVs) require greater approximation or estimations to derive SPF which in turn results in decreased accuracy of measurement. Mathematical models utilizing computer programs have been developed to approximate the DNA histogram curves and integrate the area corresponding to SPF. Two of the more popular DNA cell cycle analysis programs are those that fit the S-phase region with a second order polynomial curve approximation (polynomial model)[67] or integrate the S-phase area by dividing it into broadened rectangles through a series of Gaussian curves contained within the rectangles.[68] Neither one of these approximations is perfect. The polynomial model cannot be used with the higher CV values often obtained with solid tumors (especially nuclei extracted from paraffin) and grossly overestimates SPF in the low ranges. The rectangular model is also less accurate for estimating low SPF ranges.

We have found that the manual calculation of SPF using the rectangular method described by Baisch[69] is a more consistent and reproducible method. This method of calculation has been shown to correlate with tritiated thymidine incorporation (TLI) in human breast carcinomas.[70] TLI has been the accepted method of measuring tumor cell proliferation and breast adenocarcinomas have much lower SPF. Poor technical cell preparations with wide CV values and excessive debris compromise the manual determination of SPF but also effectively exclude application of computerized mathematical models to calculate SPF. Compared to corresponding tritiated thymidine labeling indices, FCM estimates of SPF in solid tumors usually result in higher values. Part of this difference may be due to the presence of contaminating debris in single-cell suspensions of solid tumors. Corrected SPF values obtained by mathematical subtraction of background debris are more consistent with results from thymidine labeling,[71] but these models have not been widely tested and are not presently available.

A major obstacle to the quantitation of SPF is overlapping histograms. Typicallly, the non-neoplastic cell components (e.g., inflammatory, stromal) and occasionally the diploid component of a biclonal tumor will overlap with aneuploid tumor cell populations. This is a relatively common problem which precludes accurate SPF determination when mixed cell populations are present. The use of dual marker gating on epithelial (keratin staining) or tumor cells (tumor-associated antigens) allows exclusion of non-neoplastic contaminants. This results in more accurate SPF determinations in tumors with a single stem line. In addition, the exclusion of overlapping non-neoplastic cells will often allow SPF calculation on aneuploid tumors (Fig. 11). There are rectangular models that are reported to subtract contaminating diploid SPF components which overlap with the aneuploid portion of the histogram. However, the validity of this model has not been established.

RELATIONSHIP OF PLOIDY AND SPF TO PROGNOSIS: REVIEW OF LITERATURE

Flow cytometric DNA measurements of human colon adenocarcinomas fall into two major categories. One group consists of studies of fresh or frozen unfixed tumors collected in a prospective fashion using either bare nuclei or intact cell preparations. The second group used nuclei extracted from paraffin-embedded archival specimens (usually Hedley's technique). The former approach results in cleaner dissociation of the specimen with less cellular and nuclear debris, but suffers from slow rates of patient accession and a lack of immediate and timely clinical follow-up. Conversely, paraffin-embedded material generally provides poorer quality histograms with wider CVs and varying amounts of nuclear debris. As a consequence, SPF can be measured in fewer tumors. Clinical follow-up is readily available in these retrospective studies, however, and case selection can be tailored to well-defined patient groups, tumor stages, and treatment modalities.

We attempted to identify all major studies using FCM to measure DNA in colon cancers. Many of the studies could not be included for a variety of reasons. The most frequent problem was that the data were not presented in a fashion that allowed them to be abstracted in a format allowing comparison with other studies. In many instances, staging terminology was confusing and poorly defined. Groups of stages were sometimes combined in ways which precluded translation to Dukes' stages (primarily combining Astler–Coller B1 and B2 which represent Dukes' A and B stages). In many of the studies, the sites of the adenocarcinomas were not specified. Tumor grade was mentioned in only a minority of papers and numerous other prognostic factors were only occasionally provided. In many of the reports, it was necessary to estimate 5-year survivals from survival curves. In several of the prospective studies that addressed survival, the duration of follow-up was not always clearly stated.

Prospective Analysis

Ten prospective studies of 491 tumors were found in the literature which used varying methods of disaggregation, DNA stains, and diploid control cells (Table 6). There was considerable variation in the observed frequency of abnormal (aneuploid) DNA-containing tumor cells ranging from a low of 35 percent[61] to a high of 82 percent.[64] It is noteworthy that the lowest observed frequency was obtained in a study which used collagenase to disaggregate the tumor, a method which we found to consistently give the lowest yield of aneuploid cells.[40] It should also be mentioned that the ratio of colonic to rectal tumors varied greatly and in two series the anatomic location of the tumors was not specified. The study with the highest frequency of aneuploidy had the greatest proportion of rectal tumors.[64] The wide diversity of results in these studies should lead the reader to be cautious about the interpretation of flow cytometric DNA data of colon adenocarcinomas. The average for the ten series was 64.4 percent aneuploidy and 35.6 percent diploidy a ratio which probably approximates the true distribution in a population of colon cancers (Table 6).

The reported distribution of ploidy by stage in colorectal tumors in various studies is displayed in Table 7. The observed distributions of DNA content

TABLE 6. PROSPECTIVE FLOW CYTOMETRY ANALYSIS OF COLONIC ADENOCARCINOMA

Author	No. Tumors	Colon/ Rectum	Preparation	Stain	Control	Diploid No.	(%)	Aneuploid No.	(%)
Wolley[74]	33	33/0	Enucleation	AO/PI[c]	Mucosa	20	(61)	13	(39)
Rognum[81]	85	NS	Mechanical	EB	Lymphocyte	28	(33)	57	(67)
Banner[82]	56	51/5	Enucleation	PI	Inflam. and normal cells	14	(25)	42	(75)
Teodori[91]	24	19/5	Enucleation	EB/mit	Mucosa	10	(37)	14	(63)
Melamed[92]	33	20/13	Mechanical	AO	Mucosa	15	(45)	18	(55)
Durrant[93]	31	18/13	Collagenase	EB/mit	Lymphs	20	(65)	11	(35)
Hiddemann[79]	88	43/45[a]	Mechanical	EB/mit	Mucosa	16	(18)	72	(82)
Scott[78]	30	NS[b]	Collagenase	PI	Mucosa	12	(40)	18	(60)
Emdin[94]	37	22/15	Enucleation	PI	Mucosa	14	(38)	23	(62)
Zarbo[51]	74	64/10	Mechanical	PI	Mucosa	26	(35)	48	(65)
Total	491					175 (35.6%)		316 (64.4%)	

[a]Two squamous carcinomas.
[b]Not specified.
[c]AO = acridine orange; PI = propidium iodide; EB/mit = ethidium bromide/mithramycin.

TABLE 7. PROSPECTIVE ANALYSIS OF PLOIDY: DISTRIBUTION BY STAGE

Author	Stage A		Stage B		Stage C		Stage D	
	Diploid	Aneuploid	Diploid	Aneuploid	Diploid	Aneuploid	Diploid	Aneuploid
Wolley[74]	1	0	7	2	10	11	2	0
Rognum[81]	6	10	12	27	7	14	3	11
Banner[82]	6	4	6	12	1	18	1	8
Teodori[91]	2	1	6	1	1	6	1	6
Melamed[92]	1	2	3	4	6	6	5	6
Durrant[93]	4	2	6	3	6	4	3	2
Hiddemann[79]	0	2	9	37	7*	33[a]		
Scott[78]	3	3	8	6	1	6	0	3
Emdin[94]	3	3	9	7	2	10		
Zarbo[51]	2	11	14	17	4	17	6	3
Total	28	38	80	116	45	125	20	39
(%)	(42)	(58)	(41)	(59)	(26)	(74)	(34)	(66)
Total by stage (491)	66		196		170		59	
(% of total)	(13.4)		(39.9)		(34.6)		(12.1)	
Control series (%) distribution by stage from Table 8	(13.5)		(30.4)		(34)		(22.1)	

[a]Stages C and D combined.

TABLE 8. HISTORICAL CONTROLS: DISTRIBUTION BY DUKES' STAGES[10]

Author	Total Patients	Stage A		Stage B		Stage C		Stage D	
		No.	(%)	No.	(%)	No.	(%)	No.	(%)
Eisenberg[90]	1704	176	(10)	381	(22)	659	(39)	488	(29)[a]
Jass[29]	447	60	(13)	178	(40)	209	(47)		
Chapuis[3]	709	71	(10)	251	(35)	207	(29)	180	(26)
Newland[21]	1117	117	(10.5)	407	(36.5)	337	(30)	256	(23)
Pihl[17]	878	232	(26.4)	260	(29.6)	236	(26.9)	150	(17.1)
Total	4855	656	(13.5)	1477	(30.4)	1648	(34)	1074	(22.1)

[a]Distant metastasis, excluded cases with extension to serosal surfaces or contiguous organs.

within each Dukes' stage also varied greatly. However, the total number of patients in the combined ten studies have an overall distribution by stage, comparable to that in several large historical control series of colorectal carcinomas (Table 8). The distribution by stage for the ten DNA content studies compared to the control series is as follows:

TABLE 9. DISTRIBUTION BY DUKES' STAGE[10]

	% of Total			
	A	B	C	D
DNA study population	13	40	35	12
Control series (Table 8)	13.5	30.4	34	22.1

The proportions of stage A and C tumors are about the same, while stage B tumors are increased and stage D tumors decreased in the series analyzed for DNA. The tendency to include relatively more early stage tumors in the study population may result in the observed survivals observed in comparison with the control series.

TABLE 10. DNA CONTENT BY DUKES' STAGE[10]

	% of Patients			
	A	B	C	D
Diploid	42	41	26	34
Aneuploid	58	59	74	66

The advanced stage C and D tumors had a higher proportion of aneuploid neoplasms, suggesting either a more progressive course for aneuploid tumors or the development of aneuploid cell populations as the tumor invades and progresses to a more advanced stage. Stages A and B have a higher proportion but still a minority of tumors with DNA content in the diploid range. Regardless of the reasons, there are clearly a higher proportion of aneuploid neoplasms among tumors with a more advanced stage (Table 7).

Retrospective Studies

In general, retrospective DNA studies using nuclear suspensions retrieved from paraffin blocks include larger patient populations. The seven studies with sufficient detail to be included in this review consist of approximately twice the number of patients found in the review of prospective DNA studies (Table 11). This is not surprising considering the relative ease of performing retrospective DNA studies from paraffin blocks. Varying proportions of colon and rectal tumors were noted in four of seven studies not specifying the site of the neoplasms studied. The clinical details of patient demographics, tumor site and stage, the method of selecting patients, and other relevant details were often missing in this group of studies. The disaggregation procedures were similar and the majority used propidium iodide (PI) as the DNA stain (Table 11). The frequency of aneuploidy varied from a high of 82 percent to a low of 50 percent.

TABLE 11. RESULTS OF DNA ANALYSIS FROM PARAFFIN TISSUE BLOCKS

Author	# Tumors	Colon/Rectal	Preparation	Stain	Control	Diploid No. (%)	Aneuploid No. (%)
Retrospective							
Goh[72]	203	NS[b]	50 micron 1% pepsin	PI[c]	Mucosa internal	74 (36)	129 (64)
Kokal[75]	77	47/30	30 micron .5% pepsin 30 min	PI	CRBC	24 (31)	53 (69)
Armitage[83]	134	NS	20 micron .5% pepsin 30 min	DAPI	Internal cells	62 (46)	72 (54)
Scott[84]	121	0/121	40 micron .5% pepsin 30 min	PI	NS	61 (50)	60 (50)
Bauer[76]	119	119/0	30 micron .1% pepsin	DAPI PI	Mucosa	22 (18)	97 (82)
Schutte[77]	279	NS	Trypsin	PI	NS	105 (38)	174 (62)
Visscher[73a]	95	95/0	30+ micron .5% pepsin 105 min	PI	Mucosa	56 (62)	39 (38)[a]
Total	933					404 (39)	624 (61)

[a]Right colon, stage As and B.
[b]NS = Not specified.
[c]PI = Propidium iodide.

TABLE 12. RETROSPECTIVE DNA ANALYSIS: DISTRIBUTION BY STAGE

Author	Stage A		Stage B		Stage C		Stage D	
	Diploid	Aneuploid	Diploid	Aneuploid	Diploid	Aneuploid	Diploid	Aneuploid
Goh[72]			21[a]	26[a]	3	26		
Kokal[75]	9	4	34	29	18	18	0	9
Armitage[83]	4	1	33	36	16	21	9	14
Scott[84]	9	4	34	29	18	18	0	9
Visscher[73a]	12	5	44	34	—	—	—	—
Subtotal	25	10	111	99	34	39	9	23
(%)	(71)	(29)	(53)	(47)	(47)	(53)	(28)	(72)
Total 350	35		210		73		32	
(%) of total	(10)		(60)		(21)		(9.7)	
Control series (%) distribution by stage from Table 8	(13.5)		(30.4)		(34)		(22.1)	

[a]Astler–Coller stage. Dukes' A and B combined.

The reasons for these marked variations were not clear and were seldom addressed in any of the reported studies. However, the average observed proportion of 60.7 percent aneuploid tumors was remarkably similar to the 64.4 percent observed in the prospective study summary (Table 6). The observed frequency of 60 to 64 percent appears to represent the actual proportion of aneuploid neoplasms in a large unselected population of patients with colorectal adenocarcinomas.

Retrospective studies of DNA content by stage are remarkable only for the paucity of studies with sufficient data to allow analysis by stage (Table 12). One series did not contain sufficient detail to convert Astler–Coller stage to Dukes' stage, although the two terms were used interchangeably.[72] The number of tumors with adequate staging details was remarkably small and the distribution of patients by stage varied more than in the prospective studies (Table 12). In general, more of the retrospective study cases were early stage neoplasms distributed as follows:

TABLE 13. DISTRIBUTION BY DUKES' STAGE[10]

	% of Total			
	A	**B**	**C**	**D**
DNA study population	10	60	21	9
Control series (Table 8)	13.5	30.4	34	22.1

This discrepancy suggests that preselection is present in some of the retrospective series. For example our study was confined to stage A and B tumors of the right colon treated by surgery.[73] Another study did not include any stage D patients.[72] The shift of study cases to stage B with fewer stage C tumors introduces a major selection bias that further complicates the interpretation of much of the clinical FCM data. This relatively high frequency of early stage tumors would have the potential of increasing the number of diploid tumors and observed survival. Also, the ratio of diploid to aneuploid tumors differs by stage:

TABLE 14. DNA CONTENT BY DUKES' STAGE[10]

	% of Patients			
	A	**B**	**C**	**D**
Diploid	71	53	47	28
Aneuploid	29	47	53	72

Survival by Stage

Patient survival could be extracted from three prospective and five retrospective studies (Table 15). In some reports, survival data were available and in others extrapolation from published survival curves was required. Predictably,

TABLE 15. PATIENT OUTCOME RELATED TO DNA CONTENT

Author	No. Cases	Colon/ Rectal	Survivor/Total (%)		Follow-Up
			Diploid	*Aneuploid*	
Prospective					
Wolley[74]	33	33/0	14/20 (70)	0/13 (0)	2–3 yr survival
Melamed[92]	33	20/13	8/15 (53)	12/18 (67)	2–3 yr survival
Emdin[94]	37	22/15	12/14[a] (86)	10/20 (60)	Mean F/U 30.4 mo
Subtotal			34/49 (69)	22/51 (43)	
Retrospective					
Armitage[83]	134	NA	27/62 (44)	14/72 (19)	Survival minimum 5 yr
Kokal[75]	77	47/30	24/24 (100)	34/53 (64)	Disease-free minimum survival 5 yr
Scott[84]	121	0/121	38/61 (62)	24/51 (47)	Survival minimum 15 yr
Schutte[77b]	279	NA	79/105 (75)	85/174 (49)	Survival minimum 5 yr
Visscher[73]	95	95/0[c]	34/56 (61)	20/39 (51)	Survival minimum 5 yr
Subtotal			202/308 (66)	168/386 (44)	
Total			226/350 (65)	192/449 (43)	

[a]Two patients progressing; both have wound recurrences.
[b]Calculated from survival curves.
[c]Confined to right colon, stages A and B.

prospective studies had shorter periods of follow-up compared to the 5 to 15 years of follow-up available in retrospective studies. The overall 5-year survivals for patients of all stages in the combined prospective and retrospective studies were 65 and 43 percent for the diploid and aneuploid tumors, respectively. However, the breakdown in individual studies was quite varied. Some showed differences in survival between diploid and aneuploid tumors while others did not. In one study, all patients with aneuploid tumors died[74] and in another study, all patients with diploid tumors lived.[75] Overall the data suggest that patients with diploid colorectal carcinomas have a survival advantage over those with aneuploid tumors.

Survival by stage could be evaluated in four reports, two prospective and two retrospective (Table 16). In general, these reports of DNA analyses had an increased proportion of stage B tumors and slightly higher frequencies of cancers from the other three stages when compared to historical control series (Table 8).

Analysis of survival by stage revealed some important discrepancies. The overall survival for stage A was 78 percent, compared to the 84 percent survival in control series. The survival for stage A diploid tumors was 83 percent and for aneuploid neoplasms 67 percent; however, the numbers of patients are small. In stage B, survival was 63 percent for diploid tumors and 38 percent for aneuploid tumors. These results were both considerably below the expected survival of 72 percent for stage B neoplasms (Table 18). This observation is of concern since the proportion of stage B tumors is higher in the DNA study

TABLE 16. PATIENT OUTCOME RELATED TO STAGE[10]

	Stage A		Stage B		Stage C		Stage D	
Author	**Diploid**	**Aneuploid**	**Diploid**	**Aneuploid**	**Diploid**	**Aneuploid**	**Diploid**	**Aneuploid**
Prospective								
Wolley[74]	1/1	0/0	7/7	0/2	6/10	0/11	0/2	0/0
Melamed[92]	1/1	2/2	1/3[a]	4/4	6/6	4/6	0/5	2/6
Retrospective								
Armitage[83]	3/4	0/1	19/33	12/36	4/16	1/21	1/9	1/14
Kokal[75]			21/21[b]	16/27[b]	3/3	18/26		
Total	5/6	2/3	27/43	16/42	16/32	5/38	1/16	3/20
(%)	(83)	(67)	(63)	(38)	(50)	(13)	(6)	(15)
DNA series								
Patients by stage	9		85		70		36	
(%) by stage	(4.5)		(42.5)		(35)		(18)	
Control series (%) from Table 8	(13.5)		(30.4)		(34)		(22.1)	
DNA series								
Survival by stage	7/9		43/85		21/70		4/36	
(%) survival	(78)		(51)		(30)		(11)	
Control series Survival by stage from Table 13	(84)		(72)		(38.8)		(9.9)	

[a]One death—CVA; no tumor.
[b]Astler–Coller stage; data insufficient to separate Duke's A and B staging.

TABLE 17. SURVIVAL BY STAGE

	A	B	C	D
Tumor Distribution by Stage				
FCM studies with survival data (%)	4.5%	42.5%	35%	18%
Control Studies (Table 8)	13.5%	30.4%	34%	22.1%
Survival by Stage				
FCM studies (survival)	78%	51%	30%	11%
Control series (Table 13)	84%	72%	38.8%	9.9%

TABLE 18. HISTORICAL CONTROLS: SURVIVAL RELATED TO DUKES' STAGE[10]

Author	Total Patients	Stage A		Stage B		Stage C		Stage D	
		No. of Patients (%)	% 5-year Survival[b]	No. of Patients (%)	% 5-year Survival	No. of Patients (%)	% 5-year Survival	No. of Patients (%)	% 5-year Survival
Eisenberg[90]	1704	176 (10)	79.6	381 (22)	74.4	659 (39)	(37.3)	488 (29)[a]	4.1
Jass[29]	447	60 (13)	98	178 (40)	78	C1: 169 (38) / C2: 40 (9)	40 / 10		
Chapuis[3]	709	71 (10)	62	251 (35)	55	207 (29)	29	180 (26)	6
Newland[21]	1117	117 (10.5)	89	407 (36.5)	75	337 (30)	49	256 (23)	27
Pihl[17]	878	232 (26.4)	88	260 (29.6)	76	236 (26.9)	41	150 (17)	4
Combined series	4855	656 (13.5)	84	1477 (30.4)	72	1648 (34)	38.8	1074 (22.1)	9.9

[a]Calculated from 5-year survival rates.
[b]Distant metastasis, excluded cases with extension to serosal surface or contiguous organs.

population while the survival for these stage B tumors is well below that expected from the control series (Tables 8 and 18). The reasons for these discrepancies were not addressed in the respective papers. The survival for stage C tumors was 50 percent for diploid neoplasms and 13 percent for aneuploid tumors.

Measurement of Proliferative Index

The value of SPF as a predictor of colon cancer progression is even more clouded. Very few investigators have attempted to measure the SPF of the DNA histograms (Table 19) since the majority of studies concentrated on the identification of aneuploid cell populations. Four reports included sufficient data to allow comparisons (Table 19) and in these studies aneuploid tumors had considerably higher SPF than did diploid neoplasms. This observation is consistent with studies of other cancers. Because of the close interrelationship of these two parameters, their adverse prognostic effects are difficult to analyze separately. These studies did not correct for non-neoplastic cell dilutions which were invariably included in SPF measurements of diploid range tumors. Assuming that the contaminating cells have a low SPF, this has the potential to lower the SPF of diploid range neoplasms. On the other hand, the measurement of SPF cannot often be limited to the tumor cell population in aneuploid tumors. As a consequence, the inaccurate measurement of SPF in aneuploid cells and the lower SPF in diploid cells tend to widen the gap between the two groups.

Regression analyses carried out in two studies[76,77] suggest that SPF may have a more important role than ploidy in predicting patient outcome. The paramount prognostic role of SPF determination has been suggested for breast carcinoma[70] and it would seem logical that this measure of tumor proliferation would also be important in colon cancer. However, existing studies do not have sufficient numbers of patients for careful statistical analysis and therefore the role of SPF in human colon cancer is not yet defined.

Multiple Stem Lines

The observation of multiple stem lines in human colon cancer is well established (Table 20). However, the fact that methods of specimen sampling and DNA evaluation of resected tumors were quite variable may account for some of the reported differences in results. In general, studies utilizing multiple small biopsies have broader ranges in the frequency of multiple stem lines, varying from 5 to 33 percent of total tumors studied (Table 20). The presence of diploid and aneuploid tumor cell components suggests that two stem lines are present. However, none of these studies have confirmed the epithelial, neoplastic nature of the diploid cells. The possibility that the normal DNA containing cells in these series are non-neoplastic contaminants is real and confuses the interpretation of the published data. The easiest method for documenting that diploid components are neoplastic cells is to use multiple

TABLE 19. DNA SYNTHESIS PHASE FRACTIONS.

Author	No. Tumors	No. Eval. SpF	% S = Phase Fraction					Method Calculation
			Normal Mucosa	No.	Diploid	No.	Aneuploid	
Prospective								
Tribukait[80]	77	66	7.2 ± .3	41	13.1 ± .8	74	19.1[a]	Baisch (117 of 205 samples calculated)
Hiddemann[79]	88	29	6.8 ± 1.8	16	13.9 ± 4.2	45	25.0 ± 6.4	Gohde (45 of 72 aneuploid calculated)
Emdin[94]	37	30	4.3 ± 3.1	35	7.7 ± 4.2	33	13.5 ± 6.6	Manual with pulse height analyzer
Retrospective								
Bauer[76]	120	119	NA	21	11.8 ± 1.4	76	18.2 ± 1.1	Rectangular model (119 of 120 calculated)

[a]Two groups of aneuploid values combined.

TABLE 20. OBSERVED FREQUENCY OF MULTIPLE STEM LINES IN HUMAN COLON CARCINOMAS

Author	Type of Study	No. Tumors	Diploid		Aneuploid		Types of Samples	Multiple Aneuploid Populations		
			No.	(%)	No.	(%)		No.	% Total Cases	% Aneuploid Cases
Rognum[81]	Prospective	85	28	(33)	57	(67)	5 Biopsies in 60 tumors	4	5	7.4
Tribukait[80]	Prospective	46	10	(22)	36	(78)	4 Quad biopsy 46 Tumors	15	33	42
Teodori[91]	Prospective	24	10	(42)	14	(58)	4–10 Biopsies per tumor	7	29	50
Hiddemann[79]	Prospective	88	16	(18)	72	(82)	3–15 biopsies (mean 9)	19[b]	17	26
Benner[82]	Prospective	56	14	(25)	42	(75)	1 Slice near center of tumor	10	18	24
Emdin[94]	Prospective	37	14	(38)	23	(62)	2–4 biopsies central and peripheral	7	19[c]	30
Scott[78]	Prospective	30	12	(40)	18	(60)	4 Quad biopsy	4	13	22
Bauer[76]	Retrospective	120	22	(19)	97	(81)	3 Tissue sections; 30 microns	5	4	3 (1 patient with >.1N difference)
Schutte[77]	Retrospective	279	NS[a]	(38)	NS	(62)	NS	11	3.9	6.4

[a]NS = Not specified.
[b]Corrected to exclude possible tetraploid lines.
[c]Heterogeneous defined as differences of .4c.

tumor biopsies and demonstrate monoclonal diploid and aneuploid cell populations in different samples of the tumor. Standard pathologic confirmation is required to insure that the biopsies contain tumor. If only diploid cells are found in one biopsy and other specimens contain aneuploid cells, it can be concluded that multiple stem lines probably exist. On the other hand, slices of tumor submitted for DNA analysis usually contain a large enough sample of tumor cells to include a mixture from heterogeneous stem lines if they are present. While this suggests that it is preferable to do FCM on large samples of tumor,[78] this approach is of little value if DNA analysis of tumor biopsies is to be used for planning therapy. Hiddemann[79] found that FCM of a single biopsy was representative of the tumor in only 42 percent of cases. Tribukait recognized that the number of stem lines appeared to increase with advancing stage.[80]

A careful study was performed by Scott et al,[78] in which slices and biopsies were compared for DNA content. They analyzed 261 samples from 30 fresh colorectal cancers; 12 (40 percent) of the tumors were diploid and 18 (60 percent) had aneuploid components. Nineteen (63 percent) of the 30 tumors studied had similar histograms in all biopsy specimens and the tumor was considered homogenous for DNA content. Full thickness slices were found to be representative of the tumor in 26 of the 30 tumors evaluated when compared to multiple biopsies and additional tissue slices. Major tumor heterogeneity was found in only four tumors, two of which appeared to have only small foci of aneuploid cell fractions in otherwise diploid tumors. In the remaining 28 tumors, 2 or more biopsies would have contained all stem lines in the majority of cases. In summary, DNA analysis on a single biopsy appeared to be inadequate to characterize ploidy especially on advanced stage tumors. Biopsies from four areas are probably sufficient to characterize the DNA distribution in almost all colonic carcinomas and this is recommended when DNA measurements of biopsies are to be used in planning therapy.

Correlation of DNA Content and Histological Parameters

Histological features such as tumor grade or differentiation, pattern of invasion (infiltrating versus pushing), lymphocytic response, and type of vascular invasion are associated with tumor recurrence and survival. However, the relationship of these prognostic parameters to DNA content is not clear. The majority of published studies have failed to document an association between histological grade and DNA content.[72–76,80–84] One study found increased aneuploidy in well-differentiated colon adenocarcinomas.[79] The proliferative index SPF also did not correlate with histological grade.[80,85] Table 21 summarizes the association of vascular invasion and DNA indices. Except for one study,[75] the frequency of finding any form of vascular invasion was increased in tumors with an abnormal DNA content. In this single exceptional study, there was not only a low frequency of intravascular tumor but also poor patient survival suggesting some inapparent bias in patient selection.[75]

TABLE 21. VASCULAR INVASION AND PLOIDY

Author	No. Tumors	Vascular Invasion No.	(%)	Diploid[a]	Aneuploid[a]
Wolley[74]	33	13	(39)	4/20 (20)	9/12 (75)
Banner[82]	50	38	(68)	9/14 (64)	29/42 (69)
Kokal[75]	77	4	(5)	3/24 (13)	1/50 (2)
Scott[84]	121	45	(37)	14/61 (23)	31/60 (52)
Total	281	100	(36)	30/119 (25)	70/164 (43)

[a]Number with vascular invasion/number with specified ploidy.

SUMMARY

Human colon adenocarcinomas have histological parameters that are clearly associated with prognosis. These include tumor grade, pattern of invasion, presence of lymphocytes, and vascular involvement by tumor. The latter remains controversial with respect to the relative importance of intramural and extramural vascular involvement. Some studies show a poor prognosis for intramural invasion of capillary size vascular channels by tumor.[86] On the other hand, when veins are involved by tumor, the presence of tumor in large extramural veins appears to have a much more ominous effect than intramural tumor involvement of small veins.

The results of DNA analysis of colorectal adenocarcinomas varied greatly depending on study methodology but several important points can be summarized: (1) higher stage tumors have a greater proportion of aneuploid tumors; (2) aneuploid tumors tend to have a higher growth rate (SPF) and poorer survival than diploid tumors; and (3) aneuploid tumors are associated with histological parameters indicative of a poor prognosis such as vascular invasion, but ploidy is not related to tumor grade.

One of the major problems in drawing firm conclusions about the relationship of flow cytometric DNA measurements to prognosis is great variability among the reported studies. The types of variation appear to fall into two major categories: patient selection and technical problems. The former are especially relevant in retrospective studies in which there is poor patient definition (site, grade, stage, and other standard tumor definitions) and a bias for selecting early stage tumors which have improved survivals. The latter includes a spectrum of technical problems inherent in this widely but not necessarily uniformly applied laboratory procedure. This is particularly true for DNA analysis of nuclei removed from paraffin tissue blocks. For the most part, quality control measurements including cell yields, the efficiency of extraction or disaggregation of aneuploid cells, exclusion of non-neoplastic cells, and other features characteristic of the scientific method are seldom included in studies of DNA analysis of solid tumors. Hopefully, a consensus regarding optimum technical and analytic methods will evolve, followed by the careful definition of human colon cancer cohorts. The importance of further studies is suggested by the results of this review which indicated that the presence of an aneuploid cell population is associated with a less favorable prognosis for all colorectal tumors.

Acknowledgments. The authors would like to recognize the typing skills of Gloria Johnson and the photography contribution of Nancy Peshkin. We would also like to thank Drs. Chester Herman, Raoul Braylan, and Joseph Marcus for their careful review of this manuscript and their constructive comments, which the authors feel significantly improved the quality and content of the review.

REFERENCES

1. Silverberg E: Cancer statistics. CA 37:2, 1987
2. Fisher B, Wolmark N, Rockette H, et al: Postoperative adjuvant chemotherapy or radiation therapy for rectal cancer: Results from NSABP Protocol R-01. J Natl Cancer Inst 80:21, 29, 1988
3. Chapuis PH, Dent OF, Fisher R, et al: A multivariate analysis of clinical and pathological variables in prognosis after resection of large bowel cancer. Br J Surg 72:698, 1985
4. Steinberg SM, Barkin JS, Kaplan RS, Stablein DM: Prognostic indicators of colon tumors. The gastrointestinal tumor study group experience. Cancer 57:1866, 1986
5. Fielding LP, Fry JS, Phillips RKS, Hittinger R: Prediction of outcome after curative resection for large bowel cancer. Lancet:904, 1986
6. Cohen AM, Wood WC, Gunderson LL, Shinnar M: Pathological studies in rectal cancer. Cancer 45:2965, 1980
7. Wolmark N, Cruz I, Redmond CK, et al: Tumor size and regional lymph node metastasis in colorectal cancer. A preliminary analysis from the NSABP clinical trials. Cancer 51:1315, 1983
8. Lockhart-Mummery JP: Two hundred cases of cancer of the rectum treated by perineal excision. Br J Surg 14:110, 1926–1927
9. Dukes CE: The spread of cancer of the rectum. Br J Surg 17:643, 1929
10. Dukes CE: The classification of cancer of the rectum. J Pathol Bacteriol 35:323, 1932
11. Gabriel WB, Dukes C, Bussey HJR: Lymphatic spread in cancer of the rectum. Br J Surg 23:395, 1935
12. Simpson WC, Mayo CW: The mural penetration of the carcinoma cell in the colon: Anatomic and clinical study. Surg Gynecol Obstet 68:872, 1939
13. Kirklin JW, Dockerty MB, Waugh JM: The role of the peritoneal reflection in the prognosis of carcinoma of the rectum and sigmoid colon. Surg Gynecol Obstet 88:326, 1949
14. Astler VB, Coller FA: The prognostic significance of direct extension of carcinoma of the colon and rectum. Ann Surg 139:846, 1954
15. Kyriakos M: The president's cancer, the Dukes classification and confusion. Arch Pathol Lab Med 109:1063, 1985
16. Turnbull RB Jr, Kyle K, Watson FR, Spratt J: Cancer of the colon; the influence of the no-touch isolation technic on survival rates. Ann Surg 166:420, 1967
17. Pihl E, Hughes ESR, McDermott FT, et al: 1. Carcinoma of the rectum and

rectosigmoid: Cancer specific long-term survival. A series of 1061 cases treated by one surgeon. Cancer 45:2902, 1980

18. Gastrointestinal Tumor Study Group: Adjuvant therapy of colon cancer: Results of a prospectively randomized trial. N Engl J Med 310:737, 1984

19. Wolmark N, Fisher B, Wieand HS: The prognostic value of the modifications of the Dukes C class of colorectal cancer. Ann Surg 203:115, 1986

20. Phillips RKS, Hittinger R, Blesovsky L, et al: Large bowel cancer: Surgical pathology and its relationship to survival. Br J Surg 71:604, 1984

21. Newland RC, Chapuis PH, Smyth EJ: The prognostic value of substaging colorectal carcinoma. A prospective study of 1117 cases with standardized pathology. Cancer 60:852, 1987

22. Fenoglio CM, Kaye GI, Lane N: Distribution of human colonic lymphatics in normal, hyperplastic and adenomatous tissue. Its relationship to metastasis from small carcinomas in pedunculated adenomas, with two case reports. Gastroenterology 64:51, 1973

23. Hutter RVP, Sobin LH: A universal staging system for cancer of the colon and rectum. Let there be light. Arch Pathol Lab Med 110:367, 1986

24. Riddell RH: Universal staging system for colorectal cancer. Arch Pathol Lab Med 111:312, 1987

25. Jass JR, Morson BC: A universal staging system for cancer of the colon and rectum revisited. Arch Pathol Lab Med 110:1119, 1986

26. Khankhanian N, Mavligit GM, Russell WO, Schmiek M: Prognostic significance of vascular invasion in colorectal cancer of Dukes' B class. Cancer 39:1195, 1977

27. Talbot IC, Ritchie S, Leighton M, et al: Invasion of veins by carcinoma of rectum: Method of detection, histological features and significance. Histopathology 5:141, 1981

28. Minsky BD, Mies C, Recht A, et al: Resectable adenocarcinoma of the rectosigmoid and rectum. II. The influence of blood vessel invasion. Cancer 61:1417, 1988

29. Jass JR, Atkin WS, Cuzick J, et al: The grading of rectal cancer: Historical perspectives and a multivariate analysis of 447 cases. Histopathology 10:437, 1986

30. Blenkinsopp WK, Stewart-Brown S, Blesovsky L, et al: Histopathology reporting in large bowel cancer. J Clin Pathol 34:509, 1981

31. Dukes CE, Bussey HJR: The spread of rectal cancer and its effect on prognosis. Br J Cancer 12:309, 1958

32. MacCarty WC: Factors which influence longevity in cancer. Ann Surg 76:9, 1922

33. Spratt JS, Spjut HJ: Prevalence and prognosis of individual clinical and pathologic variables associated with colorectal carcinoma. Cancer 20:1976, 1967

34. Murray D, Hreno A, Dutton J, Hampson LG: Prognosis in colon cancer. A pathologic reassessment. Arch Surg 110:908, 1975

35. Jass JR: Lymphocytic infiltration and survival in rectal cancer. J Clin Pathol 39:585, 1986

36. Jass JR, Love SB, Northover JMA: A new prognostic classification of rectal cancer. Lancet 1303, 1987

37. Carlon CA, Fabris G, Arslan-Pagnini C, et al: Prognostic correlations of operable carcinoma of the rectum. Dis Colon Rectum 28:47, 1985

38. Vindelov LL, Christensen IJ, Nissen NI: Standardization of high resolution flow cytometric DNA analysis by the simultaneous use of chicken and trout red blood cells as internal reference standards. Cytometry 5:328, 1983

39. Marcus JN, Anderson EA, O'Kane-Murphy B, Jankovich DV: (Letter to the editor) Locating the human diploid channel. Cytometry 9:275, 1988

40. Crissman JD, Zarbo RJ, Niebylski CD, et al: Flow cytometric DNA analysis of colon adenocarcinomas: A comparative study of preparatory techniques. Modern Pathology 1:198, 1988

41. Ensley JF, Maciorowski Z, Pietraszkiewicz H, et al: Solid tumor preparation for flow cytometry using a standard murine model. Cytometry 8:479, 1987

42. Ensley JF, Maciorowski Z, Pietraszkiewicz H, et al: Solid tumor preparation for clinical application of flow cytometry. Cytometry 8:488, 1987

43. Vindelov, LL: Flow microfluorometric analysis of nuclear DNA in cells from solid tumors and cell suspensions. A new method for rapid isolation and staining of nuclei. Virchows Arch B (Cell Pathol) 24:227, 1977

44. Schutte B, Reynders MMJ, Bosman FT, Blijham GH: Flow cytometric determination of DNA ploidy level in nuclei isolated from paraffin-embedded tissue. Cytometry 6:26, 1985

45. Stephenson RA, Gay H, Fair WR, Melamed MR: Effect of section thickness on quality of flow cytometric DNA content determinations in paraffin-embedded tissues. Cytometry 7:41, 1986

46. Takamatsu T, Nakanishi K, Fukada M, Fujita S: Cytofluorometry on cells isolated from paraffin sections after blocking of the background fluorescence by azocarmin G. Histochemistry 71:161, 1981

47. Oud PS, Hanselaar TGJM, Reubsaet-Veldhuizen JAM, et al: Extraction of nuclei from selected regions in paraffin-embedded tissue. Cytometry 7:595, 1986

48. Hedley DW, Friedlander ML, Taylor IW, et al: Method for analysis of cellular DNA content of paraffin-embedded pathological material using flow cytometry. J Histochem Cytochem 31:1333, 1983

49. Engelholm SA, Spang-Thomsen M, Brunner N, et al: Disaggregation of human solid tumours by combined mechanical and enzymatic methods. Br J Cancer 51:93, 1985

50. Feitz WFJ, Beck HLM, Smeets AWGB, et al: Tissue-specific markers in flow cytometry of urological cancers: Cytokeratins in bladder carcinoma. Int J Cancer 36:349, 1985

51. Zarbo RJ, Visscher D, Ma C, et al: DNA content and cell cycle kinetics of colorectal adenocarcinomas. A prospective analysis. Surg Pathol (in press)

52. Feichter GE: Pitfalls in the preparation of nuclear suspensions from paraffin-embedded tissue for flow cytometry (letter to the editor). Cytometry 7:616, 1986

53. Taylor IW, Milthorpe BK: An evaluation of DNA fluorochromes, staining techniques, and analysis for flow cytometry. I. Unperturbed cell populations. J Histochem Cytochem 28:1224, 1980

54. Hedley DW, Rugg CA, Ng ABP, Taylor IW: Influence of cellular DNA content on disease-free survival of stage II breast cancer patients. Cancer Res 44:5395, 1984

55. Collste LG, Darzynkiewicz Z, Traganos F, et al: Flow cytometry in bladder cancer detection and evaluation using acridine orange metachromatic nucleic acid staining of irrigation cytology specimens. J Urol 123:478, 1980

56. Gustafson H, Tribukait B, Esposti PL: DNA profile and tumour progression in patients with superficial bladder tumours. Urol Res 10:13, 1982

57. Ronot X, Hecquet C, Larno S, et al: G2 arrest, binucleation, and single-parameter DNA flow cytometric analysis. Cytometry 7:286, 1986

58. Barlogie B, Drewinko B, Schumann J, et al: Cellular DNA content as a marker of neoplasia in man. Am J Med 69:195, 1980
59. Joensuu H, Klemi PJ: DNA aneuploidy in adenomas of endocrine organs. Am J Pathol (in press)
60. Fu YS, Reagan JW, Richard RM: Definition of precursors. Gynecol Oncol 12:S220, 1981
61. Crissman JD, Zarbo RJ, Tyrkus M: DNA analysis of urothelial neoplasia by flow cytometry and chromosomal analysis. Lab Invest 58:20A, 1988
62. Zarbo RJ, Babu VR, Crissman JD: Flow cytometric DNA analysis of urothelial carcinomas with near-diploid karyotypes (abst). Cytometry (in press)
63. Crissman JD, Liu B, Zarbo RJ, et al: Diagnosis of urothelial neoplasia (abst). Cytometry (in press)
64. Christensson B, Tribukait B, Linder I-L, et al: Cell proliferation and DNA content in non-Hodgkin's lymphoma. Flow cytometry in relation to lymphoma classification. Cancer 58:1295, 1986
65. Hedley DW, Rugg CA, Gelber RD: Association of DNA index and S-phase fraction with prognosis of nodes positive early breast cancer. Cancer Res 47:4729, 1987
66. Tribukait B: Clinical DNA flow cytometry. Med Oncol Tumor Pharmacother 1:211, 1984
67. Dean PN: A simplified method of DNA distribution analysis. Cell Tissue Kinet 13:299, 1980
68. Dean PN, Jett JH: Mathematical analysis of DNA distributions derived from flow cytometry. J Cell Biol 60:523, 1974
69. Baisch H, Hoehde W, Linden WA: Analysis of PCP-data to determine the fraction of cells in the various phases of cell cycle. Radiat Environ Biophys 12:31, 1975
70. McDivitt RW, Stone KR, Craig RB, Meyer JC: A comparison of human breast cancer cell kinetics measured by flow cytometry and thymidine labeling. Lab Invest 52:287, 1985
71. Haag D, Feichter G, Goerttler K, Kaufmann M: Influence of systematic errors on the evaluation of the S phase portions from DNA distributions of solid tumors as shown for 328 breast carcinomas. Cytometry 8:377, 1987
72. Goh HS, Jass JR: DNA content and the adenoma-carcinoma sequence in the colorectum. J Clin Pathol 39:387, 1986
73. Visscher D, Ma C, Zarbo RJ, et al: Flow cytometric DNA analysis of right colon carcinomas. A retrospective study. Surg Pathol (in press)
74. Wolley RC, Schreiber K, Loss LG, et al: DNA distribution in human colon carcinomas and its relationship to clinical behavior. JNCI 69:15, 1982
75. Kokal W, Sheibani K, Terz J, Harada JR: Tumor DNA content in the prognosis of colorectal carcinoma. JAMA 255:3123, 1986
76. Bauer KD, Lincoln ST, Vera-Roman JM: Prognostic implications of proliferative activity and DNA aneuploidy in colonic adenocarcinomas. Lab Invest 57:329, 1987
77. Schutte B, Reynders MMJ, Wiggers T, et al: Retrospective analysis of the prognostic significance of DNA content and proliferative activity in large bowel carcinoma. Cancer Res 47:5494, 1987
78. Scott NA, Grande JP, Weiland LH, et al: Flow cytometric DNA patterns from colorectal cancers—how reproducible are they? Mayo Clin Proc 62:331, 1987
79. Hiddemann W, Von Bassewitz DB, Kleinemeier H-J, et al: DNA stemline heterogeneity in colorectal cancer. Cancer 58:258, 1986
80. Tribukait B, Hammarberg C, Rubio C: Ploidy and proliferation patterns in colo-

rectal adenocarcinomas related to Dukes' classification and to histopathological differentiation. Acta Pathol Microbiol Immunol Scand 91:89, 1983

81. Rognum TO, Thorud E, Elgjo K, et al: Large bowel carcinomas with different ploidy, related to secretory component, IgA, and CEA in epithelium and plasma. Br J Cancer 45:921, 1982

82. Banner BF, Tomas-De La Vega JE, Roseman DL, Coon JS: Should flow cytometric DNA analysis precede definitive surgery for colon carcinoma? Ann Surg 202:740, 1985

83. Armitage NC, Robins RA, Evans DF, et al: The influence of tumour DNA abnormalities in colorectal cancer. Br J Surg 72:828, 1985

84. Scott NA, Rainwater LM, Wieand HS, et al: The relative prognostic value of flow cytometric DNA analysis and conventional clinicopathologic criteria in patients with operable rectal carcinoma. Dis Colon Rectum 30:513, 1987

85. Temple WJ, Sugarbaker EV, Thornthwaite JT, et al: Correlation of cell cycle analysis with Dukes' staging in colon cancer patients. J Surg Res 28:314, 1980

86. Wiggers T, Arends JW, Schutte B, et al: A multivariate analysis of pathologic prognostic indicators in large bowel cancer. Cancer 61:386, 1988

87. Freedman LS, Macaskill P, Smith AN: Multivariate analysis of prognostic factors for operable rectal cancer. Lancet 733, 1984

88. Zhou XG, Yu BM, Shen YX: Surgical treatment and late results in 1226 cases of colorectal cancer. Dis Colon Rectum 26:250, 1983

89. Carlon CA, Fabris G, Arslan-Pagnini C, et al: Prognostic correlations of operable carcinoma of the rectum. Dis Colon Rectum 28:47, 1985

90. Eisenberg B, Decosse JJ, Harford F, Michalek J: Carcinoma of the colon and rectum: The natural history reviewed in 1704 patients. Cancer 49:1131, 1982

91. Teodori L, Tirindelli-Danesi D, Cordelli E, et al: Potential prognostic significance of cytometrically determined DNA abnormality in GI tract human tumors. Ann NY Acad Sci 468:291, 1986

92. Melamed MR, Enker WE, Banner P, et al: Flow cytometry of colorectal carcinoma with three-year follow-up. Dis Colon Rectum 29:184, 1986

93. Durrant LG, Robins RA, Armitage NC, et al: Association of antigen expression and DNA ploidy in human colorectal tumors. Cancer Res 46:3543, 1986

94. Emdin SO, Stenling R, Roos G: Prognostic value of DNA content in colorectal carcinoma. A flow cytometric study with some methodologic aspects. Cancer 60:1282, 1987

Interleukin Receptors in Lymphoid Lesions
Relevance to Diagnosis, Biology, and Therapy

James A. Strauchen

The recently discovered interleukins are a family of monokine and lymphokine hormones which, with their specific receptors, serve to regulate the immune and hematopoietic systems in a manner much akin to the endocrine system.[1] As such, this system plays a central role in the modulation of the immune response and the disorders thereof including the malignant lymphomas.[2] Interleukin 2 (IL-2), the most important of the lymphokines so far discovered, has emerged as the central mechanism for the proliferation of T lymphocytes and probably B lymphocytes and macrophages as well.[1,2]

Receptors for IL-2 have been found on the cells of several well-recognized lymphoproliferative disorders in man including adult T-cell leukemia–lymphoma associated with human T lymphocytotrophic virus (HTLV-I) infection, hairy cell leukemia, Hodgkin's disease, and a subset of non-Hodgkin's lymphoma, suggesting a possible role in the pathogenesis of these processes.[3,4] In addition, the ability in recent years to produce large amounts of these lymphokines in vitro by molecular engineering has made practical a possible role in therapy of lymphoid and non-lymphoid neoplasia.[5-7] In this chapter, the current understanding of IL-2 receptor expression in lymphoid lesions will be reviewed and possible applications to diagnosis and therapy discussed.

BIOLOGY OF INTERLEUKIN 2

Interleukin 2 (T-cell growth factor) is a 15,000 molecular weight (MW) lymphokine glycoprotein which is produced by activated T lymphocytes.[1] Interleukin 2

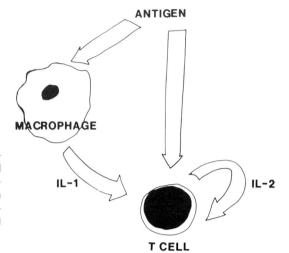

Figure 1. Activation of T cells results in the elaboration of IL-2 and the expression of specific IL-2 receptors. IL-2 receptor expression is also observed on some activated B cells, macrophages, and lymphoid tumor cells.

stimulates proliferation of activated T lymphocytes (and probably B lymphocytes and macrophages as well) by interaction with a specific cell surface receptor which is also expressed on activated T lymphocytes (Fig. 1). Activation of T lymphocytes by antigen or lectin mitogens results in secretion of IL-2 and expression of specific receptors for IL-2 creating a positive feed back loop for T-cell proliferation. Production of IL-2 and T-cell activation is also stimulated by macrophage products (monokines) IL-1 and IL-6.[1] Thus, IL-2 and its receptor constitute a major mechanism for T-cell activation and proliferation. The recent recognition of IL-2 receptors on activated B lymphocytes[7,8] and activated monocyte–macrophages[9] establishes a central role for IL-2 and its receptors in the regulation of the immune response and lymphocyte proliferation.

INTERLEUKIN 2 RECEPTORS

The biologic effects of IL-2 are mediated by interaction with a specific inducible cell surface receptor.[1,2] Receptors for IL-2 are not expressed on resting T cells, but become expressed with antigen or lectin mitogen activation.[1,2] Some in vitro T cell lines and T-cell neoplasms express IL-2 receptors at constant high levels.[2,10] Investigation of the distribution of receptors for IL-2 has been aided by the development of monoclonal antibodies specific for the IL-2 receptor, generally referred to as anti-Tac.[11,12] These monoclonal antibodies react with activated but not resting T cells and recognize an antigenic determinant (designated CD 25) located on the 55,000 MW beta chain of the IL-2 receptor.[1] Not all IL-2 receptors reactive with anti-Tac are biologically active. Studies with radiolabeled interleukin demonstrate low and high affinity receptors for IL-2. The low affinity receptors are more numerous, bind IL-2 weakly, and do not mediate biologic activity. The high affinity receptors are fewer, bind IL-2 tightly, and mediate biologic activity. It has subsequently been determined that the low affinity receptor consists only of the 55,000 MW beta chain, while the high affinity receptor consists of the beta chain and in addition a 75,000 MW alpha chain necessary for biologic activity. Although both types of receptors are recognized by anti-Tac, only the high affinity heterodimer is capable of inducing cellular proliferation.

DETECTION OF IL-2 RECEPTORS IN CLINICAL MATERIAL

IL-2 receptors are readily detectable in clinical specimens by immunohistological techniques.[3,4] A number of monoclonal antibodies to the Tac antigen are commercially available (anti-Interleukin 2 receptor, Becton-Dickinson, Mountain View, CA; anti-IL 2 R1 Coulter Immunology, Hialeah, FL). IL-2 receptor expression is readily detected in acetone-fixed fresh frozen sections by the avidin–biotin–peroxidase technique.[13] A soluble form of the receptor is also shed from activated cells and may be detected in serum by radioimmunoassay techniques.[14]

IL-2 RECEPTOR EXPRESSION IN LYMPHOPROLIFERATIVE DISEASE

Adult T-Cell Leukemia–Lymphoma

Adult T-cell leukemia–lymphoma (ATL) is the prototypical lymphoproliferative disorder associated with IL-2 receptor expression (Table 1). ATL was first reported in geographic clusters in Japan[15] and subsequently reported in the Caribbean and sporadically in the Southeastern United States and elsewhere.[16,17] ATL presents a characteristic clinical picture with a high incidence of skin and bone lesions, hypercalcemia, and circulating atypical cells of helper T-cell phenotype (Fig. 2).[16,18] ATL is regularly associated with infection by a human retrovirus, now termed HTLV-I.[18,19]

**TABLE 1. INTERLEUKIN-2 RECEPTOR EXPRESSION IN
LYMPHOPROLIFERATIVE DISORDERS**

Lymphoproliferative disorders consistently positive for IL-2 receptors (100%):
    Adult T-cell leukemia–lymphoma
    Hairy cell leukemia
Lymphoproliferative disorders frequently positive for IL-2 receptors (> 50%):
    Peripheral T-cell lymphomas
    Hodgkin's disease
    Histiocytic proliferations
Lymphoproliferative disorders sometimes positive for IL-2 receptors (< 50%):
    B-cell non-Hodgkin's lymphomas
    Cutaneous T-cell lymphomas
Lymphoproliferative disorders seldom positive for IL-2 receptor (< 10%):
    Lymphoblastic lymphoma

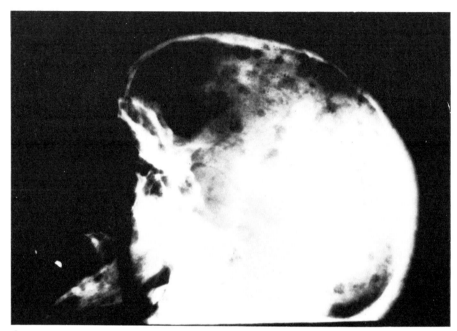

A

Figure 2. Adult T-cell leukemia–lymphoma associated with the human retrovirus HTLV-I. **A.** Skull radiograph showing lytic bone lesions. **B.** Circulating atypical cell with characteristic lobulated nucleus. **C.** Histology of an involved lymph node showing pleomorphic tumor cells of T cell type. **D.** Immunologic staining of lymph node for IL-2 receptor showing numerous intensely positive cells. (**B.** Giemsa ×1000, **C.** H&E ×450; **D.** Avidin–biotin peroxidase ×450)

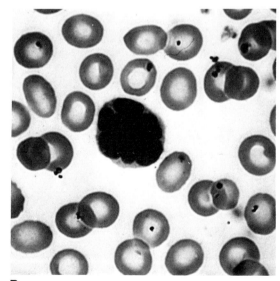

B

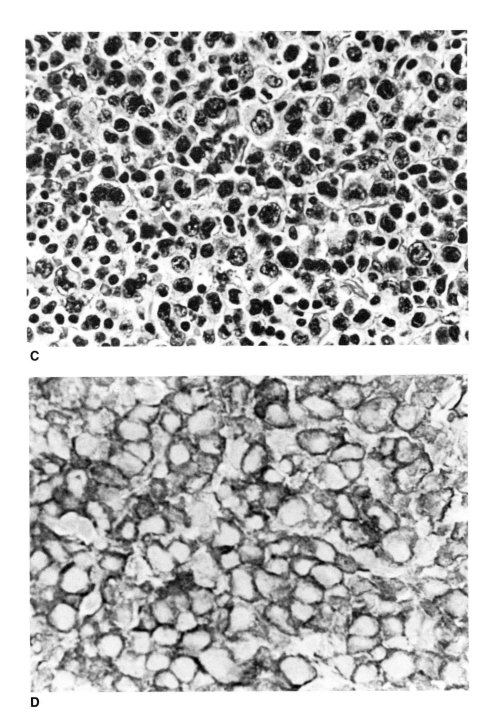

C

D

ATL cells consistently express IL-2 receptors at very high levels without prior antigen or lectin activation.[20,21] Evidence suggests that IL-2 receptor expression is mediated by the transactivator (tat) gene of HTLV-I and may be important in leukemogenesis.[21] Infection of T lymphocytes with HIV-I results in a transient polyclonal proliferation associated with IL-2 receptor expression possibly mediated by autocrine IL-2 secretion.[21] The cells of established ATL, in contrast, express IL-2 receptors at high levels, but are paradoxically not dependent on IL-2 for growth. The findings suggest a two-step model for HTLV-I-mediated leukemogenesis: an early IL-2-dependent polyclonal proliferation of T cells followed by the late emergence of an IL-2-independent neoplastic T-cell clone.[21] The model is consistent with clinical observations on the course of ATL with indolent and aggressive phases.

The diagnosis of ATL is frequently suggested by the characteristic clinical and pathologic findings.[16,18] Demonstration of Tac positivity may be helpful for confirming the diagnosis. In a recent study, Tac positivity was present in 13 of 13 HTLV-I-associated T-cell lymphomas, but in only 3 of 10 T-cell lymphomas not associated with HTLV-I.[22]

T-Cell Non-Hodgkin's Lymphomas

IL-2 receptor expression is an inconstant feature of T-cell lymphomas unassociated with HTLV-I infection. Lymphoblastic lymphoma, a disorder of immature or thymic T-cell phenotype related to acute lymphocytic leukemia does not usually express IL-2 receptors.[4] In a recent series of 23 cases of T-cell lymphoblastic lymphoma, only 1 tumor, which also expressed markers for natural killer (NK) cells, was found to be IL-2 receptor positive.[4] It is likely that the cells of lymphoblastic lymphoma which represent an immature T-cell phenotype are not competent to express this function.

T-cell lymphomas of peripheral or post-thymic phenotype, in contrast, frequently express IL-2 receptors (Fig. 3). Among peripheral T-cell lymphomas of diffuse mixed and large cell histology, receptor positivity was observed in 85 percent by Strauchen et al[3] and in 64 percent by Sheibani et al.[4] Thus, IL-2 receptor expression is common in peripheral T-cell lymphomas.

In mycosis fungoides, a T-cell lymphoma of the skin, IL-2 receptor expression is variable. Sheibani et al found receptor expression in two of five cases studied[4]; Strauchen et al found receptor expression in one case.[3] The cells of Sézary's syndrome, a chronic T-cell leukemia related to mycosis fungoides, generally lack receptor expression.[20]

IL-2 receptor expression is therefore a common feature of peripheral or post-thymic T-cell neoplasms, but it rarely occurs in prethymic or immature T-cell neoplasms. This is consistent with IL-2 receptor expression as a function of activated mature cells. IL-2 receptor expression is constant in the cells of adult T-cell leukemia–lymphoma associated with HTLV-I infection, it occurs commonly in the cells of other peripheral T-cell lymphomas, and less commonly in

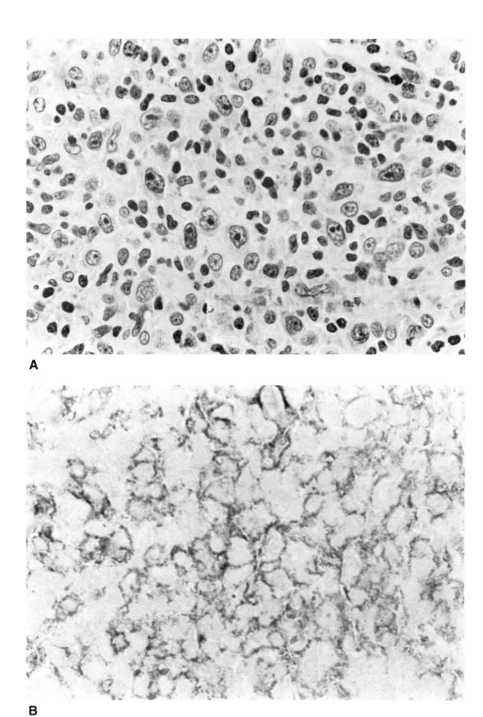

Figure 3. Non-Hodgkin's peripheral T-cell lymphoma. **A.** Histology of involved lymph node showing small and large cells. **B.** Immunologic staining for IL-2 receptors showing numerous positive cells. (**A.** H&E ×450, **B.** Avidin–biotin peroxidase ×450)

the cells of mycosis fungoides, and seldom in the cells of T-lymphoblastic lymphoma.

Hodgkin's Disease

The nature and origin of the neoplastic cell of Hodgkin's disease, the Reed–Sternberg cell and related mononuclear cells remains obscure.[23] Recent interest has focused on possible derivation from interdigitating reticular cells, a class of non-phagocytic histiocyte-like cells.[23,24] Reed–Sternberg cells demonstrate an HLA-DR (Ia)-positive null cell phenotype.[24,25] Reed–Sternberg cells in most cases are also positive for Tac (Fig. 4). Hsu et al[24] reported Tac positivity of Reed–Sternberg cells in 10 of 20 cases of Hodgkin's disease, a result also confirmed by others.[3,4] Reed–Sternberg cells express other antigens associated with cellular activation including the transferrin receptor (OK T9) and Ki 1.[23,24]

Since Tac expression is non-lineage specific, the result does not contribute to our understanding of the cellular derivation of Hodgkin's disease, but does indicate an activated cell type. It is of interest that IL-2 infusion in advanced Hodgkin's disease has resulted in dramatic albeit transient responses in two patients so treated.[26] Since much of Hodgkin's disease tissue consists of reactive lymphocytes which also express IL-2 receptors,[4] the possibility that these responses represent immunomodulation of the host response in Hodgkin's disease is likely.

Histiocytic Neoplasms

True histiocytic neoplasms frequently express receptors for IL-2,[3,4] as do activated monocyte macrophages.[9] Sheibani et al[4] reported Tac positivity in neoplastic cells of four of six cases of immunologically, cytochemically, and ultrastructurally documented true histiocytic lymphomas. Strauchen et al[3] reported positive staining for IL-2 receptors in five cases of histiocytic proliferations including true histiocytic lymphoma, fibrous histiocytoma, and granulomatous disease. The latter finding is of interest in light of data suggesting a role of IL-2 in the genesis of sarcoidosis.[27]

Hairy Cell Leukemia

Hairy cell leukemia, formerly known as leukemic reticuloendotheliosis, is a peculiar B-cell lymphoproliferative disorder of characteristic morphology which is Tac positive in nearly all cases.[28,29] IL-2 receptor expression is such a constant feature of this disorder that demonstration of Tac positivity may be of diagnostic utility (Fig. 5). Why hairy cell leukemia is so much more consistently associated with IL-2 receptor expression than other B-cell lymphomas is unclear. It is of interest that hairy cell leukemia is uniquely responsive to therapy with alpha interferon, another biologic response modifier. Hairy cells may therefore represent a unique state of B-cell differentiation associated with expression of IL-2 receptors and sensitivity to interferon.

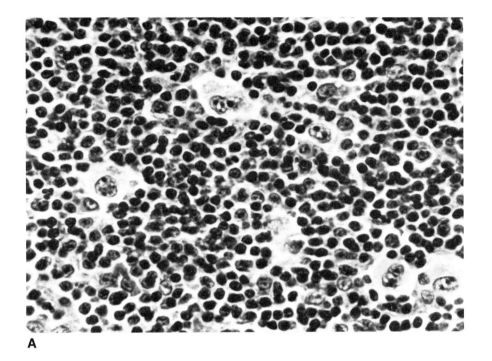

A

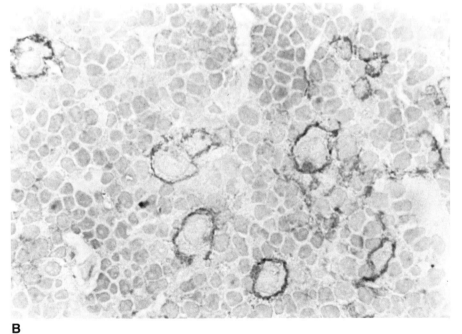

B

Figure 4. Hodgkin's disease. **A.** Section showing Reed−Sternberg cells. **B.** Immunologic staining for IL-2 receptors showing positive Reed−Sternberg cells. (**A.** H&E ×450, **B.** Avidin−biotin peroxidase ×450)

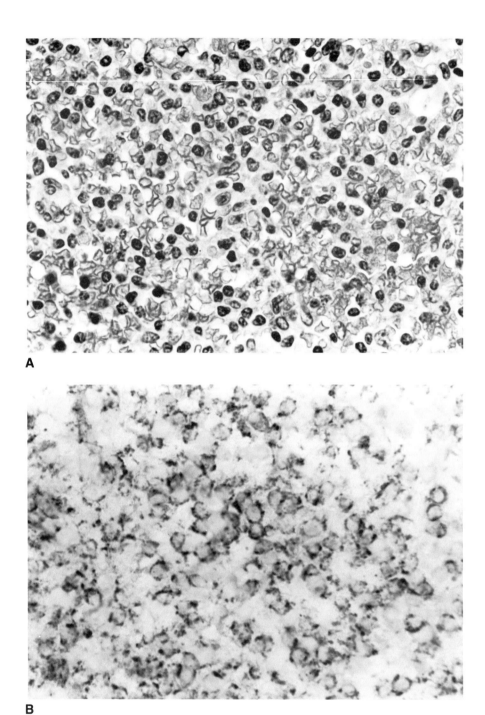

Figure 5. Hairy cell leukemia. **A.** Histology of spleen showing characteristic mononuclear cell infiltrate of the red pulp. **B.** Immunologic staining for IL-2 receptor showing diffusely positive cells. (**A.** H&E ×450, **B.** Avidin–biotin peroxidase ×450)

B-Cell Non-Hodgkin's Lymphoma

B-cell non-Hodgkin's lymphomas demonstrate inconstant expression of IL-2 receptors.[3,4] In low grade lymphomas of follicular center cell type (follicular small cleaved cell and follicular mixed small cleaved and large cell in The Working Formulation[30]), IL-2 receptor expression is generally confined to interfollicular-reactive T lymphocytes.[3,4] In some cases, a small number of IL-2 receptor-positive B lymphocytes can be demonstrated by simultaneous staining with anti-Tac and a monoclonal antibody to pan B-cell antigens.[4] In contrast, diffuse B-cell lymphomas of either low grade small lymphocytic[4] or intermediate and high grade types[3] may demonstrate significant IL-2 receptor expression on neoplastic cells (Fig. 6). Sheibani et al[4] demonstrated IL-2 receptor expression on the cells of 15 of 26 cases of diffuse small lymphocytic lymphoma (well-differentiated lymphocytic lymphoma). Simultaneous staining for pan T-cell antigens demonstrated fewer positive cells suggesting that IL-2 expression was due to the neoplastic B cells. Other series have shown a lower incidence of IL-2 receptor expression in this type of lymphoma.[3]

IL-2 receptor expression has also been reported in intermediate and high grade lymphomas. Strauchen et al[3] reported IL-2 receptors on the cells of 21 of 42 cases of intermediate and high grade B-cell lymphoma. Sheibani et al[4] reported Tac positivity on cells of 7 of 29 cases of diffuse large cell B-cell lymphoma. The significance of IL-2 receptor expression on B-cell lymphoma is unknown. IL-2 receptor expression is known to occur on physiologically activated B lymphocytes.[7,8] IL-2 receptor expression in B-cell lymphomas may reflect the state of cellular activation. However, a role in pathogenesis is not ruled out. Although IL-2 receptor expression is greater in T-cell than in B-cell lymphomas, there is sufficient overlap to preclude utility as a tool in classification.[3,4]

DIAGNOSTIC APPLICATIONS

The diagnostic utility of the demonstration of IL-2 receptor expression is limited by a lack of lineage specificity. In two lymphoproliferative disorders, adult T-cell leukemia–lymphoma associated with HTLV-I [20–22] and hairy cell leukemia[4,28,29] IL-2 receptor expression is sufficiently consistent as to have diagnostic significance. Receptor expression in other lymphoproliferative disorders is less consistent and generally not of use for diagnosis. Although IL-2 receptor expression is frequent in peripheral T-cell lymphomas, there is overlap with non-T lymphoproliferative disorders including Hodgkin's disease, histiocytic proliferations, and some intermediate and high grade B-cell lymphomas.[3,4] IL-2 receptor expression may also be seen to varying degrees in reactive and hyperplastic lymphoid proliferations (Fig. 7).[3,4] Although diffuse, intense positivity for IL-2 receptors is seen most frequently in lymphoid neoplasms, IL-2 receptor expression does not definitively distinguish neoplastic from non-neoplastic lymphoid proliferations.[3,4] Measurement of soluble IL-2 receptors in the serum may also

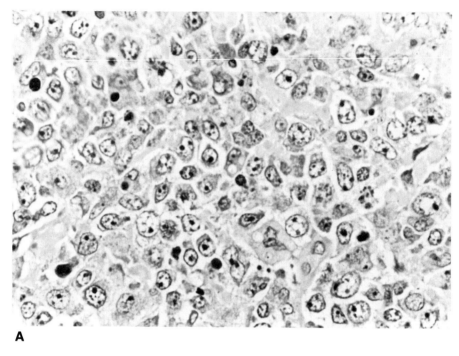

A

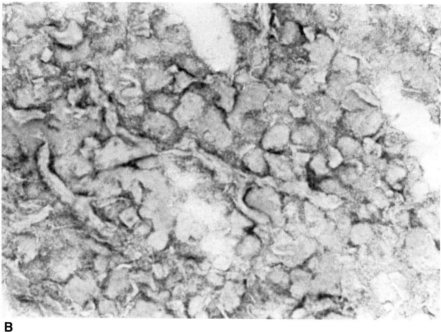

B

Figure 6. Non-Hodgkin's B-cell lymphoma. **A.** Histology showing large cell immuno-
blastic lymphoma with B-cell markers. **B.** Immunologic staining for IL-2 receptors.
Neoplastic cells are positive. (**A.** H&E ×450, **B.** Avidin–biotin peroxidase ×450)

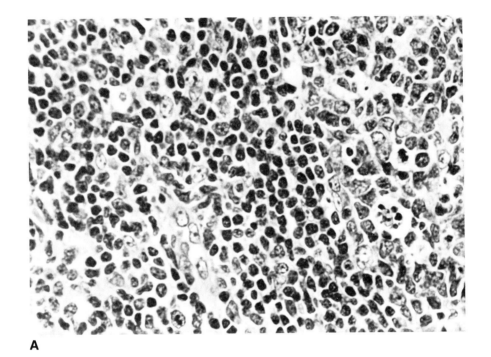

A

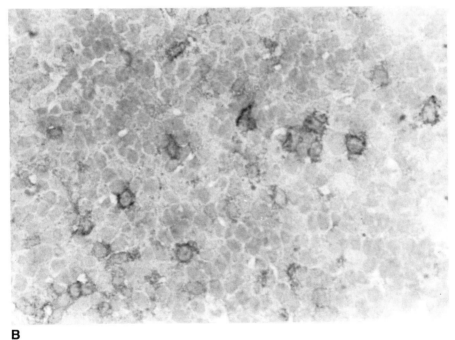

B

Figure 7. Reactive lymphoid hyperplasia. **A.** Section showing germinal center (*right*) and reactive paracortex. **B.** Immunologic staining for IL-2 receptors revealing scattered positive cells. Il-2 receptor expression is not specific to neoplasia, but may also be observed in reactive and hyperplastic conditions reflecting the physiological role of IL-2 receptors in the immune response. (**A.** H&E ×450, **B.** Avidin–biotin peroxidase ×450)

be of diagnostic and prognostic utility in some patients with lymphoproliferative disorders.[21]

THERAPEUTIC APPLICATIONS

The most exciting applications of recent discoveries with respect to IL-2 and its receptor relate to cancer therapy. Two broad approaches to therapeutic intervention have been studied: monoclonal antibodies targeted to the IL-2 receptor and adoptive immunotherapy using recombinant IL-2 with or without IL-2 activated lymphocytes (lymphokine-activated killer cells or LAK cells).

Monoclonal antibodies to the IL-2 receptor (anti-Tac) have been used experimentally in the therapy of adult T-cell leukemia and lymphoma.[21] Of five patients treated at The National Cancer Institute with anti-Tac, two had sustained responses, one lasting for 5 months.[21] Conjugates of anti-Tac with toxins or radionuclides may be even more active.[31] Since other lymphomas and Hodgkin's disease also express the IL-2 receptor, this type of therapy may have broader application. Since IL-2 receptors are expressed specifically on immunologically activated cells, anti-Tac monoclonal antibodies and conjugates may be ideal immunosuppressive agents.[32]

The ability to produce IL-2 in large quantities by recombinant DNA techniques has made feasible the exploration of possible therapeutic roles of the lymphokine. Experimental studies in animals have shown that therapy with high dose IL-2 with or without infusion of IL-2-activated lymphocytes (lymphokine-activated killer cells or LAK cells) can result in the regression of established pulmonary and hepatic metastases.[5,6]

Therapeutic trials in humans employing large doses of IL-2 alone or in combination with activated autologous lymphocytes have produced dramatic regressions in certain advanced metastatic tumors including renal cell carcinoma, malignant melanoma, and colon carcinoma.[6] IL-2 immunotherapy is believed to work by activation of a poorly defined peripheral cell population with killer cell activity.[6] Biopsy of tumor tissue in patients following therapy with IL-2 frequently demonstrates T-cell infiltration and there is evidence that expression of HLA-DR (Ia) antigens on tumor cells augments the response to IL-2.[33] Although absolute response rates to IL-2 are low (10 to 30 percent) and associated with significant toxicity, IL-2 represents the first of a new class of anticancer agents termed "biologic response modifiers." New approaches such as in vitro IL-2 activation and expansion of lymphocytes harvested directly from tumors (tumor-infiltrating lymphocytes) may produce greater activity.[34]

SUMMARY

Interleukin 2 and its receptor have emerged as a central control system in the regulation of the immune response and the proliferation of T cells, B cells, and macrophagse. IL-2 receptor expression is strongly associated with several forms of human lymphoproliferative disease including adult T-cell leukemia–lymphoma, hairy cell leukemia, Hodgkin's disease, and peripheral T-cell lymphoma in which it may play a pathogenetic role. IL-2 receptor expression may also play a role in some B-cell non-Hodgkin's lymphomas and histiocytic proliferations. Recent discoveries in immunology and advances in biotechnology have opened therapeutic possibilities for IL-2 including the use of anti-Tac monoclonal antibodies and immunoconjugates for the therapy of Tac-positive lymphoproliferative disease, the use of anti-Tac monoclonal antibodies as novel immunosuppressants, and the use of genetically engineered recombinant IL-2 and activated autologous lymphocytes in the adoptive immunotherapy of cancer. Therapeutic and diagnostic applications of IL-2 continue to be defined.

REFERENCES

1. Smith K-A: Interleukin 2: Inception, impact and implications. Science 240:1169, 1988
2. Waldmann TA: The structure, function and expression of interleukin 2 receptors on normal and malignant lymphocytes. Science 232:727, 1986
3. Strauchen JA, Breakstone BA: IL-2 receptor expression in human lymphoid lesions: Immunohistochemical study of 166 cases. Am J Pathol 126:506, 1987
4. Sheibani K, Winberg CD, Van de Velde S, et al: Distribution of lymphocytes with interleukin 2 receptors (Tac antigens) in reactive lymphoproliferative process, Hodgkin's disease and non-Hodgkin's lymphoma. Am J Pathol 127:27, 1987
5. Rosenberg SA, Lotze MT, Moul LM: Observations on the systemic administration of autologous lymphokine activated killer cells and recombinant IL-2 to patients with advanced cancer. N Engl J Med 313:1485, 1985
6. Rosenberg SA, Lotze MT, Mule JJ: New approaches to the immunotherapy of cancer using interleukin 2. Ann Int Med 108:853, 1988
7. Waldmann TA, Goldman CK, Rabb RJ, et al: Expression of interleukin 2 receptors on activated human B cells. J Exp Med 160:1450, 1984
8. Boyd AW, Fisher DC, Fox DA, et al: Structural and functional characterization of IL-2 receptors on activated human B cells. J Immunol 134:2387, 1985
9. Hermann F, Cannista SA, Levine H, Griffin JD: Expression of interleukin 2 receptor and binders of interleukin 2 by gamma interferon induced human leukemic and normal monocytic cells. J Exp Med 162:111, 1985
10. Robb RJ, Munck A, Smith KA: T cell growth factor receptors. Quantitation, specificity and biological relevance. J Exp Med 154:1455, 1981
11. Uchiyama T, Broder S, Waldmann TA: A monoclonal antibody (anti-Tac) reactive with activated and functionally mature human T cells. I. Production of anti-Tac monoclonal antibody and distribution of Tac + cells. J Immunol 126:1343, 1981
12. Uchiyama T, Nelson DL, Fleisher TA, Waldmann TA: A monoclonal antibody (anti-Tac) reactive with activated and functionally mature human T cells. II. Expression of Tac antigen on activated cytotoxic killer T cells, suppressor cells and on one of two types of helper T cells. J Immunol 126:1398, 1981

13. Hsu SM, Raine L, Fanger H: Use of avidin-biotin peroxidase complex (ABC) in immunoperoxidase techniques: A comparison between ABC and unlabelled antibody (PAP) procedures. J Histochem Cytochem 29:577, 1981

14. Rubin LA, Kurman CC, Fritz ME: Soluble interleukin-2 receptors are released from activated human lymphoid cells in vitro. J Immunol 135:3172, 1985

15. Uchiyama Y, Yodoi J, Sagawa K, et al: Adult T cell leukemia, clinical and hematologic features of 16 cases. Blood 50:481, 1977

16. Jaffe ES, Blattner WA, Blayney DW, et al: The pathologic spectrum of HTLV associated leukemia lymphoma in the United States. Am J Surg Pathol 8:263, 1984

17. Dosik H, Denic S, Patel N, et al: Adult T cell leukemia-lymphoma in Brooklyn. JAMA 259:2255, 1988

18. Broder S, Bunn PA, Jaffe E, et al: T cell lymphoproliferative syndrome associated with human T cell leukemia/lymphoma virus. Ann Int Med 100:543, 1984

19. Polesz BJ, Ruscetti FW, Gazdar AF, et al: Detection and isolation of type C retrovirus particles from fresh and cultured lymphocytes of a patient with cutaneous T cell lymphoma. Proc Natl Acad Sci USA 77:7415, 1981

20. Waldmann TA, Green WC, Sarin PS, Saxinger C: Functional and phenotypic comparison of HTLV positive adult T cell leukemia lymphoma with HTLV negative Sézary leukemia and their distribution using anti-Tac. J Clin Invest 73:1711, 1984

21. Green WC, Leonard WJ, Depper JM, et al: The human interleukin 2 receptor: Normal and abnormal expression in T cells in leukemia induced by the human T-lymphotropic retrovirus. Ann Int Med 105:560, 1986

22. Shamoto M, Suchi T, Uchiyama T: Immunoelectron-microscopic localization of Tac antigen in adult T cell leukemia-lymphoma. Am J Pathol 119:513, 1985

23. Strauchen JA: Immunopathology of Hodgkin's disease. Pathol Immunopathol Res 5:253, 1986

24. Hsu SM, Yang K, Jaffe EJ: Phenotypic expression of Hodgkin's and Reed-Sternberg cells in Hodgkin's disease. Am J Pathol 118:209, 1985

25. Strauchen JA, Dimitriu-Bona A: Immunopathology of Hodgkin's disease: Characterization of Reed-Sternberg cells with monoclonal antibodies. Am J Pathol 123:293, 1986

26. Holland JF: Personal communication

27. Pinkston P, Bietterman BB, Crystal RG: Spontaneous release of interleukin 2 by lung T lymphocytes in active pulmonary sarcoidosis. N Engl J Med 308:793, 1983

28. Hsu SM, Yang K, Jaffe ES: Hairy cell leukemia: A B cell neoplasm with a unique antigenic phenotype. Am J Clin Pathol 80:421, 1983

29. Korsmeyer SJ, Green WC, Cossman J, et al: Rearrangement and expression of immunoglobulin genes and expression of Tac antigen in hairy cell leukemia. Proc Natl Acad Sci USA 80:4522, 1983

30. Non-Hodgkin's Lymphoma Pathologic Classification Project: National Cancer Institute, Sponsored Study of Classification of Non-Hodgkin's Lymphomas: Summary and description of a working formulation for clinical usage. Cancer 45:2112, 1982

31. Kuzak RW, Atcher RW, Ganson OA, et al: Bismuth 212 labeled anti-Tac monoclonal antibody: Alpha emitting radionucleides as modalities for radioimmunotherapy. Proc Natl Acad Sci USA 86:474, 1986

32. Depper JM, Leonard WJ, Rabb RJ, et al: Blockade of the interleukin 2 receptor by anti-Tac antibody: Inhibition of human leukocyte activation. J Immunol 131:690, 1983

33. Cohen PJ, Lotfe MJ, Roberts JN, et al: The immunopathology of sequential tumor biopsies in patients with interleukin 2. Correlation of response with T cell infiltration and HLA DR expression. Am J Pathol 129:208, 1987
34. Belldegrun A, Moul LM, Rosenberg SA: Interleukin 2 expanded tumor infiltrating lymphocytes in human renal cell cancer: Isolation, characterization and antitumor activity. Cancer Res 48:206, 1988

The Role of Intraoperative Cytology in the Evaluation of Gynecologic Disease

Jacki Abrams and Steven G. Silverberg

Intraoperative cytology was first described as a rapid and useful diagnostic procedure as early as 1927 by Dudgeon and Patrick.[1] Since that time, reports of various techniques (imprints, smears, scrapes, touch-preps, and squash-preps) have been published addressing such issues as diagnostic accuracy and limitations.[2–9] Despite the obvious advantage of speed in diagnosis, it is the authors' experience that intraoperative cytology is not widely used at large hospitals in the United States. The purpose of this chapter is to familiarize practicing surgical pathologists and pathology residents with the preparatory techniques, advantages, and limitations of intraoperative cytology when used for the diagnosis of lesions of the female genital tract. The material presented in this chapter is a result of our retrospective examination of gynecologic intraoperative consultations over a 3-year period. Gynecologic specimens constitute a significant percentage of most surgical pathology practices and thereby account for a large number of intraoperative pathologic consultations.

The indications for intraoperative pathologic consultations have, over the past 5 to 10 years, expanded beyond simply an immediate therapeutic decision. In addition to rendering a primary diagnosis, evaluating resection margins, or determining the presence or absence of metastatic disease, we may be called for the following reasons: (1) determination of adequacy of diagnostic material, where a final diagnosis will be provided on permanent sections; (2) collection of material for special procedures such as hormone receptor assays, flow cytometry, or electron microscopy, or for research purposes and/or tumor banks; and (3) the demonstration of pertinent gross findings by the surgeon to the pathologist or vice versa. In the course of performing these consultations, we have found that intraoperative cytology is very useful, as an adjunct to or even as a replacement for frozen section.

ADVANTAGES OF CYTOLOGY OVER FROZEN SECTION

The most apparent value of intraoperative cytology is its speed. We find that it takes an average of 1 minute or less (using the air-dried technique) from the time of gross examination of the specimen until the slide is ready for viewing under the microscope. This compares with 5 to 10 minutes for a typical frozen section. One can therefore achieve rapid microscopic confirmation in many cases of grossly malignant appearing uterine and ovarian tumors. Additionally, one can use this technique in all situations in which a diagnosis is either known or not immediately required and the purpose of the consultation is to select tumor samples for special studies, i.e., estrogen–progesterone receptor assay on an endometrial carcinoma or flow cytometry of an ovarian tumor. Cytological techniques conserve tissue for subsequent permanent section. Thus, with a particularly small specimen or one that may be difficult to freeze or to interpret due to freeze artifact, cytology offers a major advantage over classic frozen section.

At the opposite end of the spectrum are large specimens or multiple specimens in which it is necessary to examine a number of cut surfaces. Consider a large uterine smooth muscle tumor, in which cellularity, atypia, and mitotic activity must be assessed, or multiple lymph nodes in a pelvic exenteration and/or staging procedure. Several different portions of a large tumor or several lymph nodes from a dissection specimen can be smeared and examined on a single slide in a very short period of time.

Necrotic or infected tissues also constitute an important indication for intraoperative cytology. If one performs smears rather than frozen sections on specimens from acquired immunodeficiency syndrome (AIDS) patients or, for example, in a case of tuberculous salpingitis, cryostat contamination may be prevented. In our experience, organisms such as fungi and bacteria, as well as granulomas, are easily recognized in appropriately stained cytological preparations. Examination of smears of necrotic tumor may reveal viable tumor cells which might otherwise be missed in a frozen section, due to the well-known difficulty of freezing, cutting, and interpreting necrotic tissue.

Less commonly the surgeon or gynecologist may aspirate or evacuate a cyst incidentally discovered in the pelvis. The aspiration fluid may be smeared directly on a slide, stained, and examined. Mesothelial cysts, cystic teratomas, endometriosis, and cystic carcinomas may be diagnosed in this manner.

Finally, intraoperative cytology is an excellent method for the interpretation of fine-needle aspiration cytology (FNAC). By using intraoperative cytology in conjunction with conventional frozen section, one can rapidly achieve competence in cytological diagnoses. Although the role of FNAC in the initial diagnosis of gynecological cancers is not as well established as in other organs such as breast and thyroid, its use in the follow-up of patients with known disease would certainly seem justified, according to a recent review.[10]

LIMITATIONS OF CYTOLOGICAL DIAGNOSIS

Several situations exist in which the performance of a frozen section is clearly necessary. These include the evaluation of resection margins, assessment of depth of invasion of a malignant tumor, and any situation in which a discrepancy exists between the gross impression and cytological appearance. We cannot overemphasize this last point. A borderline ovarian mucinous tumor of the endocervical type, for example, may have the classic gross appearance but show little or no cytological atypia, resembling a mucinous cystadenoma. Similarly, a serous tumor of low malignant potential may have sufficient cytological atypia to warrant a diagnosis of carcinoma; however, the presence of stromal invasion cannot be assessed cytologically and one should be conservative. In both of these situations, the gross appearance may be extremely helpful and if used in conjunction with the cytological findings one may arrive at a correct diagnosis. Frozen section may or may not be successful in identifying stromal invasion, because of the limited sampling that can be performed in the intraoperative setting. The limitation of the frozen section evaluation of the full biologic potential of tumors such as gonadal stromal tumors applies to cytological evaluation as well. As with frozen sections, the accuracy of cytological diagnosis depends primarily on careful selection of representative material, i.e., gross evaluation and proper specimen preparation. In a recent analysis of our own material, almost three times as many "false-negative" intraoperative consultations were the result of sampling error than of misinterpretation of material present on the slides.[11]

Techniques

One cannot expect to gain confidence or accuracy in cytological diagnosis if the preparation is suboptimal. Just as tissues differ with respect to freezing qualities, they differ also in fragility and "imprintability," both of which affect the cytological preparation. However, with the use of a variety of imprinting and smearing techniques combined with different fixation and staining methods, one should be able to obtain an optimal cytological preparation which includes adequate (1) cellularity, (2) fixation, and (3) nuclear–cytoplasmic detail.

Depending on the size and consistency of the tissue, cells may be obtained by touching the cut surface of the specimen to the glass slide several times or by scraping the cut surface with a scalpel blade and using the blade to gently spread the cells over the slide. With soft, fragile tissues such as lymph nodes, the touch-prep technique is adequate, while with firm specimens such as fibrotic lesions or smooth muscle tumors, it may be necessary to scrape the tissue vigorously with a blade to obtain an adequately cellular sample.

After obtaining cells, there are two options for fixation. We recommend the use of both, simultaneously, whenever possible. Slides may be alcohol fixed, which must be done immediately after obtaining cells, or air dried completely. A small hand-held hair dryer on a cool setting may aid in the latter process. With alcohol fixation, usually in 95 percent ethanol, slides may be stained with rapid modifications of either hematoxylin and eosin or the Papanicolaou method. Both of these stains are particularly useful in the identification of keratinizing squamous carcinomas. Air-dried material is stained with the Diff-Quik stain (Harleco Co.), a rapid Wright-Giemsa stain. Specimens which require the examination of multiple surfaces, such as lymph node dissections, are unsuitable for alcohol fixation because of the rapid air drying of the initial material that occurs before the entire slide is ready for staining. The air-dried technique is somewhat faster than the alcohol-fixed technique because of the short time of the Diff-Quik stain (35 seconds) and offers an advantage when multiple specimens are received at the same time.

Many other methods of preparation, fixation, and staining have been described,[2–9] but those outlined here are ones we have found simple, rapid, and easily applicable to our practice. After one masters proper preparatory technique, the final and most challenging step in intraoperative cytology is correct interpretation. The following section is designed to illustrate characteristic examples of commonly encountered lesions.

CYTOLOGICAL FEATURES OF COMMONLY ENCOUNTERED LESIONS

Non-Neoplastic Conditions

Corpus Luteum Cysts. In our experience, it is not infrequent for a gynecologist to incidentally discover a corpus luteum cyst either during a cesarean section or while doing a laparotomy for various reasons (including hemorrhage from the cyst). One can easily make the diagnosis grossly if the cyst is small and contains an inner rim of golden yellow tissue. Occasionally, the cyst may become quite large and hemorrhagic, causing the cyst wall to become thin and attenuated. A smear of the cyst lining reveals rather uniform cells with round nuclei and abundant pale, granular cytoplasm (Fig. 1). Blood and pigment-containing or foamy macrophages may be seen in the background.

Endometriosis. This condition may present as an ovarian mass or pelvic adhesions and is commonly sent for intraoperative consultation. Smears of endometriosis frequently show only hemosiderin-laden macrophages and blood (Fig. 2). We have not observed endometrial stroma often in smears of these lesions, but epithelial elements with varying degrees of atypia have been seen. In smears or frozen sections (or, for that matter, permanent sections), the epithelial elements may be absent, but the extensive sampling possible with cytological techniques increases the likelihood of their being found. As in histological sections, atypical endometriosis might be confused with malignancy, but this

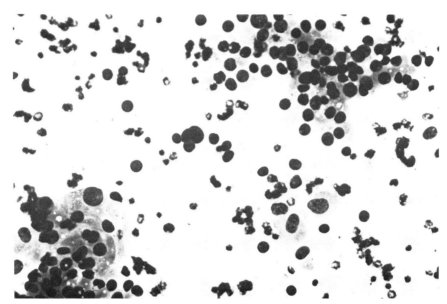

Figure 1. Corpus luteum cyst. Numerous round regular nuclei, some with abundant pale granular cytoplasm. (Diff-Quik ×300)

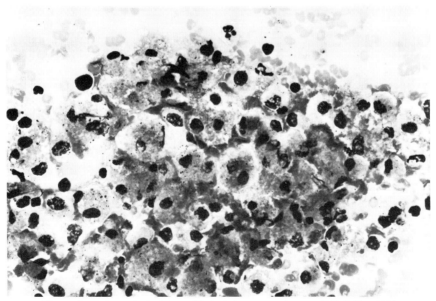

Figure 2. Endometriosis. Hemosiderin-laden macrophages. (Diff-Quik ×300)

error has not occurred in our own material because of the small numbers of atypical epithelial cells in atypical endometriosis compared with the diffuse cellularity of carcinoma. Since the two conditions may co-exist, one or the other might be missed due to sampling error (Fig. 3).

Granulomatous Inflammation. Granulomas of all etiologies are easily recognized in cytological smears as balls of cells with inconspicuous cytoplasmic borders containing numerous round-to-ovoid or elongated nuclei (Fig. 4). Foreign body giant cells from suture granulomas or caseous necrosis from tuberculosis may also be noted.

Trophoblast. When an intraoperative consultation is requested on uterine curettings in order to distinguish between an intrauterine and a possible ectopic gestation, we have found that imprints of chorionic villi will yield easily recognizable trophoblastic cells (Fig. 5). If such cells are not found, frozen section should also be performed, since one should not rely on a negative cytological finding for a diagnosis in this situation.

Ovarian Neoplasms

With the exclusion of lymph nodes, in reviewing our material the most common anatomic source was the ovary, accounting for 60 percent of all gyne-

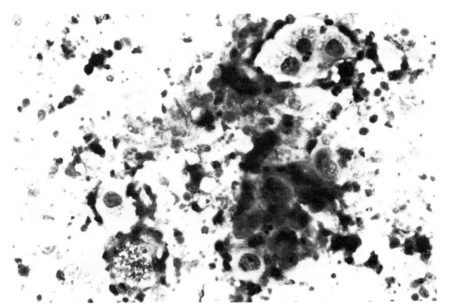

Figure 3. Atypical endometriosis. In addition to macrophages, there are clusters of atypical epithelium with enlarged cells containing prominent nucleoli. (Diff-Quik ×300)

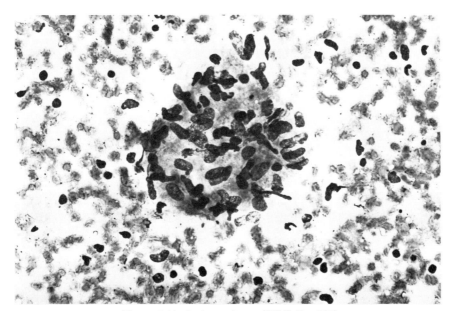

Figure 4. Vaginal granuloma. (Diff-Quik ×240)

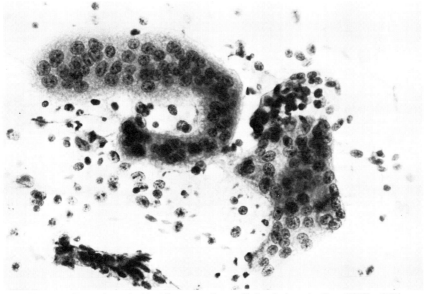

Figure 5. Syncytiotrophoblast from curettage of intrauterine abortion. (H&E ×240)

cologic specimens in which both a frozen section and cytological evaluation
were performed.

Benign Serous and Mucinous Tumors. Serous cystadenomas and cystadeno-
fibromas are characterized by cohesive, monolayered sheets of evenly spaced,
benign cells with uniform round nuclei containig small, distinct nucleoli
(Fig. 6). Mucinous cystadenomas resemble benign endocervical epithelium
when examined in routine cervical Pap smears. Cells are frequently arranged in
a honeycomb pattern with basally located nuclei and contain abundant mucin
(Fig. 7).

Serous and Mucinous Borderline Tumors and Carcinomas. With borderline
serous tumors we have observed two patterns. One consists of numerous papillary fragments composed of cells which are crowded and show some cytologically low grade pleomorphism (Fig. 8). The other, more common pattern is one
with two populations of epithelium resembling cystadenoma and carcinoma
(Fig. 9), with transitions between the two. Psammoma bodies may be seen in
borderline serous tumors but they are even more common in serous carcinomas. In addition to clusters and papillary fragments of cytologically malignant
cells, one may see numerous single malignant cells and necrosis in the background (Fig. 10).

Borderline mucinous tumors often show abundant extracellular mucin in

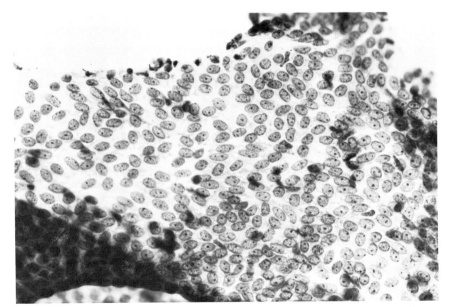

Figure 6. Serous cystadenoma. Sheet of regularly spaced benign cells with small
distinct nucleoli. (H&E ×300)

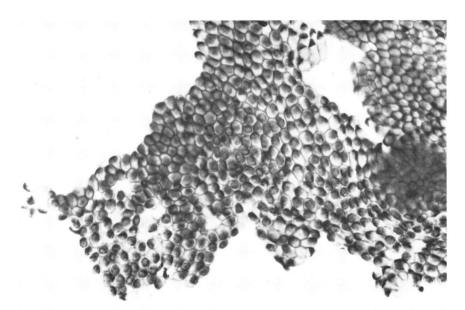

Figure 7. Mucinous cystadenoma. Note the honeycomb arrangement similar to endocervical cells seen in cervicovaginal smears. (Papanicolaou ×96)

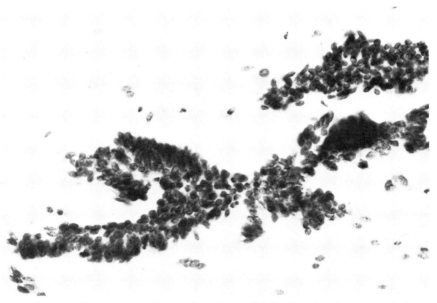

Figure 8. Serous tumor of low malignant potential. Papillary fronds composed of crowded cells with slightly atypical nuclei. (Papanicolaou ×96)

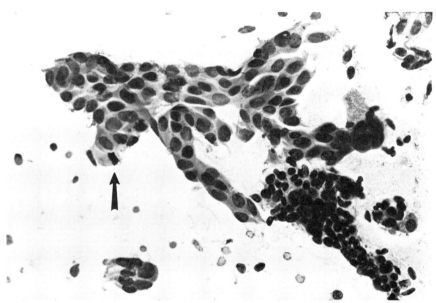

Figure 9. Serous tumor of low malignant potential. Epithelial cluster showing transition from small benign appearing cells to larger cells with nuclear atypia and mitotic figures (*arrow*). (H&E ×192)

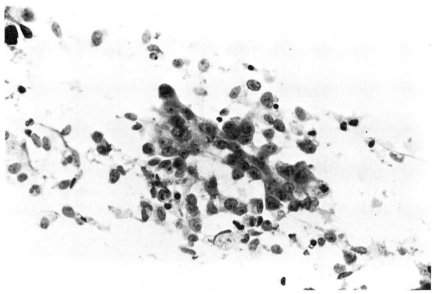

Figure 10. Serous carcinoma. Cytologically malignant cells in poorly cohesive small clusters. Numerous psammoma bodies were also present in this smear. (H&E ×192)

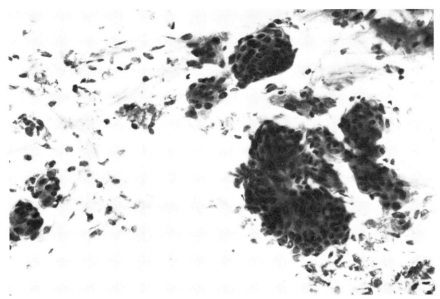

Figure 11. Mucinous tumor of low malignant potential. Clusters of atypical crowded cells with strands of extracellular mucin in the background. (H&E ×88)

the background of the smear. Groups of atypical cells with pseudostratified crowded nuclei are present within the mucin (Fig. 11). As with borderline serous tumors, the most characteristic pattern is the presence of two populations of cells, one benign and one malignant, usually with transitions within a single cluster of cells. Cytologically the malignant cells cannot be differentiated from those of a well to moderately differentiated mucinous carcinoma, but the bimorphous population is more consistent with a borderline tumor. Poorly differentiated mucinous carcinomas may be cytologically indistinguishable from other high grade carcinomas, such as endometrioid carcinoma.

Other Carcinomas. Poorly differentiated carcinomas generally cannot (and probably need not) be distinguished as to cell type in the intraoperative setting. Their malignant nature, however, is always apparent cytologically by the usual criteria (e.g., high cellularity, necrosis, lack of cohesion, high nuclear–cytoplasmic ratio, anisonucleosis, hyperchromasia, prominent nucleoli, mitotic figures). In some instances, the cell type can be suggested cytologically if voluminous clear cytoplasm (clear cell carcinoma), squamous elements (endometrioid carcinoma), or sarcomatous elements (carcinosarcoma) are found.

Mature Cystic Teratoma. Dermoid cysts of the ovary are easy to recognize grossly and are generally not a diagnostic problem. Smears of the cheesy material contained within these tumors show numerous benign squamous cells and necrotic debris (Fig. 12). As would be expected, we have also encountered

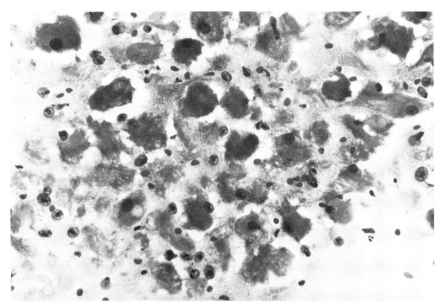

Figure 12. Mature cystic teratoma. Numerous large polygonal squamous cells, some anucleate. (Papanicolaou ×88)

glandular epithelium, fat, and brain tissue in smears from benign teratomas. We have not had the opportunity to see cytological material from an immature teratoma.

Fibroma–Thecoma. Smears from these common tumors are often quite cellular, containing numerous plump or spindled benign cells admixed with an eosinophilic fibrillar matrix representing collagen (Fig. 13). Grossly, they may resemble smooth muscle tumors or Brenner's tumors but they are readily distinguished cytologically.

Brenner's Tumor. Cytological smears of Brenner's tumors contain stromal and epithelial components. The stroma is collagenous (described above) and the epithelium consists of clusters of cells bearing some cytological resemblance to urothelium (Fig. 14). The cells are fairly uniform, with ovoid nuclei containing one small nucleolus. The distinction between a Brenner's tumor and an adenofibroma of the ovary might prove difficult on cytology alone. Cytologically, malignant Brenner's tumors resemble other high grade carcinomas.

Sex Cord–Stromal Tumors. Granulosa cell tumors of the usual (non-juvenile) type typically provide cellular smears composed of small, uniform cells, many of which contain characteristic "coffee bean" or longitudinally grooved nuclei (Fig. 15). Juvenile granulosa cell tumors do not have these nuclei and, in fact,

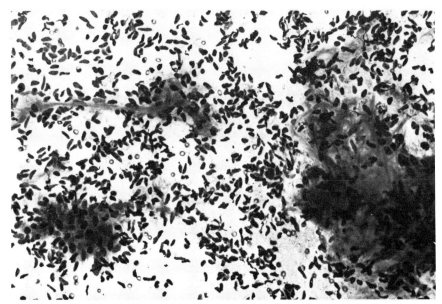

Figure 13. Ovarian fibroma. Numerous single spindled cells admixed with collagen. (Diff-Quik ×88)

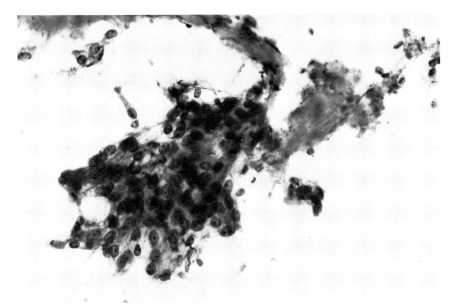

Figure 14. Brenner's tumor. Cluster of benign epithelial elements adjacent to collagenous stroma. (H&E ×300)

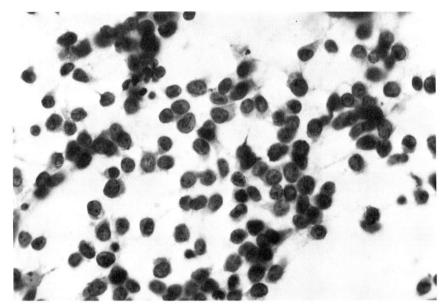

Figure 15. Granulosa cell tumor. Note longitudinal grooves in three nuclei in center of field. (H&E ×375)

may contain bizarre giant cells, making their distinction from carcinoma impossible cytologically. We have had a single Sertoli cell tumor to examine cytologically. The smear was characterized by numerous round uniform single cells and occasional tight clusters of these cells forming tubules (Fig. 16).

Small Cell Carcinoma. Smears from this uncommon tumor consist of numerous single cells with scant cytoplasm and nuclei which have a coarse chromatin pattern and occasional prominent nucleoli. Epithelial-type clustering and some cell spindling assist in the cytological distinction from *malignant lymphoma* involving the ovary. As in other sites, the diagnosis of lymphoma is more accurate by cytology than by frozen section. An example of small cell carcinoma in a young woman who presented clinically with hypercalcemia is shown in Figure 17.

Uterine Tumors

Smooth Muscle Tumors. Vigorous scraping of benign smooth muscle tumors yields a very cellular preparation composed of fairly uniform spindled cells, often devoid of cytoplasm (Fig. 18). Varying amounts of collagen may be seen in the background. If atypia or mitoses are present, the possibility of leiomyosarcoma must be considered. The gross presentation is obviously important in this differential diagnosis.

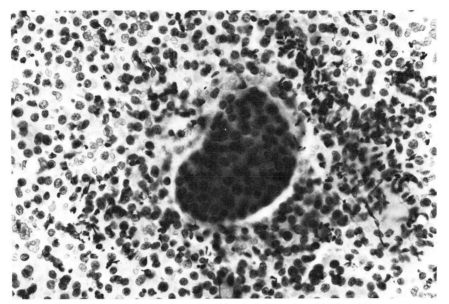

Figure 16. Sertoli cell tumor with tubule formation. (H&E ×160)

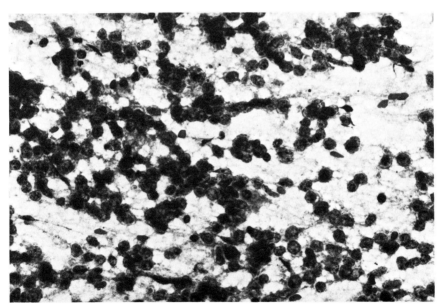

Figure 17. Small-cell carcinoma of ovary. Round-to-oval cells with coarse nuclear chromatin and little cytoplasm, growing in cords and nests and as single cells. (H&E ×300)

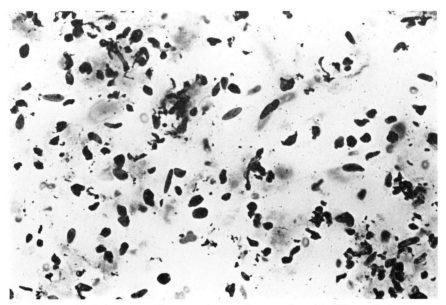

Figure 18. Leiomyoma. Numerous bare uniform oval nuclei. Other cells have retained their cytoplasm. (Diff-Quik ×192)

Endometrial and Endocervical Adenocarcinoma. Just as in routine Pap smears, these types of carcinoma may be difficult to distinguish from one another without knowledge of the gross location of the tumor (Fig. 19). The presence of benign squamous morules associated with malignant glands would certainly favor a diagnosis of endometrial carcinoma, just as voluminous mucin in tumor cells would suggest an endocervical primary. Even low grade endometrial carcinomas are clearly malignant cytologically, which sometimes makes a smear easier to interpret than a frozen section. Adenosquamous, clear cell, and serous variants are usually easy to recognize. Evaluation of depth of invasion of the myometrium and/or lymphatic space invasion in a hysterectomy specimen requires examination of frozen sections.

Endometrial Polyp. In smears, polyps frequently give rise to clusters of benign grandular epithelium as well as single large atypical spindle cells (Fig. 20). Differentiation from a low grade adenosarcoma would be difficult on cytological grounds alone.

Carcinosarcoma. We have examined only a few examples of these tumors cytologically. One may identify nests of malignant epithelial cells in close association with sarcomatous stroma (Fig. 21). We have occasionally identified rhabdomyosarcomatous and chondrosarcomatous components cytologically. The detection of these elements is obviously dependent upon sampling.

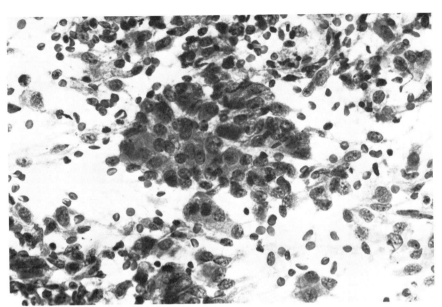

Figure 19. Endometrial adenocarcinoma. Cells are well differentiated but clearly malignant. (Papanicolaou ×300)

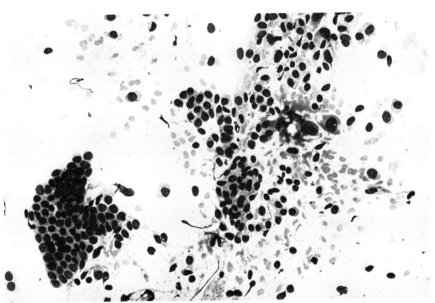

Figure 20. Endometrial polyp. Benign glandular clusters with occasional large atypical stromal cells. (Diff-Quik ×240)

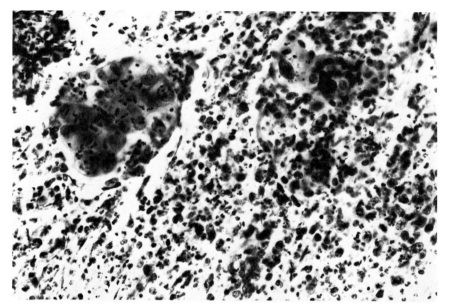

Figure 21. Endometrial carcinosarcoma. Nests of poorly differentiated carcinoma with solitary sarcomatous elements. Note necrotic debris with neutrophils in background. (H&E ×160)

Lymph Nodes

As mentioned above, one of our most frequent reasons for intraoperative gynecologic consultations is to examine pelvic and para-aortic lymph nodes in the course of surgery for cervical or endometrial cancer. We have found that microscopic foci of metastasis are more likely to be found when several cut surfaces of each lymph node are examined, and clearly it is more efficient to accomplish this cytologically (multiple nodes can be smeared and examined on a single slide using air drying with Diff-Quik staining) than by the performance of multiple frozen sections. Our accuracy rate in this situation was 94.6 percent (5.4 percent false negatives) which is at least equal to or considerably better than that reported in the literature for frozen sections.[11]

DIAGNOSTIC ACCURACY

It cannot be overemphasized that accuracy in cytological diagnosis depends on (1) careful gross examination and selection of the area to be examined microscopically, (2) proper preparation, and (3) correct interpretation. However, even in the most experienced hands errors may occur, and we have tried to highlight certain pitfalls in the preceding sections. There are few studies in the literature concerning the accuracy of intraoperative cytological diagnosis and none to date have focused solely on gynecologic disease. One of the earliest studies was published in 1969 by Sakai and Lauslahti,[2] who prospectively studied 400 cases using cytological preparations and frozen sections. All slides were examined microscopically at the time of frozen section by the same two pathologists, including a cytologist. The overall accuracy for all sites was 95.5 percent by cytology and 95.7 percent by frozen section. Only 25 cases were gynecologic specimens (ovary and uterus) and the cytological diagnosis was correct in all instances. There was one false negative by frozen section which was called strongly suspicious by cytology.

The largest series was published by Suen et al in 1978.[5] They examined 1258 specimens by frozen section and cytology. The overall accuracy for cytology was 93.6 percent. Eighty-four gynecologic specimens were examined (57 ovary and 27 uterus) and the accuracy rate was 90.5 percent. There were no false-positive diagnoses.

Lee[7] retrospectively examined 522 imprint preparations without knowledge of the gross or histological appearance of the lesions. His overall accuracy was 92.9 percent. Sixty-nine specimens were from the female genital tract (49 benign and 20 malignant) and accuracy was 100 percent. Two other studies, using cytological diagnosis compared to permanent sections,[8,9] included 22 and 28 gynecologic cases respectively. Accuracy was 100 percent in both series.

Intraoperative cytology should at least be as accurate as FNAC since the problem of inadequate sampling should be negligible. In a recent review of 238 FNACs of patients with malignant gynecologic neoplasms,[10] specificity and sensitivity were 96 and 91 percent, respectively. The authors stressed the importance of defining strict criteria for specimen adequacy.

In our own reviewed material, the overall accuracy rate (analyzed retrospectively, and excluding lymph nodes examined for metastases, which were discussed above) was 91.4 percent. There was one false-positive case, a borderline tumor diagnosed only as carcinoma (since the patient was postmenopausal there was no difference in treatment), and four false negatives (2.9 percent). Two of these were also borderline tumors, which were originally interpreted as benign; in both cases, the error was on the basis of sampling rather than misinterpretation. In the other two instances as well, small tumors (one endometrial, one a focus on the ovarian serosa) were missed grossly; thus, we had no false-negative results due to misinterpretation of cells or tissue on the slide (in many cases, frozen sections were done as well as cytological procedures). In six instances (4.3 percent), the intraoperative diagnosis was deferred (two of these cases proved to be granulosa cell tumors, while the other four followed no particular pattern), and in one additional case (0.7 percent) a Sertoli cell tumor was misinterpreted on both smear and frozen section as a granulosa cell tumor. Thus, our only significant troublesome areas in this retrospective analysis concerned the differential diagnosis of borderline and granulosa cell tumors.

The aforementioned figures can be compared to the approximate figure of 98 percent accuracy by frozen section reported in classic studies.[12-14] This figure has since been revised downward in recent surveys including larger proportions of indeterminate cases (e.g., grossly benign breast biopsies performed for mammographic abnormalities).[11] Two large series have provided information on the accuracy of frozen section specifically regarding gynecologic specimens. In the earlier series, 237 of 490 specimens, were non-cervical, and the accuracy for these specimens was 96 percent.[15] The other series[16] was from a university gynecologic hospital and included a total of 1696 consecutive operating room consultations. Excluding breast and lymph nodes (651 specimens), accuracy for "gross only" diagnoses ranged from 98.3 to 100 percent. For frozen sections, accuracy ranged from 86.9 to 100 percent, depending on the site. We agree with the opinion of these authors that little information is obtained by freezing cervical cone biopsies, and thus we do not use intraoperative cytology in their evaluation, either.

From the limited number of studies reported, it would seem that intraoperative cytological evaluation of gynecologic specimens should be as accurate as frozen sections. Since cytological evaluation may be done in less time than is necessary for the tissue to freeze, we recommend the simultaneous use of both techniques until one gains confidence and familiarity. Eventually, a high level of diagnostic accuracy may be achieved using cytology alone.

REFERENCES

1. Dudgeon LS, Patrick CV: A new method for the rapid microscopical diagnosis of tumours, with an account of 200 cases so examined. Br J Surg 15:250, 1927
2. Sakai Y, Lauslahti K: Comparison and analysis of the results of cytodiagnosis and frozen sections during operation. Acta Cytol 13:359, 1969
3. Godwin JT: Rapid cytologic diagnosis of surgical specimens. Acta Cytol 20:111, 1976
4. Bloustein PA, Silverberg SG: Rapid cytologic examination of surgical specimens. Pathol Annu 12(Part 2):251, 1977
5. Suen KC, Wood WS, Syed AA, et al: Role of imprint cytology in intraoperative diagnosis: Value and limitations. J Clin Pathol 31:328, 1978
6. Hofler H, Weybora W: A new, simple method for intraoperative fast diagnosis. Virchows Arch (Pathol Anat Histol) 382:89, 1979
7. Lee T-K: The value of imprint cytology in tumor diagnosis: A retrospective study of 522 cases in Northern China. Acta Cytol 26:169, 1982
8. Shidham VB, Dravid NV, Grover S, Kher AV: Role of scrape cytology in rapid intraoperative diagnosis: Value and limitations. Acta Cytol 28:477, 1984
9. Szczepanik E: Intraoperative cytology of tumors. Diagn Cytopathol 2:236, 1986
10. Moriarty AT, Glant MD, Stehman FB: The role of fine needle aspiration cytology in the management of gynecologic malignancies. Acta Cytol 30:59, 1986
11. Oneson RH, Minke JA, Silverberg SG: Intraoperative pathologic consultation: An audit of one thousand recent consecutive cases. (submitted)
12. Nakazawa H, Rosen P, Lane N, Lattes R: Frozen section experience in 3000 cases: Accuracy, limitations, and value in residency training. Am J Clin Pathol 49:41, 1968
13. Holaday WJ, Assor D: Ten thousand consecutive frozen sections: A retrospective study focusing on accuracy and quality control. Am J Clin Pathol 61:769, 1974

14. Lessells AM, Simpson JG: A retrospective analysis of the accuracy of immediate frozen section diagnosis in surgical pathology. Br J Surg 63:327, 1976
15. DiMusto JC: Reliability of frozen sections in gynecologic surgery. Obstet Gynecol 35:235, 1970
16. Kanbour A, Salazar H: Operating room pathology consultations in a university gynecologic hospital. Surg Gynecol Obstet 135:203, 1972

Pseudoneoplastic Lesions of the Lower Female Genital Tract

Robert H. Young and Philip B. Clement

A wide variety of non-neoplastic lesions within the female genital tract can be confused with neoplasms on clinical, gross, or microscopic examination. Tumor-like conditions involving the ovary have recently been reviewed in detail elsewhere.[1,2] This chapter will discuss a selected group of pseudoneoplastic lesions that occur in the fallopian tubes, uterus, vagina, or vulva. Emphasis is on recently described entities, older entities with new information, and lesions which pose particular diagnostic difficulty. Obviously non-neoplastic lesions (such as vulvar and vaginal cysts), human papilloma virus-related lesions, and endometrial metaplasias will not be considered.

LYMPHOMA-LIKE LESIONS OF THE CERVIX, ENDOMETRIUM, AND VULVA

Reactive lymphoid lesions in the lower female genital tract may be florid and simulate a lymphoma (Fig. 1). In a recent review of 16 lymphoma-like lesions, which are typically encountered in women of reproductive age, there were 10 in the cervix, 5 in the endometrium, and 1 in the vulva.[3] Certain clinical features favor the diagnosis of a lymphoma-like lesion. Evidence of pelvic inflammatory disease should raise the suspicion of a benign process. All five endometrial lesions had obvious microscopic evidence of chronic endometritis. One patient with a cervical lesion and one with a vulvar lesion had infectious mononucleosis. In the former case, the viral infection was not recognized until 10 days after a cervical biopsy disclosed an atypical lymphoid infiltrate. This

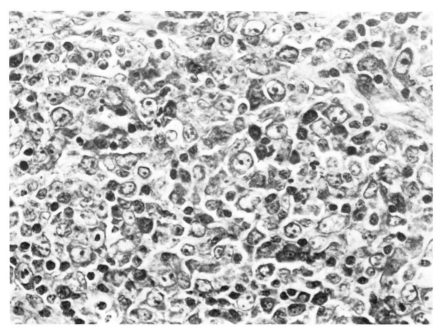

Figure 1. Lymphoma-like lesion of uterus. A dense infiltrate is composed largely of immunoblasts.

association between a lymphoma-like lesion in the female genital tract and infectious mononucleosis is consistent with the association between atypical lymphoid proliferations and infectious mononucleosis elsewhere.

Several gross and microscopic features help to distinguish lymphoma-like lesions from malignant lymphoma (Table 1).[4] Cervical lymphomas only rarely have mucosal ulceration; they often result in a barrel-shaped cervix, and they frequently extend into the paracervical tissue or vagina. The diagnosis of lymphoma of the cervix should be made with great caution if it is based solely on microscopic findings without clinical evidence of a neoplasm. In contrast, although the cervix appeared abnormal on pelvic examination in 70 percent of patients with lymphoma-like lesions, cervical enlargement was not a conspicuous feature in most cases, and diffuse enlargement was not encountered. In several cases the abnormal appearance was the result of ulceration, and the abnormality did not extend beyond the cervix in any case. Gross abnormalities, such as ulceration, are compatible with a benign process.

Microscopically, lymphoma-like lesions are typically composed of large lymphoid cells including cleaved and non-cleaved follicular center cells as well as immunoblasts (Fig. 1). A starry-sky pattern was present in 3 of the 16 ases. Mitotic activity was prominent. Plasma cells, polymorphonuclear leukocytes, and small lymphocytes characteristically are present within the infiltrate (Fig. 2), and usually extend to the endocervical epithelium (which may be

TABLE 1. COMPARISON OF FEATURES OF LYMPHOMAS AND LYMPHOMA-LIKE LESIONS

Feature	Lymphoma	Lymphoma-Like
Gross mass	Usual	Seldom
Ulceration	Seldom	Usual
Surface involvement	Seldom	Frequent
Deep invasion	Usual	Seldom
Perivascular infiltrate	Frequent	Seldom
Sclerosis	Frequent	Seldom
Large cells	Monomorphic	Polymorphic
Mitoses	Frequent	Frequent
Neutrophils, lymphocytes plasma cells in lesion	Seldom	Frequent

ulcerated.) In contrast to lymphoma-like lesions, lymphomas exhibit cellular monomorphism, a perivascular distribution of the lymphoid cells, deep invasion, and prominent sclerosis. In additional contrast, surface ulceration and intralesional acute inflammatory cells and plasma cells are rarely seen in lymphomas. There is often a spared zone of unremarkable stroma between the overlying intact epithelium and the underlying lymphoma. Immunohistochemi-

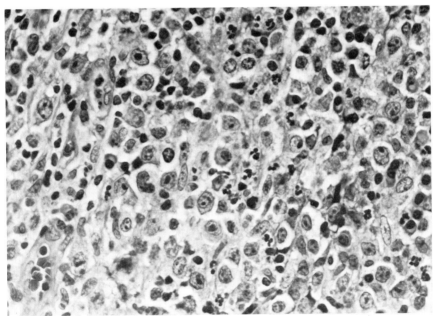

Figure 2. Lymphoma-like lesion of uterus. A polymorphous inflammatory cell infiltrate consists of large lymphoid cells, plasma cells, lymphocytes, and neutrophils.

cal stains performed in seven cases were not a significant diagnostic aid. They showed polyclonal plasma cells in six cases. Most of the atypical large cells did not stain for cytoplasmic immunoglobulin. The seventh specimen had many immunoblasts with cytoplasmic staining of polyclonal type.[3]

Ten of the 16 patients had follow-up from 6 months to 12 years. Nine were treated with procedures inadequate for the cure of malignant lymphoma, but follow-up was uneventful in all. The clinical and pathologic features of these cases suggest that they are a localized, florid lymphoid proliferation associated with chronic cervicitis or endometritis, or they reflect a generalized disorder of lymphoid cells such as infectious mononucleosis.

POSTOPERATIVE SPINDLE-CELL NODULE

In 1984, Proppe et al[5] reported the clinical and pathologic features of nine cases of a proliferative spindle-cell lesion that developed shortly after an operation on the lower genitourinary tract. The lesions resembled sarcomas (usually leiomyosarcomas) on microscopic examination, and were initially often misdiagnosed as such. Two additional examples of this lesion, which are referred to as postoperative spindle-cell nodules (PSCN), have been described.[6,7]

The 11 patients, 6 females and 5 males, ranged in age from 29 to 75 years. The PSCNs were discovered in the operative site 2.5 to 12 weeks (mean 6 weeks) after a surgical procedure involving the vagina (four cases), prostatic urethra (three cases), bladder (two cases), endocervix and endometrium (one case each). The urethral lesions were associated with hematuria or obstruction, whereas the remaining lesions were found during routine follow-up examination or within a specimen obtained by a repeat surgical procedure. Two patients treated only by local excision developed local recurrences 2 and 6 weeks later.[5] The recurrences were successfully treated by local re-excision. Of nine patients with follow-up, all were without disease 6 to 60 months after excision of the lesion.

PSCNs are soft polypoid masses that have been up to 4 cm in diameter. Microscopic examination shows intersecting fascicles of plump spindle cells (Fig. 3) often with a delicate network of small blood vessels. There is frequently ulceration with a superficial acute inflammatory cell infiltrate, and chronic inflammatory cells are seen in the deeper portions of the lesion. Small foci of hemorrhage and mild-to-moderate edema are common. Mitotic figures are often numerous with as many as 25 mitoses per 10 high power fields.[5] The cells may have plump, vesicular nuclei with one or two prominent nucleoli but they do not exhibit significant cytological atypia. The lesion may infiltrate surrounding normal tissue to a limited degree. In one nodule, ultrastructural examination of the spindle cells revealed features of fibroblasts.[5] All five spindle cell nodules that were stained immunohistochemically for desmin were positive.[8] Surprisingly, four of them also stained for cytokeratin.

Although the histological features of PSCN are readily confused with a malignancy, the association with a recent operation and the outcome of the

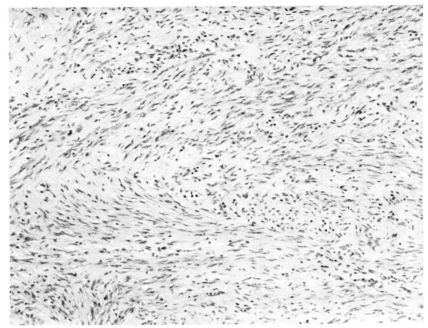

Figure 3. Postoperative spindle-cell nodule. Intersecting fascicles of spindle cells simulating the appearance of a leiomyosarcoma.

cases indicate that they are examples of a benign reactive lesion. Distinction between a PSCN and a well-differentiated leiomyosarcoma may be difficult. Histologically, the latter may be no more atypical cytologically than a PSCN, and it may be less mitotically active. It should also be remembered that the PSCN may infiltrate adjacent tissues including muscle. Both lesions may be myxoid so that the differential diagnosis of some PSCN is with the myxoid variant of leiomyosarcoma.[9] We have noted that most cases of PSCN have a prominent, very delicate network of small blood vessels, which is not a typical feature of leiomyosarcoma. Ultimately, however, distinction of a PSCN from a leiomyosarcoma depends on the clinical setting.

MISCELLANEOUS REPARATIVE AND INFLAMMATORY LESIONS

Other uncommon reparative and inflammatory pseudoneoplastic lesions have been described in the lower female genital tract in addition to lymphoma-like lesions and PSCN. On histological examination, these other reparative lesions are composed of spindle cells of fibroblastic or myofibroblastic type, chronic inflammatory cells, and histiocytes, alone or in various combinations.

Five examples of nodular (pseudosarcomatous) fasciitis have been described: three vulvar, one vaginal, and one in the round ligament of the uterus.[10-12] The gross features of only one case were described in detail, a subcutaneous vulvar mass that was 3 cm in diameter, with a gray-brown, lobulated, rubbery exterior and a homogeneous yellow-white cut surface.[12] Another vulvar lesion was a 2.5 cm in diameter, firm, mobile subcutaneous mass attached to the right ischiocavernosis muscle.[11] All five lesions exhibited the typical histological features of nodular fasciitis of soft tissues.

Two cases of uterine inflammatory pseudotumor have been reported.[13] They resembled lesions in the lung variously referred to as "inflammatory pseudotumor," "inflammatory myofibroblastic tumor,"[14] or "plasma-cell granuloma." On gross examination, solitary leiomyoma-like masses, measuring 12.5 cm and 4.5 cm, involved the myometrium. On histological examination, the lesions had mitotically inactive, spindle-shaped cells with bland nuclear features mixed with an inflammatory infiltrate rich in plasma cells (Fig. 4). In one case, the actin positivity of the spindle cells, as well as the ultrastructural features in one case, confirmed their myofibroblastic nature. Inflammatory pseudotumors must be distinguished from the recently described "uterine leiomyomas with lymphoid infiltration."[15]

Xanthogranulomatous inflammation with large numbers of foamy histiocytes may be seen in several sites in the female genital tract, and it is usually a manifestation of chronic pelvic inflammatory disease. Yellow masses (xanthogranulomas) have been described in the ovary, fallopian tube, or both (four cases)[16-19] and vagina (two cases).[20,21] One of the latter cases was of particular interest. An 81-year-old woman with recurrent vaginal polyps was thought to

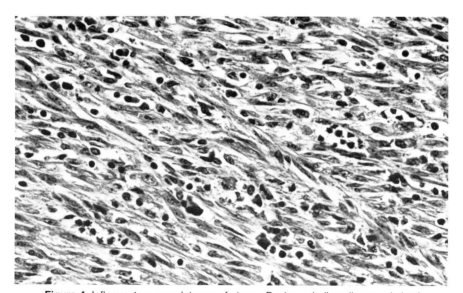

Figure 4. Inflammatory pseudotumor of uterus. Benign spindle cells are admixed with a plasma cell-rich inflammatory infiltrate.

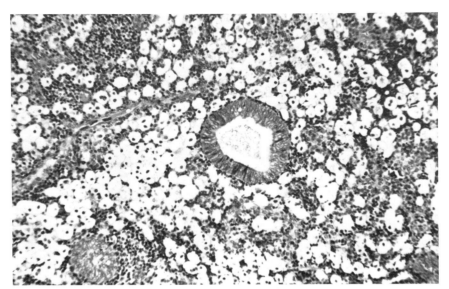

Figure 5. Xanthogranulomatous endometritis. An endometrial gland is surrounded by a stroma replaced largely by foamy histiocytes.

have a malignant tumor.[21] Microscopic examination was suggestive of a granular cell tumor, but special stains and ultrastructural examination revealed numerous intracellular bacilli. In culture, they were a pure strain of a mucoid form of *Escherichia coli*. The lesion was considered to be related to malakoplakia or Whipple's disease in which there appears to be defective clearance of bacteria.

In the uterus, seven examples of xanthogranulomatous or "histiocytic" endometritis have been described (Fig. 5); typically as a manifestation of cervical stenosis and pyometra.[22–27] In two cases, however, there was also an adenocarcinoma, one synchronous[26] and one metachronous.[27] In the latter case, xanthogranulomatous endometritis with numerous cholesterol crystals and a foreign-body giant-cell reaction was present 5 years before the diagnosis of endometrial carcinoma.[27]

Xanthogranulomatous inflammation within the uterus and fallopian tubes can be a foreign-body response to oily material, such as mineral oil, lubricants, and contrast material.[28,29] Mineral oil granulomas may cause masses measuring up to 4 cm in the cervix, endometrium, myometrium, or parametrium. A foreign-body giant-cell and fibrous reaction surrounds spaces of variable size.[28] In one case, periureteral spread of the oil resulted in fatal ureteric obstruction.[28]

The differential diagnosis of xanthogranulomatous inflammation in the fallopian tube includes "pseudoxanthomatous" salpingitis, a lesion that may be associated with pelvic endometriosis (Fig. 6).[30] The lamina propria of the tube is infiltrated by large numbers of histiocytes with abundant foamy and pigmented cytoplasm. The fine, brown pigment within the histiocytes or "pseudoxanthoma cells" is predominantly hemofuchsin (ceroid). Similar ceroid-laden histiocytes

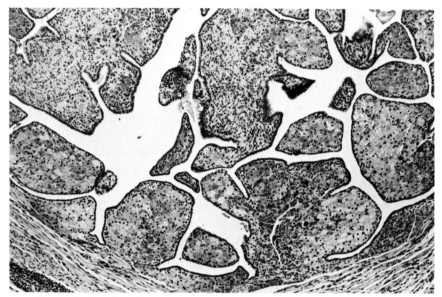

Figure 6. Pseudoxanthomatous salpingitis. The tubal plicae contain numerous pseudoxanthoma cells. The patient had ovarian endometriosis.

within the tubal mucosa, so-called "pigmentosis tubae," have been described following pelvic irradiation.[31]

Malakoplakia rarely involves the reproductive system, usually, but not exclusively, in postmenopausal women. Twenty-three cases have been described.[32–38] They involved one or more sites, including the vagina (seven cases), endometrium (seven cases), cervix (five cases), fallopian tube and broad ligament (five cases), ovary (three cases), and vulva and Bartholin's glands (three cases). Several cases recurred,[34] and one case in the endometrium had a co-existent endometrial adenocarcinoma.[33] The gross and histological appearance, including the presence of diagnostic Michaelis–Guttman bodies, are similar to malakoplakia elsewhere.[39]

A final pseudoneoplastic lesion in this group was a mass in the vaginal apex composed of spindle cells in a storiform pattern.[40] The lesion mimicked a fibrous histiocytoma except for the presence of a foreign-body reaction to polarizable material. It was interpreted as a reactive fibrohistiocytic proliferation similar to the silica-induced lesions described in soft tissues.[41]

MICROGLANDULAR HYPERPLASIA OF ENDOCERVICAL GLANDS

In the late 1960s, a series of reports described an endocervical lesion characterized by an epithelial proliferation that was often confused with adenocarcinoma.[42–47] This lesion is now widely known as "microglandular hyperplasia" (MGH) (Figs. 7 through 11). MGH is usually related to progesterone stimula-

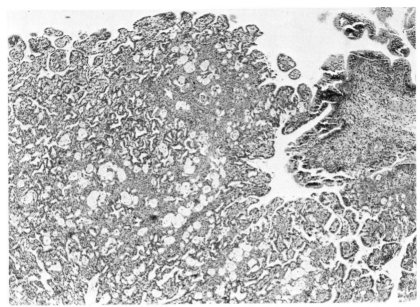

Figure 7. Microglandular hyperplasia of cervix. The lesion, which forms a polyp, is composed of small, closely packed glands. Some normal endocervical epithelium is seen at the top right.

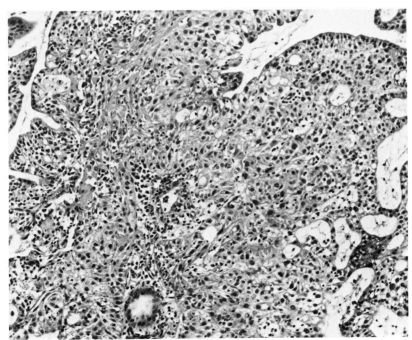

Figure 8. Microglandular hyperplasia of cervix. Most of the field shows a solid cellular proliferation with the more typical features of microglandular hyperplasia present only at the periphery.

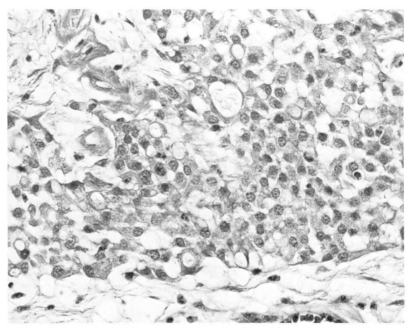

Figure 9. Microglandular hyperplasia of cervix. Most of the cells in this field have moderately abundant eosinophilic cytoplasm. A few cells, however, have vacuolated cytoplasm and eccentric nuclei simulating the signet-ring cells of an adenocarcinoma.

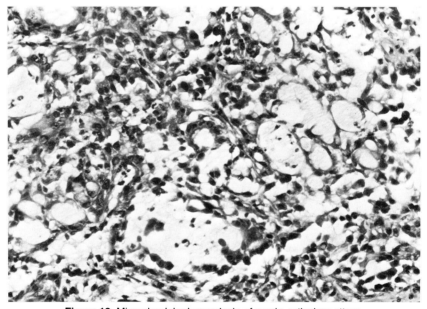

Figure 10. Microglandular hyperplasia of cervix, reticular pattern.

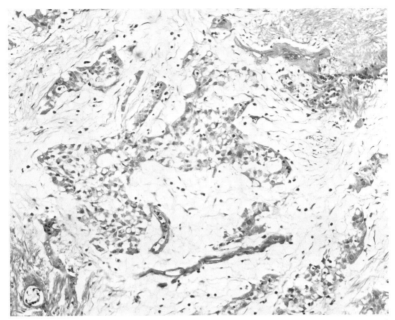

Figure 11. Microglandular hyperplasia of cervix. Irregular nests and clusters of cells are dispersed in a myxoid stroma simulating infiltration of a carcinoma.

tion. It is most commonly seen in users of oral contraceptives (67 percent of the cases) and less commonly during pregnancy (7 percent of the cases).[42–56] Occasionally, however, MGH is seen in a patient receiving only estrogen[45,53,54] or in a patient in whom none of the aforementioned associations is present. The lesion is usually in young women (mean, 33.5 years), but approximately 6 percent of the reported cases have occurred in postmenopausal women.

A patient with MGH is usually asymptomatic, but she may complain of abnormal vaginal bleeding or discharge. Most commonly, MGH is an incidental microscopic finding in as many as 24 percent of cone biopsies.[49] This figure rises to 44 percent in those using oral contraceptives.[49] It may be visible as a polypoid friable lesion or an erosion. Rarely, there is extensive gross involvement of the cervix.[47,50]

Histologically, microglandular hyperplasia typically consists of closely packed glands (Fig. 7) that vary from small and round to irregular and cystically dilated. They usually contain a basophilic or eosinophilic secretion that stains for mucin and often contains many acute inflammatory cells. The glands are closely packed, but occasionally they are separated by scant fibrous stroma that rarely is extensively hyalinized.[56] Inflammatory cells, both acute and chronic but mainly the former, are often conspicuous in the stroma. The cells lining the glands and cysts are usually low columnar, cuboidal, or flat, with faintly basophilic or granular cytoplasm. Occasionally they have abundant eosinophilic cytoplasm (Fig. 9), and rarely they are so-called hobnail cells.[56] Subnuclear vacuoles are sometimes present and may be conspicuous. The vacuoles stain positively for mucin but are negative for glycogen. The nuclei of the cells are almost always small and regular with fine chromatin. Nucleoli are occasionally visible, and hyperchromatic nuclei with a degenerative appearance are sometimes seen. Mitoses are generally rare, but counts up to one mitotic figure per ten high power fields may be seen.[56]

Less common patterns of MGH include reticular (Fig. 10) and solid (Fig. 8).[54,56] In the former, the cells, some of which may be spindle shaped, are loosely dispersed in an edematous stroma. In the latter, there are sheets of cells without gland formation. Some cells within the solid foci have pale cytoplasm and eccentric nuclei (Fig. 9) simulating the signet-ring cells of an adenocarcinoma.[56]

In occasional cases of MGH, the relationship of the proliferating cells to the stroma may cause diagnostic difficulty. Small nests, cords, and large aggregates of cells are irregularly distributed in a myxoid stroma, imparting a pseudoinfiltrative pattern (Fig. 11).[56] However, these cells lack cytological atypia and usually merge with foci of typical MGH.

The major tumor to be distinguished from MGH is clear cell carcinoma. Both lesions may have tubular, cystic, and solid patterns, but the papillary pattern of clear cell carcinoma is not encountered in MGH. The solid foci of clear cell carcinoma usually consist of cells with abundant, clear, glycogen-rich cytoplasm, whereas those of MGH very rarely have conspicuous clear cytoplasm and lack glycogen. Although some clear cell carcinomas may have relatively bland cytological features with low mitotic rates, and some cases of MGH may have atypia and rare mitoses, the atypia and mitotic rates in clear cell carcinoma generally exceed those of MGH.

MISCELLANEOUS PSEUDONEOPLASTIC LESIONS OF ENDOCERVICAL GLANDS

In addition to MGH, the endocervical epithelium may proliferate in a variety of settings and produce diverse microscopic appearances. Some may be confused with an in situ or invasive adenocarcinoma. Perhaps the most common lesion is a florid papillary proliferation in chronic endocervicitis (Fig. 12). This appearance is well known, and it is unlikely to cause diagnostic problems. The differential diagnosis includes the rare well-differentiated endocervical adenocarcinomas with a prominent papillary or villoglandular pattern that may be underdiagnosed as a benign proliferation.[57] Parenthetically, a similar papillary proliferation lined by endocervical-type epithelium may be seen in vaginal adenosis, so-called papillary adenosis (Figs. 13 and 14).

Another common finding in endocervical glands that may cause some diagnostic difficulty is florid squamous metaplasia. Particular difficulty may be posed by cases in which the involved glands are deep in the wall, closely packed, and irregularly distributed (Fig. 15). However, the bland cytology of

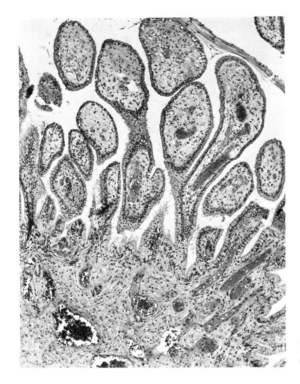

Figure 12. Prominent papillae in case of chronic endocervicitis.

the metaplastic squamous cells and awareness of this phenomenon should avoid a serious diagnostic error.

The Arias–Stella reaction was seen in the endocervical glands of 9 percent of gravid hysterectomy specimens in one study.[58] The lesion involves only one or two glands. Glands in any part of the endocervical canal may be affected, but superficial glands are a more common site than deep glands.[58] Epithelium within endocervical polyps may also be affected.[59] The cytological features are similar to those within endometrial glands. They include stratified cells with abundant vacuolated cytoplasm and enlarged, pleomorphic, hyperchromatic nuclei that impart a hobnail appearance to some cells (Fig. 16). Optically clear nuclei may be seen.[58] Mitoses are rare or absent.[60] Arias–Stella changes may be mistaken for adenocarcinoma in situ (ACIS) or clear cell carcinoma particularly in a biopsy or cytology specimen. Such diagnoses should therefore be made with caution during pregnancy. Clear cell carcinoma, however, will typically be associated with a mass, and histological examination will reveal features inconsistent with the Arias–Stella reaction including the presence of invasion plus tubular, papillary, and solid patterns. ACIS, in contrast to the Arias–Stella reaction, usually exhibits uniformly atypical nuclei and numerous mitotic figures. ACIS usually lacks marked cytoplasmic vacuolation, hobnail cells, or optically clear nuclei.

Fluhmann suggested the designation "tunnel cluster" for a common alter-

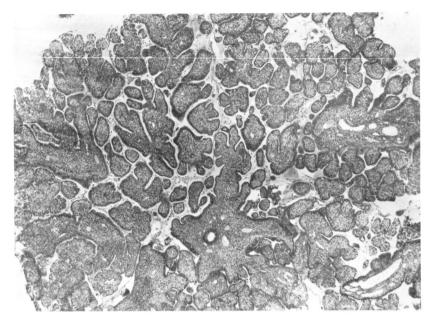

Figure 13. Papillary adenosis of vagina.

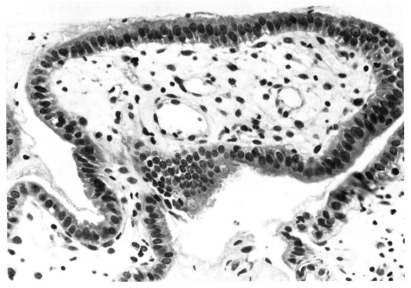

Figure 14. Papillary adenosis of vagina. A papilla is lined by low columnar epithelial cells devoid of atypia.

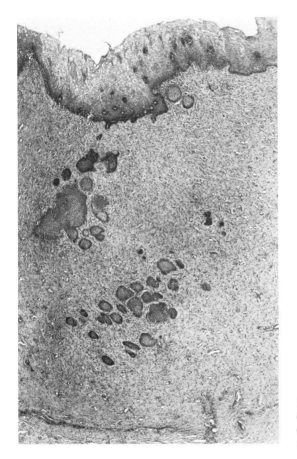

Figure 15. Squamous metaplasia of cervix. Note relatively deep location of metaplastic squamous nests in cervical stroma.

ation of the endocervical glands that is an incidental finding on histological examination (Fig. 17).[61,62] He demonstrated tunnel clusters in the transformation zone of 8 percent of adult women, 13 percent of postmenopausal women, and 40 percent of women in the first trimester. They were not seen before the age of 30. These are discrete, 0.5 to 5 mm, rounded foci composed of 20 to 50, oval, round or irregular, closely packed tubules of varying size (Fig. 17).[61,62] The tubules, which may be cystically dilated, are separated from each other by scanty fibrous tissue, and the cluster is surrounded by the normal, superficial endocervical stroma. The tubules are lined by endocervical cells which may be normal columnar, cuboidal, or flattened. Only one or two tunnel clusters are usually seen, although in rare cases, there are large numbers in a confluent arrangement.[61] We have seen one florid example in which the epithelial cells lining the tubules exhibited mild nuclear atypia and occasional mitotic figures (Fig. 18) prompting the diagnosis of adenoma malignum ("minimal deviation adenocarcinoma") by several consultants. Tunnel clusters, however, lack the infiltrative pattern, stromal desmoplasia, and deep invasion of adenoma ma-

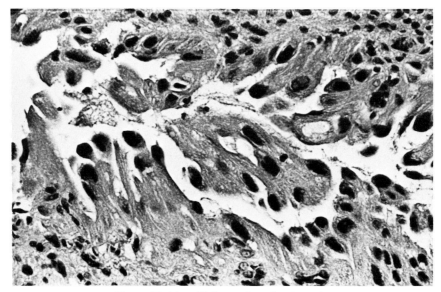

Figure 16. Arias–Stella reaction of endocervix.

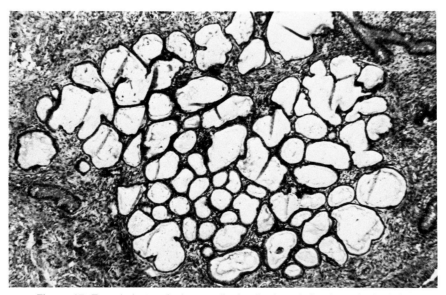

Figure 17. Tunnel cluster. A circumscribed collection of closely packed tubular structures are lined by cuboidal to flattened epithelium.

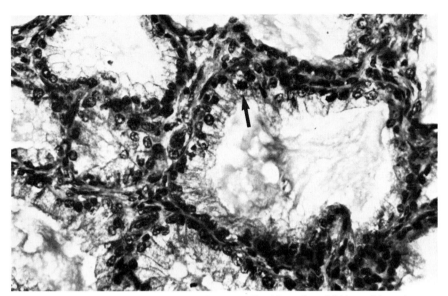

Figure 18. Tubules within a tunnel cluster are lined by cells exhibiting mild atypia; note a mitotic figure (*arrow*).

lignum. Fluhmann concluded that tunnel clusters represent an involutionary stage of normal endocervical glands (clefts) and have no clinical significance.[61] There is no evidence to suggest that they represent a hyperplastic or premalignant change. Therefore, the proposed alternate designation of "adenomatous hyperplasia"[62] should be avoided.

We have recently encountered two examples of an apparently hitherto undescribed pseudoneoplastic process of the endocervical glands.[63] In both cases, gross examination of the uterus, removed for uterine leiomyomas and prolapse respectively, revealed numerous mucin-filled cysts up to 1 cm in diameter. The cysts were scattered irregularly in the endocervix from the mucosa almost to the serosa (Fig. 19). Histologically, the cysts were lined by benign columnar (Fig. 20), cuboidal, or flattened endocervical epithelium devoid of mitotic activity. In one case, the non-cystic endocervical glands were normal in appearance and location, whereas in the other case, many of the superficial glands were arranged in tunnel clusters. In both cases, a diagnosis of adenoma malignum was considered by the referring pathologist. The characteristic features of adenoma malignum, however, were not present. The cysts were interpreted as deeply situated, but otherwise typical, Nabothian cysts. Non-cystic endometrial-type glands also may be encountered occasionally as an incidental microscopic finding deep in the endocervical wall (Fig. 21).[64] The lack of both atypia and an associated stromal reaction should facilitate their distinction from adenocarcinoma.

Two final lesions merit brief consideration in the differential diagnosis of

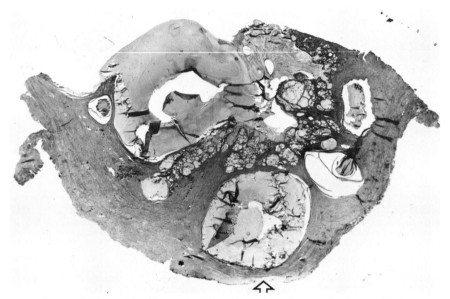

Figure 19. Deep Nabothian cysts with endocervical stroma extend almost to the serosa (*arrow*).

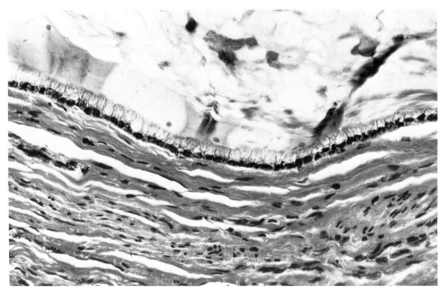

Figure 20. Deep Nabothian cyst. Cyst is lined by bland appearing columnar epithelium.

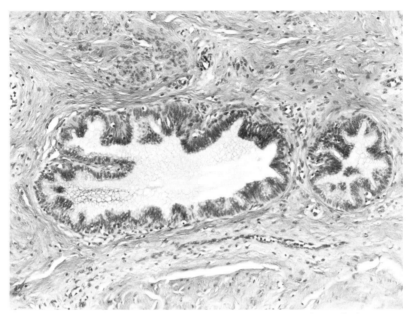

Figure 21. Glands lined by endometrial-type epithelium deep in cervical stroma lack significant atypia.

endocervical ACIS. Cytomegalovirus (CMV) infection, which is usually an incidental histological finding within the endocervix, has large basophilic intranuclear inclusions in the affected endocervical epithelial cells, and in some cases, endothelial cells.[65–68] Immunohistochemical staining for CMV antigen may be confirmatory.[67] Two cases in the literature,[65,66] and another in our experience, were associated with florid follicular cervicitis. The intranuclear inclusions, as well as cytoplasmic inclusions, are sufficiently characteristic that confusion with ACIS is unlikely (Fig. 22). In contrast to ACIS, the cells involved by CMV are singly disposed within normal endocervical columnar cells (Fig. 22).

Radiation to the cervix can cause markedly atypical nuclear changes that can be mistaken for ACIS, particularly if the pathologist is unaware of this history.[69] In contrast to ACIS, however, the bizarre nuclear features following radiation are more variable from one cell to another and lack mitotic activity (Fig. 22). Radiation-induced vascular and stromal changes, including postradiation fibroblasts, may also be present.[69]

ATYPICAL HYPERPLASIA OF MESONEPHRIC REMNANTS

Mesonephric remnants within the wall of the cervix have been well known since Meyer[70] reported them in 27 percent of the specimens he studied. The remnants usually consist of the main mesonephric duct surrounded by variable numbers of

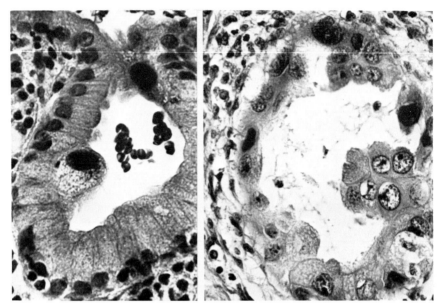

Figure 22. (*Left*) Cytomegalovirus infection of endocervical glands. Note occasional endocervical columnar cells containing characteristic intranuclear inclusions and granular cytoplasmic inclusions. (*Right*) Postradiation atypia of endocervical glands. Cells lining endocervical gland exhibit bizarre, hyperchromatic nuclei.

small, round, but occasionally cystically dilated, tubules (Figs. 23 through 25). The tubules are lined by low cuboidal epithelial cells usually lacking atypia and containing densely eosinophilic hyaline secretions (Fig. 24).[71–73]

It is not widely recognized that mesonephric remnants can exhibit florid hyperplasia and atypia to the extent that they may be easily confused with adenocarcinoma.[74,75] In one study of 44 mesonephric lesions of the cervix, 27 were regarded as mesonephric remnants, 11 were considered hyperplastic, and 6 were thought to represent atypical mesonephric hyperplasia[74]. The mesonephric remnants consisted of a main branching duct, usually lying 3 to 6 mm beneath the surface of the endocervical epithelium, surrounded by clusters of small tubules. The hyperplastic lesions had larger clusters due to proliferation and crowding of the tubules, but an orderly pattern about the main mesonephric duct was maintained. In the atypical cases, the tubular proliferation was more florid. The tubules displayed a more haphazard arrangement as they deeply and diffusely involved the cervical stroma simulating infiltration by a well-differentiated adenocarcinoma. An associated stromal reaction, however, was absent. The epithelium of the tubules in these six lesions was cuboidal-to-columnar with varying degrees of nuclear atypism and mitotic activity up to one to two per ten high power fields. Hysterectomy was performed in 20 patients including 2 who received postoperative radiation. Cervical conization was the sole therapy in 23, and 1 patient received no treatment after her biopsy. In 38

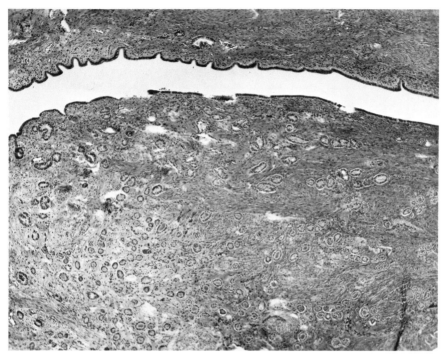

Figure 23. Mesonephric hyperplasia. A mesonephric duct is surrounded by a florid proliferation of mesonephric tubules.

patients with follow-up, all were without evidence of disease from 1.6 to 16.7 years (median, 4.7 years) after diagnosis, including the 6 atypical cases and the 17 patients in whom the mesonephric proliferation extended to the surgical margins.

Mesonephric adenocarcinomas occur[76,77] with such rarity that the diagnosis should be made with caution and only after florid mesonephric hyperplasia has been excluded. In contrast to mesonephric hyperplasia, a mesonephric carcinoma is likely to produce a grossly visible lesion. There is typically irregular destructive invasion by the glands with an associated stromal reaction. Severe nuclear atypicality and prominent mitotic activity, of course, favor malignancy.

Mesonephric hyperplasia should be distinguished from both adenoma malignum[78–85] and clear cell adenocarcinoma of the cervix.[86,87] The glands in adenoma malignum are much more irregular in size and shape than the tubules of mesonephric hyperplasia, and at least some of them are more dilated than the small tubular glands of mesonephric hyperplasia. In addition, they are lined by tall columnar mucinous cells in contrast to the cuboidal non-mucinous epithelial cells of the tubules. Adenoma malignum also has an edematous or desmoplastic stromal reaction. The tubules in mesonephric hyperplasia might be confused with the tubular glands that are present in many clear cell adenocarcinomas of

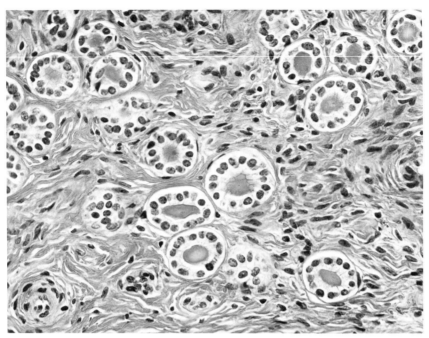

Figure 24. Mesonephric hyperplasia. Mesonephric tubules contain eosinophilic secretion and are lined by cytologically bland cuboidal cells.

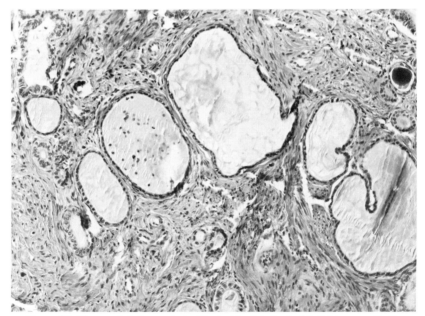

Figure 25. Mesonephric hyperplasia. Most of the tubules in this field are cystically dilated.

the cervix.[86,87] The tubules in mesonephric hyperplasia rarely undergo cystic dilation imparting a low power appearance that may mimic the tubulocystic pattern of clear cell carcinoma. In contrast to mesonephric hyperplasia, at least some of the cells lining the glands and cysts of clear cell carcinoma have conspicuous clear cytoplasm or are hobnail cells. Additionally, clear cell carcinomas with a pure tubular pattern are uncommon. They are usually associated with diffuse and papillary patterns, which are not compatible with a diagnosis of mesonephric hyperplasia. Glycogen stains may be helpful in the differential diagnosis as the cells in clear cell carcinoma are glycogen rich in contrast to those of mesonephric hyperplasia.

FIBROEPITHELIAL POLYPS WITH STROMAL ATYPIA

In 1966, Norris and Taylor[88] drew attention to the occasional presence of atypical stromal cells within fibroepithelial polyps of the lower female genital tract that sometimes caused the polyps to be misdiagnosed as sarcoma botryoides. Several reports have subsequently appeared.[89–98] Most occur in the vagina, but occasionally they arise in the cervix or vulva.[88,95,97] The polyps typically occur in women in the reproductive age group, but rarely they are in children. Approximately 25 percent of the women have been pregnant. The patients may be asymptomatic or have postcoital bleeding.

The polyps are usually 4 cm or less in greatest dimension. Microscopic examination shows intact squamous epithelium. The underlying stroma is edematous or myxoid, and it contains scattered mesenchymal cells, some of which have irregular, enlarged, hyperchromatic nuclei, resembling reactive fibroblasts (Fig. 26). The cells have granular eosinophilic cytoplasm and delicately branched, sharply tapered cytoplasmic processes. Cross-striations and longitudinal fibrils are absent. Although mitoses may be present, and even abnormal,[88,96] they are usually few.

The major differential diagnosis in these cases is sarcoma botryoides. Sarcoma botryoides of the vagina typically occurs in young children under 5 years of age and is rare in older women, whereas atypical polyps of the vagina have only very rarely been encountered in children. It should be mentioned that sarcoma botryoides of the cervix occurs in an older age group than its vaginal counterpart (mean age, 18 years).[99] Age differences are not, therefore, as helpful in cervical cases. The absence of a cambium layer is an important point of distinction from sarcoma botryoides, although a cambium layer may be present only focally in the latter. Sarcoma botryoides, at least focally, has closely packed small cells with hyperchromatic nuclei and other cells with eosinophilic cytoplasm containing cross-striations. Fibroepithelial polyps lack these features.

Occasionally, atypical cells similar to those seen in some fibroepithelial polyps are an incidental finding in the superficial stroma of the cervix, vagina, and vulva.[95,100] Similar cells rarely occur in the stroma of otherwise typical endometrial polyps.

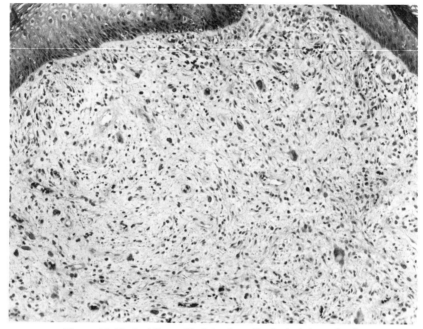

Figure 26. Vaginal fibroepithelial polyp with atypical stromal cells.

ECTOPIC DECIDUA

Decidual reaction in the lower female genital tract is sometimes encountered within the endocervical stroma and lamina propria of the fallopian tube. It is usually an incidental histological finding in pregnant women[101-104] or, rarely, in newborns.[105] During pregnancy, a similar reaction occurs in the submesothelial stroma of the pelvic cavity, including that of the uterine corpus and fallopian tubes.[103,106]

Cervical decidual reaction was detected on histological examination in 36 percent of antepartum cervical biopsies in one study,[101] and in 31 percent of gravid hysterectomy specimens in another.[102] The decidual cells resemble eutopic decidua. They are usually confined to microscopic foci within the loose subepithelial cervical stroma or within the stroma of endocervical polyps (Fig. 27).[102,107] Attenuation, erosion, or ulceration of the overlying epithelium is common. The decidual reaction typically disappears by the eighth postpartum week.[101] Ectopic decidual reaction has been documented within the lamina propria of the fallopian tubes in from 5 to 8 percent of pregnant women at term[103,104] and, rarely, in women receiving exogenous progestins.[108]

Rare cases of a florid decidual reaction in the cervix[107,109-113] and vagina[111,114] have taken the form of grossly visible masses during the first, second, or third

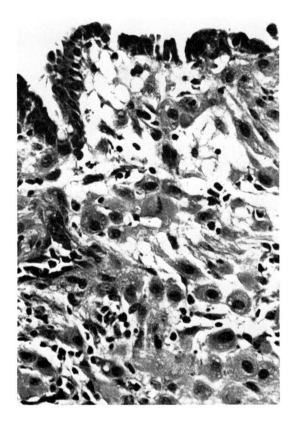

Figure 27. Ectopic decidual reaction of endocervical stroma.

trimester. Some cases have had antepartum bleeding. Pelvic examination reveals a polypoid, nodular, or ulcerating mass, up to 6 cm, that mimics a malignant tumor. Histological examination of a biopsy specimen has usually provided the correct diagnosis but, in occasional cases, focal atypia of the decidual cells has resulted in diagnoses of carcinoma[111] or malignant lymphoma.[113] The mitotic inactivity and bland nuclear features of most decidual cells, however, should facilitate distinction from a neoplasm. Ectopic decidua in postpartum patients may undergo hyalinization (Fig. 28) which sometimes serves to obscure its nature.

PROLIFERATIVE LESIONS OF THE FALLOPIAN TUBE

Varying degrees of hyperplasia and/or atypia of the tubal epithelium may be seen in a number of settings including patients with functioning ovarian tumors and excess estrogen production. The epithelial hyperplasia has occasional mitotic figures, but it is unaccompanied by cytological atypia. Such changes may

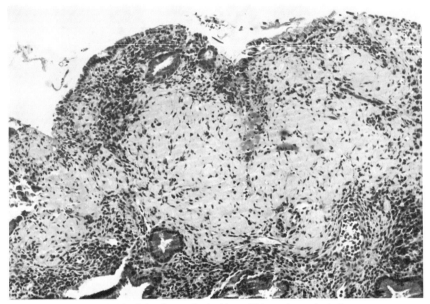

Figure 28. Hyalinized ectopic decidua within endocervical stroma.

be the only pathologic evidence of estrogen excess if the endometrium is not available for microscopic examination. More commonly, epithelial hyperplasia is an incidental finding, or it is present in a tube that is the site of acute or chronic inflammation.[115–119] In one study, 18.5 percent of 124 unselected surgically resected fallopian tubes showed proliferative changes of the epithelium such as nuclear stratification and atypia.[117] In half of these cases, there was salpingitis. Some authors have designated examples of atypical hyperplasia unassociated with inflammation as carcinoma in situ, but there is no evidence that these lesions progress to carcinoma. One study, however, has shown an association of tubal hyperplasia with malignant tumors in the upper genital tract.[120] Some cases of hyperplasia associated with inflammation may have marked atypia, and the appearance may simulate that of an in situ or invasive adenocarcinoma (Fig. 29).[115–119] These cases may pose considerable diagnostic difficulty and are the major focus of this discussion.

Pseudocarcinomatous changes have long been recognized in tuberculous salpingitis,[121] but are also seen with other forms of bacterial salpingitis.[118] Atypical proliferative changes may involve the mucosa, muscularis, or serosa alone or in combination. The hyperplastic mucosal changes include the formation of papillae and a cribriform glandular pattern (Fig. 29) in which the lining cells exhibit mild-to-moderate nuclear pleomorphism, hyperchromatism, and mitotic activity. The proliferative mucosa may protrude into the lumen of the tube and simulate an exophytic tubal carcinoma. As exemplified by salpingitis isthmica nodosa, the tubal epithelium has a propensity to invaginate into the

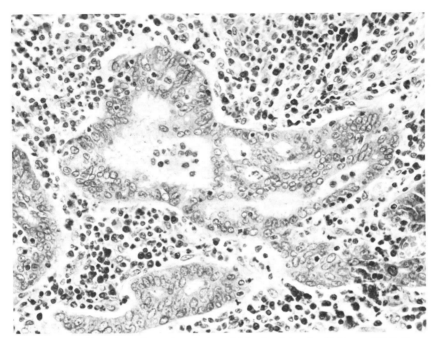

Figure 29. Pseudocarcinomatous lesion of fallopian tube. A cribriform pattern is present. Note marked inflammation.

underlying muscularis. Accordingly, in cases of hyperplasia associated with inflammation, small gland-like structures may be present in the lamina propria and muscle. In such cases, the glands, particularly when irregularly distributed and associated with a stromal response accompanying the inflammation, may mimic invasive adenocarcinoma. Pseudoglandular hyperplasia of the overlying mesothelial cells, which become incorporated within subserosal inflammatory and fibrotic tissue, may lead to an erroneous interpretation of transmural extension of a carcinoma.

A number of differences between carcinomas and pseudocarcinomatous inflammatory lesions facilitate the differential diagnosis. From the clinical viewpoint, carcinoma of the tube is usually a disease of older women, whereas the pseudocarcinomatous lesions are often seen in young women with pelvic inflammatory disease. The great majority of carcinomas are grossly evident, are not associated with significant inflammation, and exhibit severe nuclear atypia. In contrast, pseudocarcinomatous changes simulating carcinoma are incidental microscopic findings associated with overt inflammatory manifestations, and they do not usually exhibit severe cytological atypia. If atypical mesothelial proliferation is a component of the lesion, the mesothelial cells are often lined up in rows and generally exhibit mild nuclear atypia.

Heat artifact (prolonged intraoperative cautery or heating of the specimen

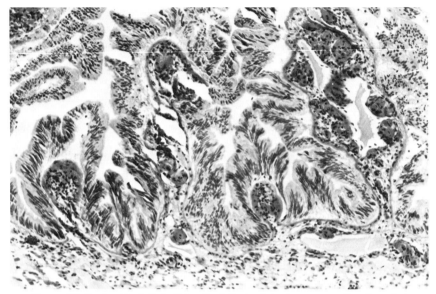

Figure 30. Heat artifact. Cells lining the fallopian tube have a peculiar elongated appearance.

inadvertently after surgical removal) may produce an appearance of marked cellular stratification and pseudoatypia,[122] simulating carcinoma (Fig. 30).

Mucinous or squamous metaplasia may occur in the tubal epithelium. Mucinous metaplasia may be associated with mucinous tumors of the cervix, ovary, or both, and it is particularly common in patients with the Peutz–Jeghers syndrome.[123–127] These changes are unlikely to cause diagnostic difficulty. Nonetheless, care should be taken to distinguish benign mucinous metaplasia from spread of a well-differentiated mucinous carcinoma of the endometrium or cervix[127] along the surface of the tubal epithelium.

Another apparently metaplastic process was designated by Saffos and her associates[128] as "metaplastic papillary tumor of the fallopian tube." They described four examples that were incidental findings in pregnant and postpartum women. The lesion involves only part of the circumference of the mucosa and is characterized by small papillae lined by large epithelial cells with abundant eosinophilic cytoplasm (Fig. 31). The cells may contain mucin and have large oval vesicular nuclei. Mitotic figures are rare. Although the exact nature of this lesion is not certain, its microscopic size, lack of invasion, and bland or only slightly atypical nuclei suggest a benign, possibly non-neoplastic process. These features should allow distinction from primary carcinoma of the tube.

Finally, the fallopian tube epithelium may exhibit a focal Arias–Stella-like change in as many as 16 percent of cases of ectopic tubal pregnancy.[129]

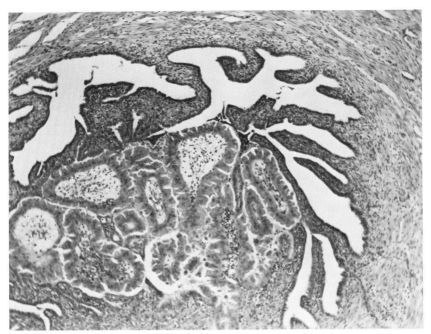

Figure 31. Metaplastic papillary tumor of fallopian tube.

PROLAPSE OF FALLOPIAN TUBE INTO VAGINA AFTER HYSTERECTOMY

Prolapse of the fallopian tube into the vagina occasionally occurs after a hysterectomy. Approximately 80 percent of the cases have been after vaginal hysterectomy.[130–138] On clinical examination, a lesion simulating granulation tissue is visible at the vaginal apex and is often painful on biopsy. Microscopic examination shows glandular epithelium surrounded by abundant inflammatory cells. A villous pattern often suggests the plicae of the tube (Fig. 32), but sometimes the plicae are blunted, and their tubal nature is not immediately apparent (Fig. 33). The presence of smooth muscle of the tubal muscularis can sometimes aid in the correct diagnosis. In a unique case, a fallopian tube prolapsed into the urinary bladder, clinically mimicking a carcinoma.[139]

MELANOTIC LESIONS

The endocervix is the most common non-cutaneous site for the blue nevus; approximately 50 cases have been described.[140,141] Only one vaginal case has been reported,[142] although another lesion, mentioned by Norris and Taylor,[143]

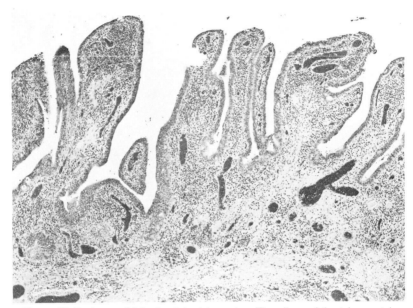

Figure 32. Prolapse of fallopian tube into vagina. The plicae of the tube contain numerous inflammatory cells.

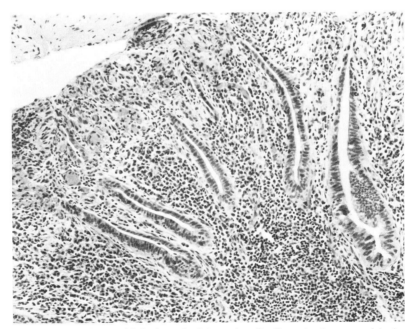

Figure 33. Prolapse of fallopian tube into vagina. Papillary structures consistent with plicae were inapparent in this case rendering diagnosis more difficult.

may represent an additional example. The former lesion was clinically diagnosed as a malignant melanoma. Endocervical blue nevi are almost always an
incidental gross or microscopic finding within hysterectomy or cervical biopsy
specimens of adults. One, or occasionally several, flat, blue-to-black, ill-defined
lesions involve the endocervical mucosa, most frequently its posterior aspect.
The lesions usually do not exceed 4 mm in diameter, but two examples have
measured 1.5 and 2.0 cm, respectively.[140] The histological appearance resembles that of cutaneous blue nevi, consisting of melanin-laden polygonal and
spindle cells with dendritic processes. They are arranged in irregular clusters
within the superficial endocervical stroma (Fig. 34). The cells are argyrophilic,
argentaffinic, and immunoreactive for S-100 protein.[140] Little difficulty should
be encountered in distinguishing blue nevi from malignant melanoma. The
epithelial pigmentation, junctional activity, and malignant cytological features
of melanoma are absent in blue nevus. A unique case with the histological
features of a cellular blue nevus involved the cervix, vagina, and hymenal ring
in a 19-year-old black woman.[144]

Benign melanotic pigmentation ("melanosis") has been described in the
squamous epithelium of the cervix (four cases),[145–148] vagina (four cases),[143–149] or
cervix and vagina (one case).[150] Irregular areas of mucosal pigmentation are
commonly seen on clinical examination, although some have been recognized
only histologically.[149] Microscopic examination reveals a proliferation of benign
melanocytes within the basal layer as well as melanin pigmentation of the basal
cells. The melanocytic proliferations were associated with elongated rete pegs
in one case from the cervix[145] and one from the vagina.[143] The lesions resembled

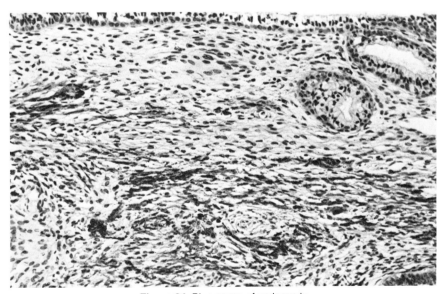

Figure 34. Blue nevus of endocervix.

a benign cutaneous lentigo.[147] In another case, melanocytic proliferation was not identified, and the pigmentation was confined to the basal cells resembling a cutaneous ephelis.[149]

Acknowledgment. Most of the material illustrated comes from the consultation files of Dr. Robert E. Scully. We are grateful to Dr. Scully for allowing us to use this material.

REFERENCES

1. Clement PB: Non-neoplastic lesions of the ovary. In Kurman RJ (ed): Blaustein's Pathology of the Female Genital Tract. New York, Springer Verlag, 1987, pp. 471–515
2. Young RH, Scully RE: Non-neoplastic disorders of the ovary. In H Fox (ed): Haines and Taylor, Obstetrical and Gynecological Pathology. New York, Churchill Livingstone, 1987, pp. 519–541
3. Young RH, Harris NL, Scully RE: Lymphoma-like lesions of the lower female genital tract. A report of 16 cases. Int J Gynecol Pathol 4:289, 1985
4. Harris NL, Scully RE: Malignant lymphoma and granulocytic sarcoma of the uterus and vagina. A clinicopathologic analysis of twenty-seven cases. Cancer 53:2530, 1984
5. Proppe KH, Scully RE, Rosai J: Postoperative spindle cell nodules of genitourinary tract resembling sarcomas. A report of eight cases. Am J Surg Pathol 8:101, 1984
6. Kay S, Schneider V: Reactive spindle cell nodule of the endocervix simulating uterine sarcoma. Int J Gynecol Pathol 4:255, 1985
7. Clement PB: Postoperative spindle cell nodule of the endometrium. A case report. Arch Pathol Lab Med 112:566, 1988
8. Wick MR, Young RH, Mills SE, et al: Immunohistochemical features of spindle cell nodules and inflammatory pseudotumors of the genitourinary tract. Lab Invest 48:103A, 1988
9. King ME, Dickersin GR, Scully RE: Myxoid leiomyosarcoma of the uterus. A report of six cases. Am J Surg Pathol 6:589, 1982
10. Allen PW: Nodular fasciitis. Pathology 4:9, 1972
11. Roberts W, Daly JW: Pseudosarcomatous fasciitis of the vulva. Gynecol Oncol 11:383, 1981
12. Gaffney EF, Majmudar B, Bryan JA: Nodular fasciitis (pseudosarcomatous fasciitis) of the vulva. Int J Gynecol Pathol 1:307, 1982
13. Gilks CB, Taylor GP, Clement PB: Inflammatory pseudotumor of the uterus. Int J Gynecol Pathol 6:275, 1987
14. Dehner LP: Extrapulmonary inflammatory myofibroblastic tumor: The inflammatory pseudotumor as another expression of the fibrohistiocytic complex. Lab Invest 54:15A, 1986
15. Ferry JA, Harris NL, Scully RE: Uterine leiomyomas with lymphoid infiltration simulating lymphomas. (submitted)
16. Minkowitz S, Friedman F, Henniger G: Xanthogranuloma of the ovary. Arch Pathol 80:209, 1965

17. Pace EH, Voet RL, Melancon JT: Xanthogranulomatous oophoritis: An inflammatory pseudotumor of the ovary. Int J Gynecol Pathol 3:398, 1984
18. Kunakemakorn P, Ontai G, Balin H: Pelvic inflammatory pseudotumor: A case report. Am J Obstet Gynecol 126:286, 1986
19. Shalev E, Zuckerman H, Rizescu I: Pelvic inflammatory pseudotumor (xanthogranuloma). Acta Obstet Gynecol Scand 61:285, 1982
20. Gidwani GP, Ballard LA Jr, Jelden GL, Lavery IC: Xanthogranuloma of the vagina. Cleve Clin Q 46:163, 1979
21. Strate SM, Taylor WE, Forney JP, Silva FG: Xanthogranulomatous pseudotumor of the vagina: Evidence of a local response to an unusual bacterium (mucoid *Escherichia coli*). Am J Clin Pathol 79:637, 1983
22. Kohn R, Reif A: "Pseudoxanthomatoese" endometritis. Zentralbl Allg Pathol 110: 281, 1967
23. Budny NN: Pyometra with massive foam cell reaction: A case report. Am J Obstet Gynecol 112:126, 1972
24. Barua R, Kirkland JA, Petrucco OM: Xanthogranulomatous endometritis: Case report. Pathology 10:161, 1978
25. Buckley CH, Fox H: Histiocytic endometritis. Histopathology 4:105, 1980
26. Pounder DJ, Iyer PV: Xanthogranulomatous endometritis associated with endometrial carcinoma. Arch Pathol Lab Med 109:73, 1985
27. Pounder DJ, Iyer PV: Benign senile pyometra, endometrial cholesterol granulomas and adenosquamous carcinoma. Aust NZ J Obstet Gynecol 25:139, 1985
28. Campbell JS, Nigam S, Hurtig A, et al: Mineral oil granulomas of the uterus and parametrium and granulomatous salpingitis with Schaumann bodies and oxalate deposits. Fertil Steril 15:278, 1964
29. Elliott GB, Brody H, Elliott KA. Implications of "lipoid salpingitis". Fertil Steril 16:541, 1965
30. Clement PB, Young RH, Scully RE: Necrotic pseudoxanthomatous nodules of the ovary and peritoneum in endometriosis. Am J Surg Pathol 12:390, 1988
31. Herrera GA, Reimann BEF, Greenberg HL, Miles PA: Pigmentosis tubae, a new entity: Light and electron microscopic study. Obstet Gynecol 61:80S, 1983
32. Aikat BK, Radhakrishnan VV, Rao MS: Malakoplakia: A report of two cases with review of the literature. Indian J Pathol Microbiol 16:64, 1973
33. Tesluk H, Munn RJ: Malacoplakia of the uterus (letter). Arch Pathol Lab Med 108:692, 1984
34. Chen KTK, Hendricks EJ: Malakoplakia of the female genital tract. Obstet Gynecol 65:84S, 1985
35. Paquin ML, Davis JR, Weiner S: Malacoplakia of Bartholin's gland. Arch Pathol Lab Med 110:757, 1986
36. Klempner LB, Giglio PG, Niebles A: Malacoplakia of the ovary. Obstet Gynecol 69:537, 1987
37. Kawai K, Fukuda K, Tsuchiyama H: Malacoplakia of the endometrium. An unusual case studied by electron microscopy and a review of the literature. Acta Pathol Jpn 38:531, 1988
38. Chadha S, Vuzevski VD, ten Kate FJW: Malakoplakia of the endometrium: A rare cause of postmenopausal bleeding. Eur J Obstet Gynec Reprod Biol 20:181, 1985
39. McClure J: Malakoplakia. J Pathol Bact 140:275, 1983
40. Snover DC, Phillips G, Dehner LP: Reactive fibrohistiocytic proliferation simulating fibrous histiocytoma. Am J Clin Pathol 76:232, 1981

41. Weiss SW, Enzinger FM, Johnson FB: Silica reaction simulating fibrous histiocytoma. Cancer 42:2738, 1978
42. Taylor HB, Ivey NS, Norris HJ: Atypical endocervical hyperplasia in women taking oral contraceptives. JAMA 202:185, 1967
43. Kyriakos M, Kempson RL, Konikov NF: A clinical and pathologic study of endocervical lesions associated with oral contraceptives. Cancer 22:99, 1968
44. Anderson WR, Levine AJ: The contraceptive polyp: A diagnostic dilemma. J Iowa Med Soc 58:585, 1968
45. Graham J, Graham R, Hirabayashi K: Reversible "cancer" and the contraceptive pill. Report of a case. Obstet Gynecol 31:190, 1968
46. Candy MD, Abell MR: Progestogen-induced adenomatous hyperplasia of the uterine cervix. JAMA 203:323, 1968
47. Govan ADT, Black WP, Sharp JL: Aberrant glandular polypi of the uterine cervix associated with contraceptive pills: Pathology and pathogenesis. J Clin Pathol 22:84, 1969
48. Carbia E, Rubio-Linares G, Alvarado-Duran A, Lopez-Llera M: Histologic study of the uterine cervix during oral contraception with ethynodiol diacetate and mestranol. Obstet Gynecol 35:381, 1970
49. Nichols TM, Fidler HK: Microglandular hyperplasia in cervical cone biopsies taken for suspicious and positive cytology. Am J Clin Pathol 56:424, 1971
50. Wilkinson E, Dufour DR: Pathogenesis of microglandular hyperplasia of the cervix uteri. Obstet Gynecol 47:189, 1976
51. Moltz L, Becker K: Cribriform polypoid adenomatous (atypical) hyperplasia of the endocervical glands of the uterus under hormonal contraception. Eur J Obstet Gynec Reprod Biol 7:331, 1977
52. Robboy SJ, Welch WR: Microglandular hyperplasia in vaginal adenosis associated with oral contraceptives and prenatal diethylstilbestrol exposure. Obstet Gynecol 49:430, 1977
53. Tsukada Y, Piver MS, Barlow JJ: Microglandular hyperplasia of the endocervix following long-term estrogen treatment. Am J Obstet Gynecol 127:888, 1977
54. Leslie KO, Silverberg SG: Microglandular hyperplasia of the cervix: Unusual clinical and pathological presentations and their differential diagnosis. Prog Surg Pathol 5:95, 1984
55. Chumas JC, Nelson B, Mann WJ, et al: Microglandular hyperplasia of the uterine cervix. Obstet Gynecol 66:406, 1985
56. Young RH, Scully RE: Atypical forms of microglandular hyperplasia of the cervix simulating carcinoma: A report of five cases and review of the literature. Am J Surg Pathol (in press)
57. Young RH, Scully RE: Cervical papillary adenocarcinoma of villoglandular type: A clinicopathological analysis of 13 cases. Cancer (in press)
58. Schneider V: Arias–Stella reaction of the endocervix. Frequency and location. Acta Cytol 25:224, 1981
59. Cariana DJ, Guderian AM: Gestational atypia in endocervical polyps: The Arias–Stella reaction. Am J Obstet Gynecol 95:589, 1966
60. Cove H: The Arias–Stella reaction occurring in the endocervix in pregnancy. Recognition and comparison with adenocarcinoma of the endocervix. Am J Surg Pathol 3:567, 1979
61. Fluhmann CF: Focal hyperplasia (tunnel clusters) of the cervix uteri. Obstet Gynecol 17:206, 1961

62. Sherrer CW, Parmley T, Woodruff JD: Adenomatous hyperplasia of the endocervix. Obstet Gynecol 49:65, 1977

63. Clement PB, Young RH: Deep Nabothian cysts of the uterine cervix: A possible source of confusion with adenoma malignum. (submitted)

64. Noda K, Kimura K, Ikeda M, Teshima K: Studies on the histogenesis of cervical adenocarcinoma. Int J Gynecol Pathol 1:336, 1983

65. Rose L: Incidental finding of cytomegalovirus inclusions in cervical glands. Am J Obstet Gynecol 95:956, 1966

66. Goldman RL, Bank RW, Warner NE: Cytomegalovirus infection of the cervix: An "incidental" finding of possible clinical significance. Report of a case. Obstet Gynecol 34:326, 1969

67. Zhao Y: Cytomegalovirus infection of the uterine cervix. Report of two cases. Chin Med J 95:467, 1982

68. Brown S, Senekjian EK, Montag AG: Cytomegalovirus infection of the uterine cervix in a patient with acquired immunodeficiency syndrome. Obstet Gynecol 71:489, 1988

69. Kraus FT: Irradiation changes in the uterus. In Norris HJ, Hertig AT (eds): The Uterus. Baltimore: Williams & Wilkins, 1973, pp. 457–488

70. Meyer R: Beitrag zur Kenntnis des gartnerschen Ganges beim Menschen. Z Geburtshilf. Gynaekologie 59:234, 1907

71. Huffman JW: Mesonephric remnants in the cervix. Am J Obstet Gynecol 56:23, 1948

72. Sneeden VD: Mesonephric lesions of the cervix. A practical means of demonstration and a suggestion of incidence. Cancer 11:334, 1958

73. Mackles A, Wolfe SA, Neigus I: Benign and malignant mesonephric lesions of the cervix. Cancer 11:292, 1952

74. Shah KH, Kurman RJ, Scully RE, Norris HJ: Atypical hyperplasia of mesonephric remnants in the cervix. Lab Invest 42:53A, 1980

75. Ayroud Y, Gelfand MM, Ferenczy A: Florid mesonephric hyperplasia of the cervix: A report of a case with review of the literature. Int J Gynecol Pathol 4:245, 1985

76. Valente PT, Susin M: Cervical adenocarcinoma arising in florid mesonephric hyperplasia: Report of a case with immunocytochemical studies. Gynecol Oncol 27:58, 1987

77. Buntine DW: Adenocarcinoma of the uterine cervix of probable wolffian origin. Pathology 11:713, 1979

78. McKelvey JL, Goodlin RR: Adenoma malignum of the cervix. A cancer of deceptively innocent histological pattern. Cancer 16:549, 1963

79. Silverberg SG, Hurt WG: Minimal deviation adenocarcinoma ("adenoma malignum") of the cervix: A reappraisal. Am J Obstet Gynecol 121:971, 1975

80. Young RH, Welch WR, Dickersin GR, Scully RE: Ovarian sex cord tumor with annular tubules. Review of 74 cases including 27 with Peutz–Jeghers syndrome and four with adenoma malignum. Cancer 50:1384, 1982

81. McGowan L, Young RH, Scully RE: Peutz–Jeghers syndrome with "adenoma malignum" of the cervix. A report of two cases. Gynecol Oncol 10:125, 1980

82. Kaku T, Enjoji M: Extremely well-differentiated adenocarcinoma ("adenoma malignum") of the cervix. Int J Gynecol Pathol 2:28, 1983

83. Kaminski PF, Norris HJ: Minimal deviation carcinoma (adenoma malignum) of the cervix. Int J Gynecol Pathol 2:141, 1983

84. Michael H, Grawe L, Kraus FT: Minimal deviation endocervical adenocarcinoma:

Clinical and histologic features, immunohistochemical staining for carcinoembryonic antigen, and differentiation from confusing benign lesions. Int J Gynecol Pathol 3:261, 1984

85. Steeper TA, Wick MR: Minimal deviation adenocarcinoma of the uterine cervix ("adenoma malignum"). An immunohistochemical comparison with microglandular endocervical hyperplasia and conventional endocervical adenocarcinoma. Cancer 58:1131, 1986

86. Nordqvist SRB, Fidler WJ Jr, Woodruff JM, Lewis JL Jr: Clear cell adenocarcinoma of the cervix and vagina. A clinicopathologic study of 21 cases with and without a history of maternal ingestion of estrogens. Cancer 37:858, 1976

87. Kaminski PF, Maier RC: Clear cell adenocarcinoma of the cervix unrelated to diethylstilbestrol exposure. Obstet Gynecol 62:720, 1983

88. Norris HJ, Taylor HB: Polyps of the vagina. A benign lesion resembling sarcoma botryoides. Cancer 19:227, 1966

89. Elliott GB, Reynolds HA, Fidler HK: Pseudo-sarcoma botryoides of cervix and vagina in pregnancy. J Obstet Gynaec Br Cwlth 74:728, 1967

90. Burt RL, Prichard RW, Kim BS: Fibroepithelial polyp of the vagina. A report of five cases. Obstet Gynecol 47:52s, 1976

91. Chirayil SJ, Tobon H: Polyps of the vagina: A clinicopathological study of 18 cases. Cancer 47:2904, 1981

92. Davies SW, Makanje HH, Woodcock AS: Pseudo-sarcomatous polyps of the vagina in pregnancy. Case report. Br J Obstet Gynaec 88:566, 1981

93. O'Quinn AG, Edwards CL, Gallager HS: Case report. Pseudosarcoma botryoides of the vagina in pregnancy. Gynecol Oncol 13:237, 1982

94. Miettinen M, Wahlstrom T, Vesterinen E, Saksela E: Vaginal polyps with pseudosarcomatous features. A clinicopathologic study of seven cases. Cancer 51:1148, 1983

95. Elliott GB, Elliott JDA: Superficial stromal reactions of lower genital tract. Arch Pathol 95:100, 1973

96. Mitchell M, Talerman A, Sholl JS, et al: Pseudosarcoma botryoides in pregnancy. Report of a case with ultrastructural observations. Obstet Gynecol 70:522, 1987

97. Cachaza JA, Caballero JJL, Fernandez JA, Salido E: Endocervical polyp with pseudosarcomatous pattern and cytoplasmic inclusions: an electron microscopic study. Am J Clin Pathol 85:633, 1986

98. Maenpaa J, Soderstrom KO, Salmi T, Ekbad U: Large atypical polyps of the vagina during pregnancy with concomitant human papilloma virus infection. Eur J Obstet Gynecol Reprod Biol 27:65, 1988

99. Daya D, Scully RE: Sarcoma botryoides of the uterine cervix in young women. A clinicopathologic study of 13 cases. Gynecol Oncol 29:290, 1988

100. Clement PB: Multinucleated stromal giant cells of the uterine cervix. Arch Pathol Lab Med 109:200, 1985

101. Johnson LD: Dysplasia and carcinoma in situ in pregnancy. In Norris HJ, Hertig AT (eds): The Uterus. Baltimore, Williams & Wilkins, 1973, pp. 382–412

102. Schneider V, Barnes LA: Ectopic decidual reaction of the uterine cervix. Frequency and cytologic presentation. Acta Cytol 25:616, 1981

103. Tilden IL, Winstedt R: Decidual reactions in fallopian tubes. Histologic study of tubal segments from 144 post-partum sterilizations. Am J Pathol 19:1043, 1943

104. Hellman LM: The morphology of the human fallopian tube in the early puerperium. Am J Obstet Gynecol 57:154, 1949

105. Linhartova A: Unusual lesions of the uterine cervix. Int J Gynecol Obstet 10:34, 1972

106. Zaytsev P, Taxy JB: Pregnancy-associated ectopic decidua. Am J Surg Pathol 11:526, 1987

107. Bowles HE, Tilden IL: Decidual reactions of the cervix. West J Surg Obstet Gynecol 59:168, 1951

108. Mills SE, Fechner RE: Stromal and epithelial changes in the fallopian tube following hormonal therapy. Hum Pathol 11:583, 1983

109. Hennessy JP: Unusual decidual reaction of the cervix. Am J Obstet Gynecol 46:570, 1943

110. Klein J, Domeier LH: An unusual decidual reaction in the cervix. Am J Obstet Gynecol 51:423, 1946

111. Lapan B: Deciduosis of the cervix and vagina simulating carcinoma. Am J Obstet Gynecol 58:743, 1949

112. Orr CJB, Pedlow PRB: Deciduosis of the cervix manifesting as antepartum hemorrhage and simulating carcinoma. Am J Obstet Gynecol 82:884, 1961

113. Armenia CS, Shaver DN, Modisher MW: Decidual transformation of the cervical stroma simulating reticulum cell sarcoma. Am J Obstet Gynecol 89:808, 1964

114. Mathie JG: Vaginal deciduosis simulating carcinoma. J Obstet Gynaecol Br Emp 64:720, 1957

115. Dougherty CM, Cotten NM: Proliferative epithelial lesions of the uterine tube. I. Adenomatous hyperplasia. Obstet Gynecol 24:849, 1964

116. Pauerstein CJ, Woodruff JD: Cellular patterns in proliferative and anaplastic disease of the fallopian tube. Am J Obstet Gynecol 96:486, 1966

117. Moore SW, Enterline HT: Significance of proliferative epithelial lesions of the uterine tube. Obstet Gynecol 45:385, 1975

118. Mostoufizadeh M, Scully RE: Pseudocarcinomatous lesions of the fallopian tube. Lab Invest 48:61a, 1983

119. Stern J, Buscema J, Parmley T, et al: Atypical epithelial proliferations in the fallopian tube. Am J Obstet Gynecol 140:309, 1981

120. Stern J, Buscema J, Parmley T, et al: Atypical epithelial proliferations in the fallopian tube. Am J Obstet Gynecol 140:309, 1981

121. Puflett D: Tuberculosis salpingitis resembling adenocarcinoma. Med J Aust 2:149, 1972

122. Cornog JL, Currie JL, Rubin A: Heat artifact simulating adenocarcinoma of fallopian tube. JAMA 214:1118, 1970

123. Costa J: Peutz–Jeghers syndrome. Case presentation. Obstet Gynecol 50:15s, 1977

124. Gloor E: Un cas de syndrome de Peutz–Jeghers associé a un carcinoma mammaire bilateral. A un adénocarcinoma du col utérin et a des tumeurs des cordons sexuels a tubules annéles bilaterales dans les ovaires. Schweiz Med Wochenschr 108:717, 1978

125. Berger G, Frappart L, Berger F, et al: Tubules anneles de l'ovaire, metaplasie mucipare de l'endocol et syndrome de Peutz–Jeghers. Arch Anat Cytol Pathol 29:353, 1981

126. LiVolsi VA, Merino MJ, Schwartz PE: Coexistent endocervical adenocarcinoma and mucinous adenocarcinoma of ovary: A clinicopathologic study of four cases. Int J Gynecol Pathol 1:391, 1983

127. Young RH, Scully RE: Mucinous ovarian tumors associated with mucinous adeno-

carcinomas of the cervix. A clinicopathological analysis of 16 cases. Int J Gynecol Pathol 7:99, 1988

128. Saffos RO, Rhatigan RM, Scully RE: Metaplastic papillary tumor of the fallopian tube: A distinctive lesion of pregnancy. Am J Clin Pathol 74:232, 1980

129. Birch HLV, Collins CG: Atypical changes of genital epithelium associated with ectopic pregnancy. Am J Obstet Gynecol 81:1198, 1961

130. Sapan IP, Solberg NS: Prolapse of the uterine tube after abdominal hysterectomy. Obstet Gynecol 42:26, 1973

131. Ellsworth HS, Harris JW, McQuarrie HG, et al: Prolapse of the fallopian tube following vaginal hysterectomy. JAMA 224:891, 1973

132. Silverberg SG, Frable WJ: Prolapse of fallopian tube into vaginal vault after hysterectomy. Arch Pathol 97:100, 1974

133. Carmichael DE: Prolapse of the fallopian tube into the vaginal vault. Am J Obstet Gynecol 125:266, 1976

134. Novendstern J: Prolapse of fallopian tube after abdominal hysterectomy. Am J Obstet Gynecol 135:1120, 1979

135. Thomson JD: Fallopian tube prolapse after abdominal hysterectomy. Aust NZ J Obstet Gynaec 20:187, 1980

136. Wolfendale M: Exfoliative cytology in a case of prolapsed fallopian tube. Acta Cytol 24:545, 1980

137. Bilodeau B: Intravaginal prolapse of the fallopian tube following vaginal hysterectomy. Am J Obstet Gynecol 143:970, 1982

138. Wheelock JB, Schneider V, Goperlund DR: Prolapsed fallopian tube masquerading as adenocarcinoma of the vagina in a postmenopausal woman. Gynecol Oncol 21:369, 1985

139. Anastasiades KD, Majmudar B: Prolapse of fallopian tube into urinary bladder, mimicking bladder carcinoma. Arch Pathol Lab Med 107:613, 1983

140. Patel DS, Bhagavan BS: Blue nevus of the uterine cervix. Hum Pathol 16:79, 1985

141. Casadei GP, Grigolato P, Cabibbo E: Blue nevus of the endocervix. A study of five cases. Tumori 73:75, 1987

142. Tobon H, Murphy AI: Benign blue nevus of the vagina. Cancer 40:3174, 1977

143. Norris HJ, Taylor HB: Melanomas of the vagina. Am J Clin Pathol 46:420, 1966

144. Rodriguez HA, Ackerman LV: Cellular blue nevus. Clinicopathologic study of forty-five cases. Cancer 21:393, 1968

145. Schneider V, Zimberg S, Kay S: The pigmented portio: Benign lentigo of the uterine cervix. Diagn Gynecol Obstet 3:269, 1981

146. Deppisch LM: Cervical melanosis. Obstet Gynecol 62:525, 1983

147. Dundore W, Lamas C: Benign nevus (ephelis) of the uterine cervix. Am J Obstet Gynecol 152:881, 1985

148. Barter JF, Mazur M, Holloway RW, Hatch KD: Melanosis of the cervix. Gynecol Oncol 29:101, 1988

149. Nigogosyan G, de la Pava S, Pickren JW: Melanoblasts in vaginal mucosa. Origin for primary malignant melanoma. Cancer 17:912, 1964

150. Tsukuda Y. Benign melanosis of the vagina and cervix. Am J Obstet Gynecol 124:211, 1976

Serous Surface Carcinoma of the Ovary and Peritoneum
A Flow Cytometric Study

Michael L. Rutledge, Elvio G. Silva, Donia McLemore, and Adel El-Naggar

Serous surface carcinoma (SSC) of the ovary is a malignant neoplasm that predominantly involves the surface of the ovary, with little or no parenchymal invasion. Typically, the ovaries are not enlarged and the bulk of the tumor is spread throughout the pelvic and abdominal peritoneum (stage III). Despite absent or minimal parenchymal invasion, several reports have indicated that SSC carries a distinctly poorer prognosis than serous ovarian carcinomas that deeply invade and replace the ovarian parenchyma.[1-3] One reason for this poorer prognosis might be that SSC represents a multifocal disease[2] that results from a field phenomenon whose effects escape current surgical and chemotherapeutic treatments. Advanced SSC could be the result of multiple, independent pertioneal and/or ovarian primary tumors. In contrast, advanced conventional serous ovarian carcinomas are thought to consist of a single primary tumor with multiple metastases to the ovaries and peritoneum. Flow cytometric (FCM) DNA analyses of conventional ovarian carcinomas show a remarkable spatial homogeneity of tumor DNA content within the same patient,[4] such that tumors in the ovaries and peritoneum have identical DNA patterns (i.e., diploid tumor tissue in both the ovary and peritoneum).

Therefore, we undertook a multiple-site analysis of tumor DNA content in our patients with SSC to determine whether the extent of spatial variability of DNA was similar to that seen in non-SSC ovarian carcinomas. We retrospectively analyzed paraffin-embedded tumor samples from at least two separate sites for each of 26 patients with stage III SSC of the ovary and/or peritoneum to

*Supported in part by a grant from the M.D. Anderson Cancer Center Research Project Fund.

determine the prognostic significance of tumor ploidy and the tumors' degree of DNA heterogeneity.

MATERIALS AND METHODS

Pathologic materials from patients diagnosed between 1971 and 1983 as having SSC of the ovary and/or peritoneum were drawn from the files of the University of Texas M.D. Anderson Cancer Center Department of Pathology. The hematoxylin and eosin-stained sections and surgical pathology reports of the 59 cases were reviewed by 2 of us (MLR, EGS). Patients selected met the following criteria: (1) ovaries not enlarged (< 4 cm), (2) minimal or no microscopic ovarian parenchymal invasion. Cases with focal deep invasion were included. Cases showing diffuse replacement of the ovarian parenchyma by the neoplasm were excluded. (3) predominant serous histology; (4) adequate ovarian tumor samples and availability of embedded material; (5) presence of abdominal peritoneal disease (stage III); and (6) at least 36 months of clinical follow-up. Twenty-six patients were chosen, including 2 patients without ovarian involvement.

Assignment of histological grade was done by examination of all available sections from both ovarian and peritoneal tumors, using a modification of grade 1, 2, and 3 (well, moderately, poorly differentiated) architectural method of Czernobilsky.[5] For example, if the architectural serous pattern was either a grade 1 or 2 but significant nuclear pleomorphism was seen in sections from at least two separate sites, then the grade was advanced by one. Thus, a moderately differentiated serous carcinoma with significant nuclear pleomorphism was assigned to grade 3. Clinical and follow-up information was obtained from medical records and clinicians' files. All patients had undergone total abdominal hysterectomy, bilateral salpingo-oophorectomy, and debulking of tumor. Grossly identifiable tumor was removed in all but six patients. All patients had received combinations of chemotherapeutic agents, including cyclophosphamide, cisplatin, doxorubicin, and hexamethylmelamine. Survival was defined as the period from the first laparotomy to death from cancer or until the last follow-up visit. The mean follow-up period was 48.3 months.

Tissue for flow cytometry was processed, with some modifications, as previously described.[6] Blocks were chosen to ensure that tumor cells represented at least 75 percent of the tissue processed; the remaining non-neoplastic cells served as diploid cell markers. Blocks were processed to sample tumor from one or both ovaries, if both were involved, and from the peritoneum. From each site, 5000 cells were analyzed on an Epic V flow cytometer equipped with an argon–ion laser. The percentage of cells in G_0/G_1 was calculated with the integrated statistical analysis on the Epic V.

Analyses of the DNA histograms were carried out using the method of Rodenburg et al.[8] Those histograms with a single G_0/G_1 peak and a coefficient of variation (CV) of less than 5.5 percent were classified as diploid. All other patterns were considered non-diploid. Those patterns with a diploid and an additional G_0/G_1 peak were termed aneuploid. Those preparations with a single G_0/G_1 peak and a CV greater than 5.5 percent were classified as periploid. Tumor ploidy was further quantitated by the DNA index, which is the ratio of the DNA content of the aneuploid G_1 cells to that of the diploid G_1 cells. The tumors in a given patient were considered heterogeneous if there were separate aneuploid and diploid deposits or if the DNA indices of two aneuploid deposits differed by more than 0.3.

RESULTS

A comparison of patient outcome, histological grade, and flow cytometric data is shown in Table 1. Of the 26 patients studied, 18 (70 percent) died of disease, with a mean survival of 25.7 months. Four patients are alive with residual disease (mean survival, 47 months), and four are clinically free of tumor (mean survival, 72 months). Histologically, all but two of the SSC tumors were high grade by virtue of their solid growth pattern and extensive nuclear pleomorphism (Fig. 1). Two largely papillary carcinomas with less severe nuclear alterations (Fig. 2) were classified grade 2. Examination of histological findings for relationships with the DNA content measured by FCM and with patient outcome did not show recognizable correlations.

Overall, there were 4 diploid (15 percent), 2 periploid (8 percent), and 20 aneuploid tumors (77 percent) as indicated by FCM analysis. Eight of the aneuploid tumors exhibited DNA spatial variability and are discussed in additional detail. Three patients with diploid tumors (75 percent) died of disease, while the remaining patient with a diploid tumor is a long-term, disease-free survivor. Among the 22 patients with non-diploid tumors (2 periploid and 20 aneuploid), 15 (68 percent) died of disease. The mean survival of patients who had only diploid tumors was 54 months (range, 22 to 111 months), compared with 34 months for those with non-diploid tumors (range, 1 to 63 months). Both patients with periploid DNA patterns were alive at the end of the study. Among

TABLE 1. PATIENT OUTCOME AND FCM RESULTS

DNA Content	Clinical Status			Histological Grade (No. of Cases)			Totals (%)
	NED[a]	AWD	DOD	1	2	3	
Homogenous							
Diploid	1	0	3	0	0	4	4 (15)
Periploid	1	1	—	0	0	2	2 (8)
Aneuploid	2	1	9	0	1	11	12 (46)
Heterogeneous							
Aneuploid	0	2	6	0	1	7	8 (31)
Totals (%)	4 (15)	4 (15)	18 (70)	0	2 (8)	24 (92)	26 (100)

[a]NED = no evidence of disease; AWD = alive with disease; DOD = died of disease.

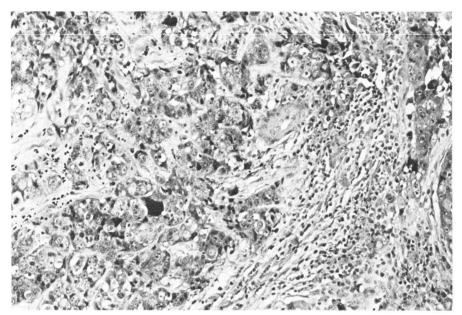

Figure 1. Grade 3 serous surface carcinoma. (H&E ×125)

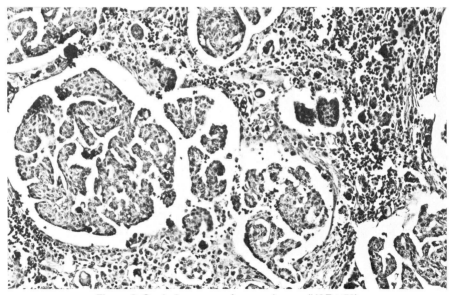

Figure 2. Grade 2 serous surface carcinoma. (H&E ×50)

the 18 patients who died of disease, 15 (83 percent) had aneuploid tumors, whereas 88 percent of the survivors had either aneuploid or periploid tumors. The mean DNA index for the homogeneously aneuploid tumors was 1.6 (range, 1.1 to 2.1).

Of the 26 patients, 18 had tumors that were homogeneous with respect to spatial DNA content, including 4 with diploid, 2 with periploid, and 13 with aneuploid tumors. A total of 46 sites were tested in these 18 patients (mean, 2.5 sites per patient; range, 2 to 4). The mean survival for this group was 32.8 months (range, 6 to 111 months). The remaining eight patients had heterogeneous tumor DNA (Table 2) and a mean survival of 32.8 months (range, 6 to 63 months). Two of these patients (25 percent) are alive with clinical evidence of disease, and the other six died of disease after a mean survival of 20.1 months. Five of the patients with tumor heterogeneity had separate diploid and aneuploid deposits. Differences were noted between ovarian and peritoneal tumors (Table 2, Cases 7 and 8) and between bilateral ovarian tumors (Cases 1 through 6). In addition, Case 6 (Fig. 3) had two different aneuploid tumors (left ovary, DNA index 1.3; omentum, DNA index 1.8) and a diploid tumor (right ovary). Two cases (3 and 4) each had aneuploid tumors with different DNA indices at the sites tested (ovaries). Among the 8 patients with DNA heterogeneity, a total of 18 separate sites were tested (mean 2.3; range 2 to 3), with a mean DNA index of 1.4 (range, 1.2 to 2.2).

DISCUSSION

The use of flow cytometry as an independent, prognostic variable in advanced ovarian cancer has been documented.[7-9] Retrospective studies using paraffin-embedded tissues have yielded results equivalent to those with freshly pre-

TABLE 2. CASES OF SSC TUMOR HETEROGENEITY

			Site		
			Peritoneal Sites		Clinical Status
	Left	Right			
Case	Ovary	Ovary	#1	#2	(Survival in Mo)
1	1.3	1.0			AWD (43)[a]
2	1.7	1.0			AWD (36)
3	1.4	1.7			DOD (10)
4	1.7	2.0			DOD (10)
5	1.8	1.0			DOD (28)
6	1.3	1.0	1.8		DOD (60)
7	1.0	1.0	1.0	2.2	DOD (6)
8	1.0	1.0	1.5		DOD (10)

[a]AWD = alive with disease; DOD = died of disease.

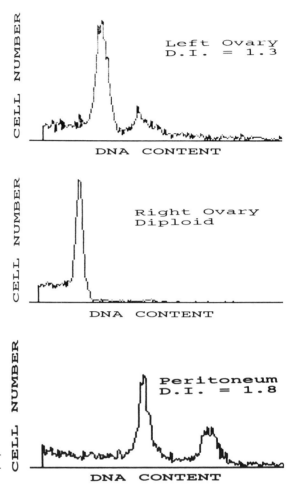

Figure 3. Tumor DNA heterogeneity in SSC (Case 6) as determined by flow cytometry.

pared tissue,[8] although the technical resolution of embedded tissues is inferior. In order to study the DNA patterns of the relatively uncommon SSC of the ovary and/or peritoneum in sufficient numbers, we used paraffin-embedded tissues. We were able to obtain acceptable results as compared with those of previous studies using archival materials. Like the investigators in another study of ovarian carcinomas,[8] however, we encountered cases (periploid) in which the coefficient of variation of the G_0/G_1 peak in an otherwise diploid DNA pattern was suboptimal (> 5.5 percent).

Interestingly, the overall outcome for our study group with stage III SSC of the ovary and/or peritoneum differs from outcomes in previously reported series.[1-3] These earlier studies uniformly noted a poorer prognosis and shorter survival for patients with SSC as compared with patients with non-SSC ovarian carcinomas, although long-term survivors have been reported.[10] Our follow-up remains incomplete, but 8 of our 26 patients (31 percent), have survived at least 3 years since diagnosis. This is in contrast to the 11 to 31 percent (dependent on tumor size and grade) 3-year survival of stage III ovarian carcinomas reported by Malkasian et al.[11] This issue is obviously not resolved. The idea that a predominantly non-invasive (surface) carcinoma should carry a worse prognosis than does one of similar histology and extent that invades and destroys the underlying parenchyma is difficult to reconcile.

One part of our study analyzed the correlation between tumor DNA content and patient outcome. We found a high incidence of tumor DNA aneuploidy (77 percent) among the 26 patients studied. This incidence of aneuploidy is lower than the 87 percent aneuploidy found using fresh tissue as samples from conventional serous carcinomas of various stages as described by Friedlander et al[7] but higher than the 40 percent seen in a study by Rodenburg et al[8] of paraffin-embedded tumor from patients with advanced ovarian carcinoma. In our study group, an aneuploid tumor DNA pattern had little prognostic significance, as this pattern was widely dispersed among patients who died of disease and those alive at this report. Even a diploid tumor DNA pattern carried little significance, as 75 percent of patients with a diploid pattern died of disease. Perhaps the DNA content of SSC of the ovary and/or peritoneum would prove prognostically useful in lower stage cases. However, such cases have rarely been reported.[1–3]

The other part of our study analyzed samples of tumor taken at the initial laparatomy from several different sites in each patient. We were interested in the hypothesis that the SSC is a multifocal neoplasm,[2] and might therefore express heterogeneity in its DNA content. Previous studies have provided ample evidence that the tumor DNA content of non-SSC ovarian carcinomas are remarkably homogenous from site to site (i.e., ovary and omentum) within a given patient. The 97 patients in 3 combined series (Table 3) show an 11 percent incidence of tumor heterogeneity among various histological types of ovarian carcinoma.[4,8,9] This spatial stability of a crude genotypic trait (cellular DNA content) is remarkable given the known heterogeneity of phenotypic expression (i.e., histological appearance) of these neoplasms. Thus the finding of a high percentage (31 percent) of tumor DNA heterogeneity among our 26

TABLE 3. STUDIES OF SPATIAL VARIABILITY OF TUMOR DNA IN CONVENTIONAL (NON-SSC) OVARIAN CARCINOMA

Study	No. Cases	Cases with Spatial Variability (%)
Rodenburg et al[8]	48	6 (12.5)
Iversen et al[9]	23	1 (4.3)
Friedlander et al[7]	24	3 (12.5)
Totals	95	10 (10.5)

patients indicates that the fundamental basis of the more common, non-SSC ovarian carcinomas and SSC of the ovary and/or peritoneum may differ.

Examples of tumor DNA heterogeneity have been found in a variety of other human malignancies, including colorectal,[12] lung,[13] and renal[14] carcinomas. Tumor DNA heterogeneity was found to be an important prognostic factor in lung carcinomas,[13] but the mean survival for the SSC patients with homogeneous DNA patterns who died of disease differed little (32.8 months) from that among the group with tumor DNA heterogeneity (32.8 months). This finding would indicate, however, the need to adequately sample these tumors in order to obtain a representative picture of the tumor DNA pattern.

The concept of tumor heterogeneity is well established,[15,16] and both genotypic and phenotypic variations within a given tumor have been described. It is possible that the higher incidence of tumor DNA heterogeneity among our patients with SSC simply implies that they, like those with other neoplasms that consist of a known primary with secondary metastases, possess this characteristic as a part of their tumor progression. The lower incidence of DNA pattern heterogeneity (Table 3) in the more closely related non-SSC ovarian carcinomas (which also have primary and metastatic tumors) more convincingly argues for the supposition that a higher percentage of cases of SSC of the ovary and/or peritoneum are multifocal, independent primaries.

ADDENDUM

Since this manuscript was accepted for publication, another study has been published showing that SSC has a worse prognosis than conventional invasive serous ovarian carcinomas. [Mills SE, Andersen WA, Fechner RE, Austin MB: Serous surface papillary carcinoma: A clinicopathologic study of 10 cases and comparison with stage III–IV ovarian serous carcinoma. Am J Surg Pathol 12:827, 1988.

REFERENCES

1. Gooneratne S, Sassone M, Blaustein A, Talerman A: Serous surface papillary carcinoma: A clinicopathologic study of 16 cases. Int J Gynecol Pathol 1:258, 1982
2. August CZ, Murad TM, Newton M: Multiple focal extraovarian serous carcinoma. Int J Gynecol Pathol 4:11, 1985
3. White PF, Merino MJ, Barwick KW: Serous surface papillary carcinoma of the ovary: A clinical, pathologic, ultrastructural, and immunohistochemical study of 11 cases. Pathol Annu 20(Pt.1):403, 1985
4. Friedlander ML, Taylor IW, Tattersall MHN: Cellular DNA content: A stable feature in epithelial ovarian cancer. Br J Cancer 49:173, 1984
5. Czernobilsky B: Primary epithelial tumors of the ovary. In Blaustein A (ed): Pathology of the Female Genital Tract. New York, Springer-Verlag, 1982, p. 518

6. McLemore DD, Wall TJ, Stephens LC, Jardine JH: Processing of paraffin-embedded tissues for flow cytometry. J Histotechnol 10:109, 1987
7. Friedlander ML, Taylor IW, Russell P, et al: Ploidy as a prognostic factor in ovarian cancer. Int J Gynecol Pathol 2:55, 1983
8. Rodenburg CJ, Cornelisse CJ, Heintz PAM, et al: Tumor ploidy as a major prognostic factor in advanced ovarian cancer. Cancer 59:317, 1987
9. Iversen OE, Skaarland E: Ploidy assessment of benign and malignant ovarian tumors by flow cytometry. A clinicopathologic study. Cancer 60:82, 1987
10. Chen KTK, Flam MS: Peritoneal papillary serous carcinoma with long-term survival. Cancer 58:1371, 1986
11. Malkasian GD Jr, Melton LJ III, O'Brien PC, Greene MH: Prognostic significance of histologic classification and grading of epithelial malignancies of the ovary. Am J Obstet Gynecol 149:274, 1984
12. Emdin SO, Stenling R, Roos G: Prognostic value of DNA content in colorectal carcinoma: A flow cytometric study with some methodological aspects. Cancer 60:1282, 1987
13. Tirindelli-Danesi D, Teodori L, Mauro F, et al: Prognostic significance of flow cytometry in lung cancer: A 5-year study. Cancer 60:844, 1987
14. Ljungberg B, Stenling R, Roos G: Flow cytometric DNA analysis of renal-cell carcinoma. Anal Quant Cytol Histol 9:505, 1987
15. Heppner GH: Tumor heterogeneity. Cancer Res 44:2259, 1984
16. Rubin H: Cancer as a dynamic developmental disorder. Cancer Res 45:2935, 1985

Adenoid Cystic Carcinoma of the Breast
A Morphologically Heterogeneous Neoplasm

Paul Peter Rosen

Adenoid cystic carcinoma (ACC) of the breast constitutes less than 0.1 percent of mammary carcinomas,[1] but it has engendered a disproportionate amount of interest. Perhaps this is due to the favorable prognosis of the tumor and its structural resemblance to neoplasms of the same name that arise in the salivary glands or rarely in the skin, lung, and other sites. Although ACC of the breast is usually depicted with the characteristic cylindromatous growth pattern, it is in fact a structurally diverse tumor. The purpose of this chapter is to describe the morphological heterogeneity and clinical aspects of mammary ACC.

MATERIALS AND METHODS

The majority of the 23 patients described here are derived from diagnostic consultations. Also included are a few women who received their primary treatment at Memorial Sloan–Kettering Cancer Center. Clinical information was obtained from physicians, hospital records, and the patients. Pathologic data are based on a review of the pathology reports and histological sections. In virtually all consultation cases, the submitting pathologist made a diagnosis of adenoid cystic carcinoma or considered this in the differential diagnosis.

RESULTS

Gross Pathology

The measured gross size was known for 16 tumors and ranged from 0.5 to 8.0 cm (mean, 2.2 cm; median 2.2 cm). Low grade tumors tended to be smaller

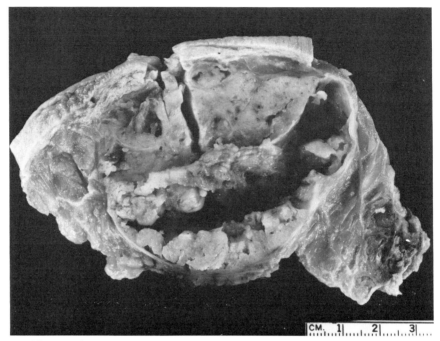

Figure 1. Gross photograph showing a well-circumscribed margin and cystic central degeneration in an 8-cm high grade ACC. This 65-year-old woman remains well 7.5 years after mastectomy.

(range, 0.5 to 2.8 cm; mean, 1.6 cm; median, 2.0 cm) than high grade tumors (range, 1.5–8.0 cm; mean, 3.5 cm; median, 2.7cm).

Gross descriptions were available for 15 tumors. Fourteen had a circumscribed and/or nodular configuration, including four tumors in the high grade group (Fig. 1). Gross cyst formation was noted in one low grade and one high grade tumor. When color was mentioned, it was most often pink, tan, or grey.

Microscopic Pathology

Despite the gross circumscribed appearance of virtually all tumors in the series, about half of the lesions had an invasive growth pattern when examined microscopically. In most instances in which the tumor invaded the surrounding breast, there were one or more central nodules which accounted for the gross findings (Fig. 2). Microcystic areas, not appreciated grossly, were seen in five lesions. These appeared to have been formed as a result of cystic dilation of glands in the tumor rather than as a result of degenerative changes in the tumor. Perineural invasion was found in one tumor and there were intra-lymphatic tumor emboli at the periphery of another ACC. In a number of other cases, shrinkage artifacts simulated lymphatic invasion. On the basis of his-

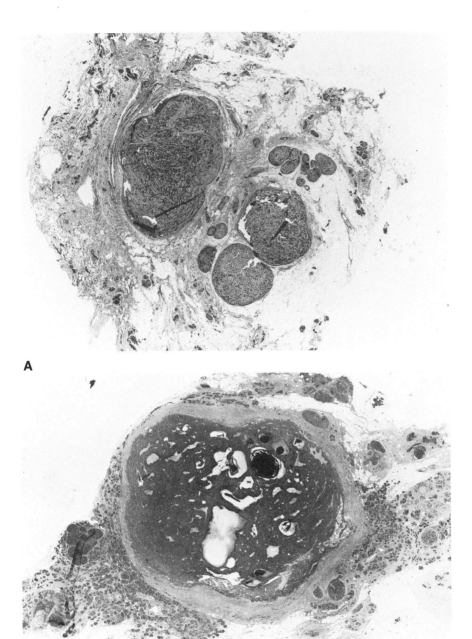

Figure 2. A. Low magnification photograph of the histological section of an entire low grade ACC demonstrating a multinodular configuration. Note slight cystic changes in two nodules. The patient is a 51-year-old woman treated by partial mastectomy and axillary disection. She was well 5 year later. **B**. Low magnification photograph of a histological cross-section of a low grade ACC from a 59-year-old woman who is well 3 years after mastectomy. In addition to the central circumscribed nodule of solid carcinoma with cystic areas, there is an invasive component extending laterally into the surrounding breast.

tological features described below, 18 tumors were classified as low grade and 5 were high grade.

Low Grade ACC. Low grade carcinomas exhibited the typical adenoid cystic growth pattern (Fig. 3) which features gland or tubule formation (the adenoid component) and varying amounts of stromal or basement membrane material (the cylindromatous component). Within a given tumor, there was often heterogeneity in the distribution of these elements. Some microscopic fields, which consisted largely of the glandular or adenoid pattern, had a prominent cribriform appearance (Fig. 4). In other areas, the presence of abundant stroma or basement membrane material and sparse glands resulted in a superficial similarity to ordinary duct carcinoma (Fig. 5). Also seen in some but not all tumors were foci of sebaceous, syringomatous (Fig. 6), adenomyoepitheliomatous (Fig. 7), and squamous differentiation (Fig. 7). Solid growth was absent or only a minor component in low grade ACC.

High Grade ACC. The most distinctive microscopic feature of these tumors is their growth largely as solid nodules with a poorly formed adenoid cystic growth

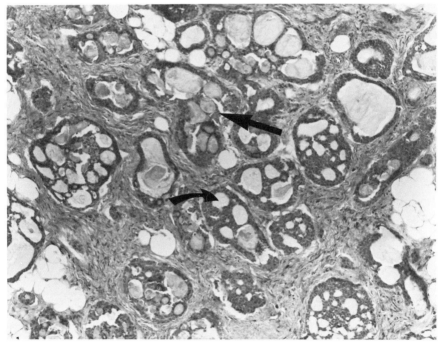

Figure 3. Low grade ACC from a 66-year-old woman. Seven years after mastectomy she is well. Note true glandular lumens (*curved arrow*) and cylinders (*straight arrow*) composed of basement membrane material.

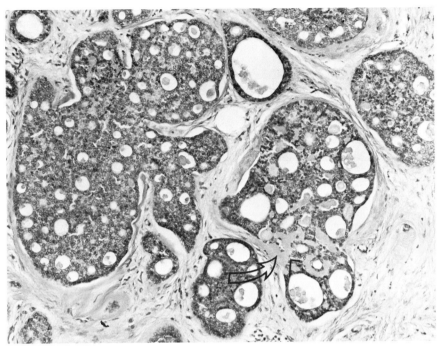

Figure 4. Low grade ACC with prominent cribriform areas. Note cylindromatous elements in a gland on the right (*arrow*).

pattern. The tumor cells throughout these lesions are cytologically poorly differentiated, tending to have sparse cytoplasm and relatively large, hyperchromatic nuclei. Intraductal carcinoma was evident in a minority of all ACC but on occasion this was a prominent feature of high grade tumors with extensive intralobular and intraductal growth in surrounding breast tissue. One tumor had extensive areas of cribriform and compact, nearly solid growth as well as a typical ACC component (Fig. 8). Another lesion was characterized by prominent basaloid features (Fig. 9).

Clinical Data

Age. Age at diagnosis ranged from 25 to 67 years with a median of 53 and mean of 56 years. The age distributions of low grade and high grade types of ACC were similar.

Laterality and Location in Breasts. The right breast was affected in 12 cases (52 percent) and the left in 11 cases (48 percent). One patient had concurrent contralateral intraductal carcinoma. The location of the lesion in the breast was described in 12 cases. Six were central or subareolar, three were in the inner quadrants, and three were located in outer quadrants. The distribution of lat-

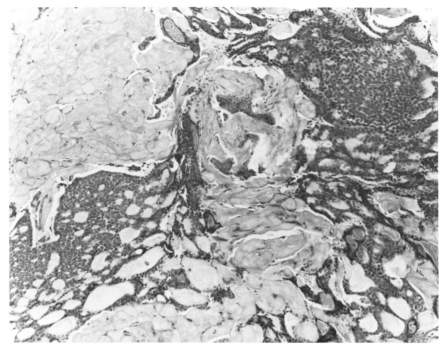

Figure 5. Distorted glandular elements in dense sclerotic stroma of an ACC. This pattern can be mistaken for ordinary invasive duct carcinoma, especially in a small incisional or needle biopsy sample. (Same patient as Figure 3.)

erality and of location was not appreciably different between low and high grade lesions.

Clinical Presentation and Findings. A palpable mass was found in 16 cases. The tumor was tender in two and a third patient described discomfort. The clinical diagnosis of two tumors was fibroadenoma. A patient who presented with bloody nipple discharge was regarded clinically as having a papilloma. Mammograms were reportedly negative in two cases. Duration of the tumor was stated in nine cases, ranging from 1 month to 9 years. The median duration was 24 months and the mean was 32 months. Six tumors were present for at least 1 year before excision. There was no apparent difference in duration between low and high grade lesions.

Hormone Receptor Analysis. Results of estrogen (ER) and/or progesterone (PR) receptor analysis were available in six cases. ER (15 fmol) and PR (17 fmol) were positive in one low grade tumor. Negative ER (5 fmol) and positive PR (19 fmol) were reported in another low grade lesion. Negative ER and PR were found in two other low grade ACC and 2 high grade ACC.

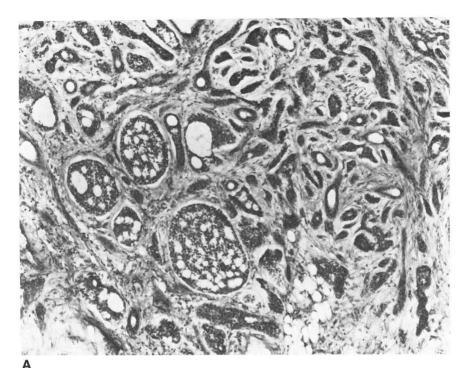

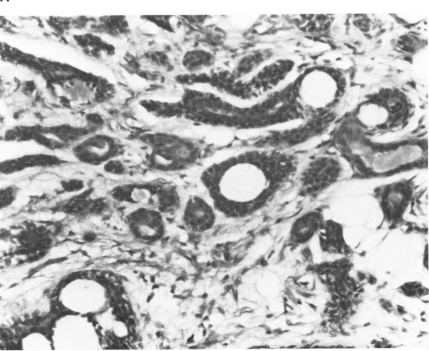

Figure 6. A. Low power view of an ACC with prominent syringomatous features. Three characteristic adenoid cystic glands are evident to the left. Four years after mastectomy this 53-year-old patient was well. B. Note the comma-shaped syringomatous tubule.

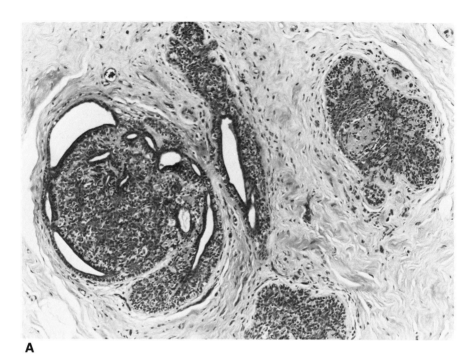

A

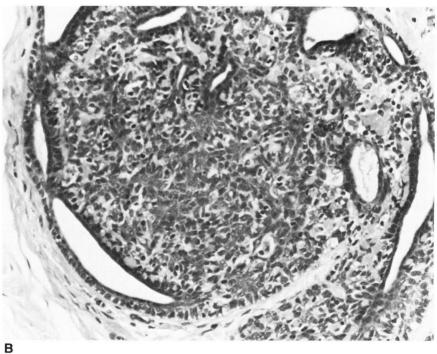

B

Figure 7. Three patterns of in situ growth in ACC associated with a low grade ACC. **A.** Intraductal carcinoma with adenomyoepitheliomatous pattern on the left and focal squamous differentiation on the right. **B.** Magnified view of adenomyo-epitheliomatous hyperplasia in duct. *(continued)*

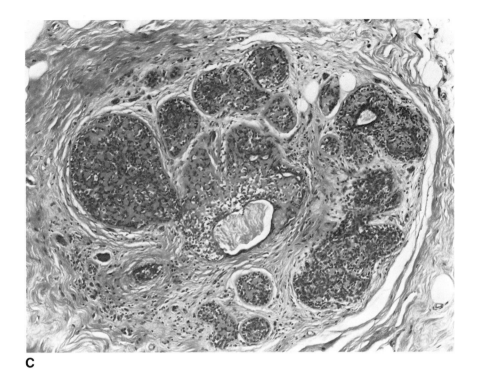

C

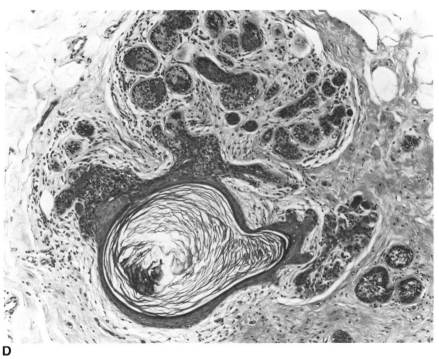

D

Figure 7 (cont.) C. Solid intralobular carcinoma with a prominent cylindromatous pattern. **D.** Squamous metaplasia in a terminal duct and adjacent lobule showing cylindromatous growth. (Same patient as Figure 2).

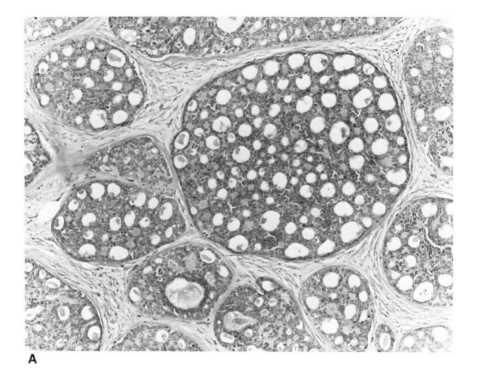

A

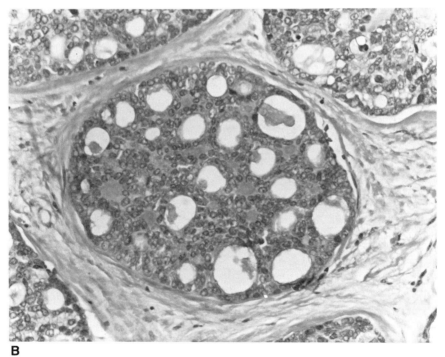

B

Figure 8. A. Prominent cribriform pattern in a high grade ACC. **B.** A portion of a gland demonstrating inconspicuous cylindromatous features. (*continued*)

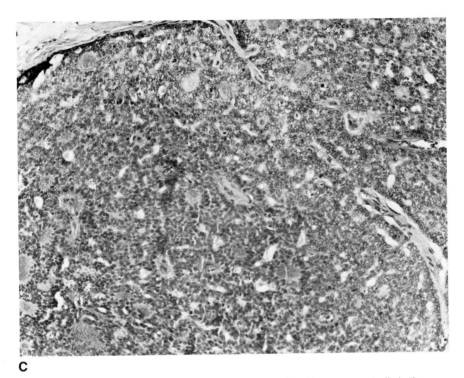

C

Figure 8 (cont.) C. The nearly solid compact growth pattern seen centrally in the same tumor. Cylindromatous and cribriform elements are quite inconspicuous. The patient is a 38-year-old woman who is well 2 years after mastectomy.

Treatment and Follow-Up. The following primary surgical procedures were performed: excisional biopsy, 2; partial mastectomy, 1; partial mastectomy and lymph node dissection, 2; simple mastectomy, 4; simple mastectomy and lymph node biopsy, 3; and modified radical mastectomy, 11. Lymph nodes were negative in 16 cases in which they were examined. Residual ACC was found in 7 of 18 mastectomy specimens, including 6 of 11 modifed radical and 1 of 7 simple mastectomies. Residual carcinoma remained in the breast after excision of five low grade ACC, four of which had a microscopically invasive growth pattern, and in two mastectomies for high grade lesions.

Follow-up ranged from 14 to 155 months with the mean and median of 56 and 53 months, respectively. All patients remain well, there having been no local or systemic recurrences of the ACC. Concurrent contralateral intraductal carcinoma diagnosed in a 49-year-old woman was treated by modified radical mastectomy at the same time that a simple mastectomy was performed for a 2-cm ACC. A 53-year-old woman was treated for primary ocular melanoma 3 years after mastectomy for ACC.

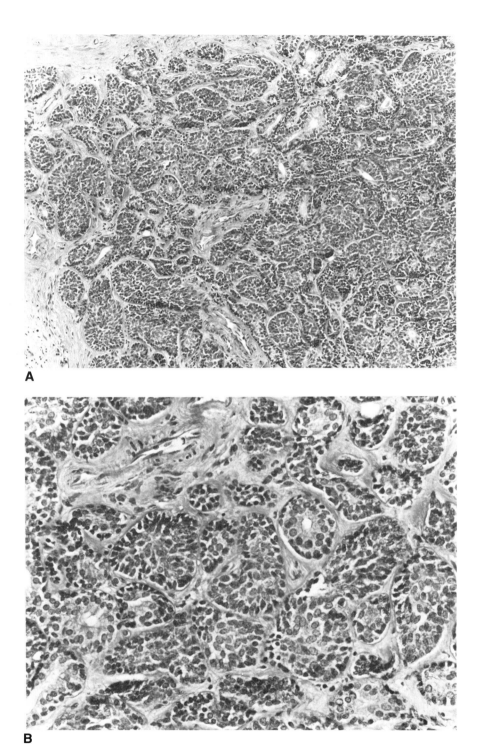

Figure 9. A. This high grade ACC has prominent alveolar growth. **B.** Note the basaloid orientation of cells in tumor glands. The 53-year-old patient had a modified radical mastectomy and was well 12 years later.

DISCUSSION

Clinical Features of Adenoid Cystic Carcinoma

Our data on the clinical presentation of ACC are entirely consistent with published observations. The age distributuion of ACC is similar to that of breast carcinoma in general with reported cases between 38 and 81 years of age. The mean age in larger series has varied from 50 to 64 years of age. The disease occurs predominantly in women but occasional cases have been described in men.[4,18] There is no predilection with respect to laterality and ACC is not associated with bilaterality.

Typically, ACC presents as a mass which may be tender, as noted in three of our cases, none of which had perineural invasion. Any part of the breast may be involved, but a disproportionate number of ACC cases are found in the central or subareolar region. Despite this location, however, nipple discharge is rarely present. While recent onset is usually described, ACC has been reported to be present for intervals up to 15 years prior to treatment.[2,3] The longest interval in the present series was 9 years.

Estrogen and progesterone receptors have been previously reported to be negative in ACC[8,19] with one exception[20] and the same result was obtained in four of six cases studied biochemically in our series. However, we have documented one tumor with positive estrogen and progesterone receptors and another with positive progesterone and negative estrogen receptors. The latter two were of low grade lesions with no special distinguishing morphological features.

Published data on the prognosis of ACC are based almost entirely on patients who were treated by surgery.[1-9] With few exceptions, mastectomy has proven curative, although chest wall recurrence has been documented after a simple mastectomy[12] and there have been a small number of reports that described systematic metastases after mastectomy.[5,11,13,14] The lungs have been involved in all cases that had metastases. Pulmonary metastases have been clinically apparent as late as 9 years after primary treatment. Axillary lymph node metastases were mentioned in two instances.[11,16] Very few deaths due to metastatic ACC have been reported[11,13] and documentation of the diagnosis of ACC is not convincing in one of these cases.

Recurrence may occur in the breast after local excision.[4,5,9,17] The time to recurrence in the breast varied from less than 1 year[5] to more than 20 years.[17] Axillary lymph nodes resected after recurrence in the breast were negative in three cases and the disease was reportedly controlled by further surgery in all seven cases of local recurrence.

The majority of ACC appear well circumscribed or nodular on gross inspection. This may be misleading, however, since there is often microscopic peripheral extension into the surrounding breast as invasive and/or as in situ carcinoma. Multinodularity is a further problem since small nodular foci at the periphery may be grossly inapparent. Because we found that most patients who had a local recurrence in the breast had tumors with peripheral invasion, such lesions should be treated by generous wide excision if mastectomy is not to be performed.

Ultimately, the treatment of patients with ACC will be determined by the conditions in a particular case. Small circumscribed low grade lesions can probably be managed by excision alone. In many cases, however, the tumor is likely to extend microscopically beyond the grossly palpable tumor. Wider excision, possibly quadrantectomy, is indicated for relatively large tumors that have an invasive growth pattern. The role of radiotherapy as an adjunct to breast-conserving therapy is not established for this type of tumor. Mastectomy should be considered for invasive lesions when a cosmetically satisfactory excision cannot be achieved, especially when there is a high grade component. A low axillary dissection should be included with the mastectomy and should be performed separately if a high grade lesion is being treated by excisional surgery.

Pathology of Adenoid Cystic Carcinoma

The classic microscopic growth pattern of ACC consists of a combination of glandular and cylindromatous elements. Electron microscopic studies[4,5,8,19] and immunohistochemistry[21] reveal that the non-glandular component is formed from reduplicated basal lamina. Although some heterogeneity of growth pattern is encountered in most ACC, the nature of the lesion is usually evident if one has adequate histological sections available. Small samples which emphasize predominantly gland-forming regions may be mistaken for cribriform duct carcinoma. On the other hand, densely sclerotic areas seen out of context resemble ordinary duct carcinoma. In this latter circumstance, one may suspect ACC if the stroma has a laminar or nodular configuration. While this issue can be addressed by electron microscopy or immunohistochemistry, excisional biopsy is the preferred method for definitive diagnosis. The specimen obtained by fine-needle aspiration biopsy may also have features suggestive of ACC.[8]

It is also possible that some conventional, less favorable forms of mammary carcinoma may be incorrectly diagnosed as ACC. In one recent review,[1] such misclassification occurred in about half of 27 cases recorded by the Connecticut Tumor Registry as ACC. The majority of misclassified cases were duct carcinomas with a prominent cribriform intraductal component. Problems were also encountered in distinguishing adenoid cystic from papillary and mucinous carcinomas. In the present series, the adenoid cystic pattern was recognized by submitting pathologists in virtually all cases.

Various growth patterns that have been described in ACC of salivary glands[22] have also been noted when these tumors occur in the breasts.[15,19] These configurations have been described as cribriform, solid, glandular (tubular), reticular, or trabecular and basaloid. In the present series, we also noted adenomyoepitheliomatous and syringomatous areas as further evidence of structural diversity. An attempt to subclassify ACC on the basis of these patterns will require a large number of cases and presently would have little clinical significance in view of the very favorable prognosis overall for these tumors. The distinction between low and high grade lesions in the present series was prompted by the study of Roe et al[19] in which ACC were stratified into three grades on the basis of the proportion of solid growth (I, no solid elements; II, less than 30 percent solid; III, more than 30 percent solid). Tumors with a solid component tended to be larger than those which lacked this feature and these patients were more likely to have recurrences. The one patient who developed metastases had a grade III tumor.

In the present series, lesions referred to as high grade because of a substantial solid component also tended to be larger, but they did not differ otherwise in regard to such features as patient age, laterality, duration prior to treatment, hormone receptors, and the presence of residual carcinoma in a mastectomy specimen. Since no patient had axillary metastases or has thus far developed a recurrence, our data did not reveal a prognostic difference between low and high grade tumors.

Collagenous Spherulosis (Adenoid Cystic Hyperplasia)

An unusual benign condition also to be considered in the differential diagnosis of ACC is a peculiar type of duct proliferation which we have referred to as "adenoid cystic hyperplasia." Recently the term "collagenous spherulosis"[23] has been recommended. This lesion consists of round, acellular deposits of stromal material among the epithelial cells (Fig. 10). Since the epithelial proliferation is usually also gland forming, the resulting complex bears a resemblance to ACC. There is a tendency for the spherule material to have a stellate or laminar structure but there have not yet been immunohistochemical or electron microscopic studies which would establish how much basal lamina is present. Thus far, it has been determined that spherules contain elastin, collagen, and PAS-positive material. Foci of duct hyperplasia with collagenous spherulosis may be found in association with a wide spectrum of other lesions. It has been present coincidentally in breast tissue obtained from patients with benign breast disease and also in patients who have carcinoma. The carcinomas have been ductal but none have had ACC. Sclerosing adenosis and papillomatosis are commonly associated hyperplastic changes.

A review of hyperplastic duct lesions seen in our consultations during 1 year revealed collagenous spherulosis in 1.7 percent of the cases. Usually it was an incidental finding. The age distribution was quite broad since our youngest patient was 22 and the oldest was 74. We have not undertaken a systematic follow-up but no subsequent carcinoma has been found in several patients traced 5 to 10 years after an excisional biopsy contained collagenous spherulosis among other benign proliferative changes. Others have reported similar results[23] and on this basis collagenous spherulosis must be considered a hyperplastic condition with little precancerous potential. It is hoped that wider recognition of this lesion will prevent inappropriate diagnoses of ACC and make it possible to acquire more information about its clinical significance.

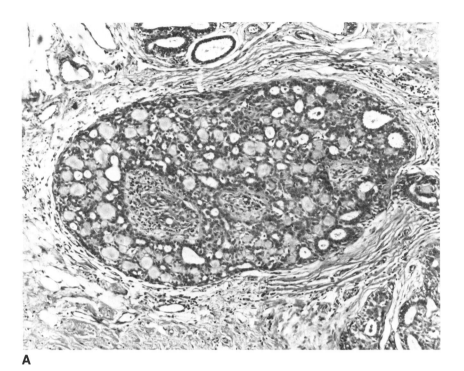

A

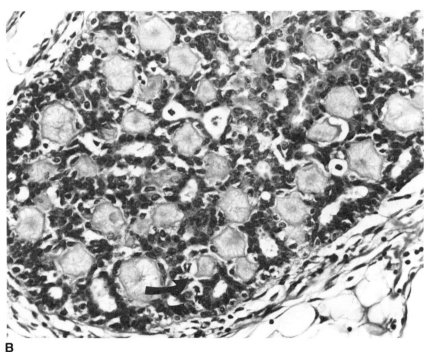

B

Figure 10. Collagenous spherulosis. **A.** A hyperplastic duct found in a breast biopsy from a 22-year-old woman. **B.** At high magnification, the spherules of this case have a radial structure centrally and a peripheral dense laminar border. Hyperplastic myoepithelial cells are apparent in proximity to some spherules (*arrow*).

Acknowledgments. We are indebted to the patients, their families, and their physicians whose help has made this study possible. The following physicians are acknowledged: J. Barrow, M. Bilous, H. Bogaars, E. Breakell, E. Casper, A DePalo, A. Fracchia, H. Gerber, J. Griffin, J. Hammer, W. Hartley, W. Jacobson, P. Kiessling, K. Kostroff, S. Leyser, R. Martin, R. McPherson, A. Michel, C. Moddrell, T. Moran, F. Nime, P. Parshley, W. Poston, M. Praeger, W. Recant, G. Robbins, T. Rudy, C. Schmidt, G. Shead, J. Smith, C. Soechtig, K. Wagner, O. Warr, T. Wentz, W. Wetzel, J. White, and D. Will. The manuscript was prepared by Mrs. Sandra Franklin. Mr. Kin Kong made the photographs.

REFERENCES

1. Sumpio BE, Jennings TA, Sullivan PD, Merino MJ: Adenoid cystic carcinoma of the breast. Data from the Connecticut Tumor Registry and a review of the literature. Ann Surg 205:295, 1987
2. Galloway JR, Woolner LB, Clagett OT: Adenoid cystic carcinoma of the breast. Surg Gynecol Obstet 122:1289, 1966
3. Anthony PP, James PD: Adenoid cystic carcinoma of the breast: Prevalence, diagnostic criteria and histogenesis. J Clin Pathol 28:647, 1975
4. Qizilbash AH, Patterson MC, Oliveira KF: Adenoid cystic carcinoma of the breast: Light and electron microscopy and a brief review of the literature. Arch Pathol Lab Med 101:302, 1977
5. Peters GN, Wolff M: Adenoid cystic carcinoma of the breast: Report of 11 new cases. Cancer 52:680, 1982
6. Friedman BA, Oberman HA: Adenoid cystic carcinoma of the breast. Am J Clin Pathol 54:1, 1970
7. Koss LG, Brannan CD, Ashikari R: Histologic and ultrastructural features of adenoid cystic carcinoma of the breast. Cancer 26:1271, 1970
8. Zaloudek C, Oertel YC, Orenstein JM: Adenoid cystic carcinoma of the breast. Am J Clin Pathol 81:297, 1984
9. Cavanzo FJ, Taylor HB: Adenoid cystic carcinoma of the breast. An analysis of 21 cases. Cancer 24:740, 1969
10. Harris M: Pseudoadenoid cystic carcinoma of the breast. Arch Pathol Lab Med 101:307, 1977
11. Verani RR, Vander Bel-Kahn J: Mammary adenoid cystic carcinoma with unusual features. Am J Clin Pathol 59:653, 1976
12. Wilson WB, Spell JP: Adenoid cystic carcinoma of breast: A case with recurrence and regional metastases. Ann Surg 166:861, 1967
13. Nayer HR: Cylindroma of the breast with pulmonary metastases. Dis Chest 31:324, 1957
14. Lim SK, Kovi J, Warner OG: Adenoid cystic carcinoma of breast with metastasis: A case report and review of the literature. JAMA 71:329, 1979
15. Orenstein JM, Dardick I, Van Nostrand AWP: Ultrastructural similarities of adenoid cystic carcinoma and pleomorphic adenoma. Histopathology 9:623, 1985
16. Wells CA, Nicholl S, Ferguson DJP: Adenoid cystic carcinoma of the breast: A case with axillary lymph node metastasis. Histopathology 10:415, 1986
17. Lusted D: Structure and growth patterns of adenoid cystic carcinoma of the breast. Am J Clin Pathol 54:419, 1970

18. Hjorth S, Magnusson PH, Blomquist P: Adenoid cystic carcinoma of the breast. Acta Chir Scand 143:155, 1977
19. Ro JY, Silva EG, Gallager HS: Adenoid cystic carcinoma of the breast. Hum Pathol 18:1276, 1987
20. Kern WH: Morphologic and clinical aspects of estrogen receptors in carcinoma of the breast. Surg Gynecol Obstet 148:240, 1979
21. d'Ardenne AJ, Kirkpatrick P, Wells CA, Davies JD: Laminin and fibronectin in adenoid cystic carcinoma. J Clin Pathol 39:138, 1986
22. Azumi N, Battifora H: The cellular composition of adenoid cystic carcinoma. An immunohistochemical study. Cancer 60:1589, 1987
23. Clement PB, Young RH, Azzopardi JG: Collagenous spherulosis of the breast. Am J Surg Pathol 11:411, 1987

Diagnostic Histology of Myocardial Disease in Endomyocardial Biopsies and at Autopsy

J.T. Lie

Heart disease continues to be the leading cause of death and morbidity in the developed countries the world over. For the practicing pathologist, proficiency in diagnostic cardiac histology assumes even greater importance now that endomyocardial biopsy has become a commonly used investigative tool to document morphologically different cardiac disorders, to monitor therapeutic responses and drug toxicity, and to detect allograft rejection in heart transplantation.[25,73]

   This chapter offers a pictorial survey of normal and abnormal cardiac histology as an aid to pathologists in the diagnosis of common and uncommon forms of heart disease. It focuses on the typical histological findings as well as highlighting the subtleties and pitfalls for which one needs to be watchful. Almost all the salient changes described and illustrated herein can be elicited in well-stained hematoxylin and eosin (H&E) sections. Special stains are needed only rarely.

NORMAL CARDIAC HISTOLOGY, VARIATIONS, AND ARTIFACTS

Normal Histology and Variations

The heart is a muscular pump with the contractile atrial and ventricular myocardium formed by a syncytium-like and spirally layered arrangement of cardiac myocytes that take their origin from the fibrous skeleton of the heart. Only the conduction fibers of the atrioventricular bundles (of His) bridge the fibrous skeleton as they traverse from the atrial septum to the ventricular septum by penetrating the right fibrous trigone (central fibrous body).

The striated muscle fibers of the vertebrate heart differ in several respects from those of skeletal muscle.[10] Cardiac myocytes are not syncytial, as was formerly thought, but are made up of separate cellular units joined end-to-end by surface specialization, the *intercalated disks*, that run transversely across the myocytes. The fibers are not simple cylindrical units, but they branch out and connect with adjacent fibers to form a complex three-dimensional network. The elongated nuclei are centrally located instead of immediately beneath the sarcolemma.

The myocardium is perfused by a rich network of capillaries. The number of capillaries per unit area is unchanged in hypertrophied hearts.[58] It has been calculated that 36 percent of the circumference of each cardiac myocyte is within 200 nm of a capillary, and that the ratio of capillaries to myocytes is 1:1.

The normal adult ventricular myocyte has a width of 10 to 15 μm and a length of 80 to 100 μm. The atrial myocytes are similar in length, but more slender (6 to 12 μm), less orderly aligned, and contain specific atrial granules.[23] Because cardiac myocytes branch freely, their cross-sections appear somewhat irregular in outline and size when compared with the corresponding longitudinally oriented fibers (Fig. 1a and 1b). In cardiac hypertrophy, an increase in volume of the heart muscle takes place with an increase up to four to five times the thickness of individual fibers. There is a concomitant characteristic increase in the size and number of hyperchromatic nuclei (Fig. 1c and 1d).

The regenerative capacity of cardiac muscle is insignificant, and healing takes place by the formation of fibrous scar tissue. In the newborn, cardiac myocyte division ceases toward the end of the first week and nuclei only divide from 6 to 15 postnatal days. Cell volume increases from about 15 days onward when about 80 percent of the cardiac myocytes are binucleated. This gives rise to the crowded appearance of an elevated nucleus or cell ratio density in a neonatal heart compared with that of a young adult (Fig. 2).

The normal right ventricular myocardium almost invariably shows focal areas of fiber disarray and corrugated wavy fibers (Fig. 3). They may represent histological markers of hypertrophic cardiomyopathy[80] and acute myocardial ischemia,[11] respectively, if found in the ventricular septum or left ventricular free wall. However, their presence in the right ventricle has little diagnostic value.

Saphir[68] drew attention to the intercalated disks in human hearts. They are scarcely noticeable in sections of non-dilated hearts stained with H&E, but they become visibly prominent in sections of dilated hearts. *Segmentation* refers to separation of cardiac myocytes in the line of the intercalated disks, whereas *fragmentation* means apparent fracture of myocytes at some point between the disks. Both are essentially the same process,[30] namely, an artifact of rigor mortis, and they become more prominent with lengthening postmortem intervals (Fig. 4a). Putrefaction and antemortem sepsis with gas-forming microorganisms are the most common cause of lacy or "bubbly" myocardium (Fig. 4b), not to be confused with myocytolysis or true vacuolar degeneration.

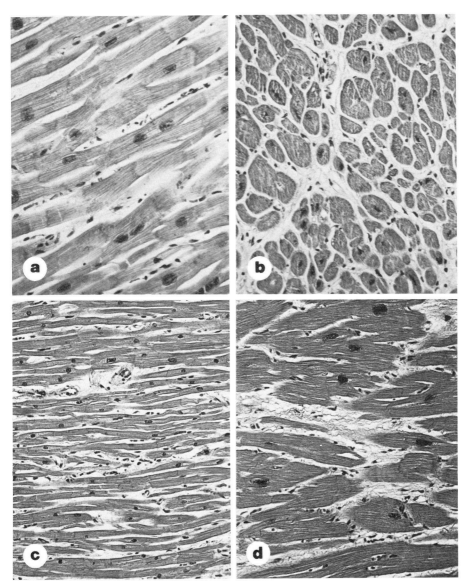

Figure 1. Normal histology and variations of cardiac myocytes. **a.** Longitudinally oriented cardiac myocytes with central nuclei. **b.** Irregular outline and size of normal cardiac myocytes in cross-sections. **c.** Normal cardiac myocytes are dwarfed by (**d**) hypertrophied myocytes photographed at the same magnification.

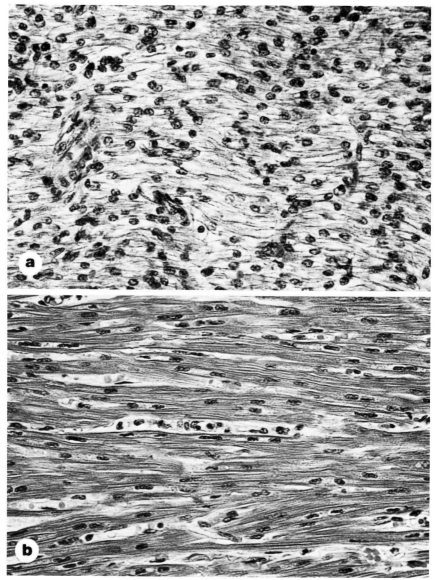

Figure 2. Comparison of cardiac myocytes in **a** newborn and **b** young adult. The former have a crowded appearance because the myocyte fibers are closely aligned and 80 percent of myocytes are binucleated.

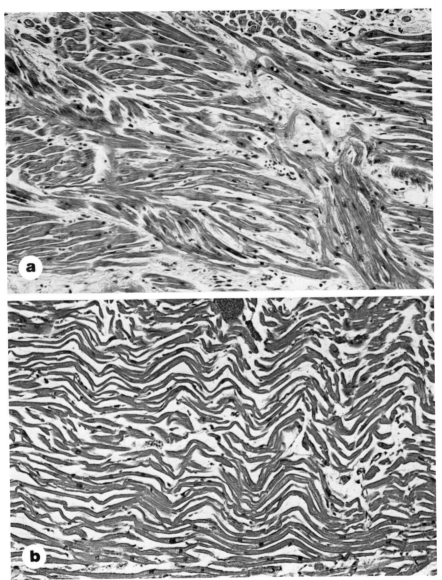

Figure 3. a. Fiber disarray (a common finding in hypertrophic cardiomyopathy) and (**b**) wavy fibers (indicative of acute ischemia) are commonplace in normal right ventricular myocardium and have no diagnostic value.

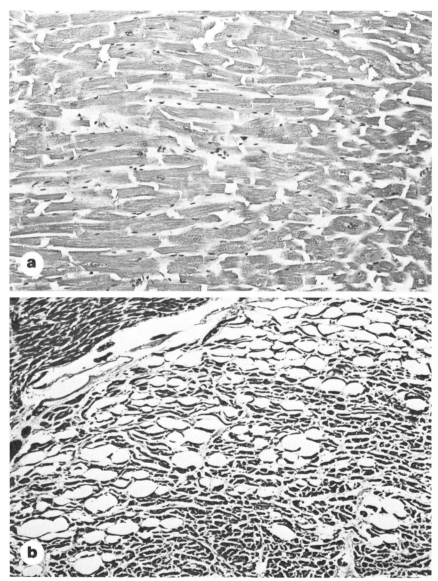

Figure 4. a. Fractured cardiac myocytes with separation occurring mostly at the intercalated disks is an artifact of rigor mortis, delayed refrigeration, and tissue fixation. **b.** Lacy or "bubbly" myocardium caused by gas-forming microorganisms.

Fatty Infiltration, Myocytolysis, Basophilic Degeneration, and Calcification

Fatty infiltration denotes excessive deposits of adipose tissue in locations where it normally exists. In the heart, fatty infiltration in the right ventricular free wall is commonplace and distributed transmurally. Fatty infiltration is found less

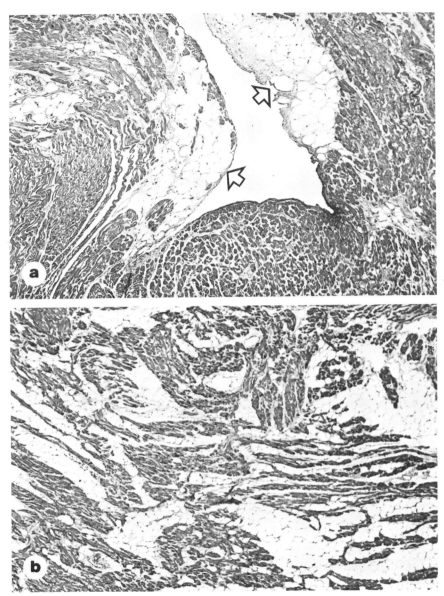

Figure 5. a. Subendocardial fatty infiltration (*arrows*) in normal left ventricular myocardium. **b.** Transmural fatty infiltration in normal right ventricular myocardium.

commonly in the ventricular septum and left ventricular free wall, usually in the subendocardial muscle (Fig. 5). Thus, a right-heart endomyocardial biopsy with tissue samples containing fat cannot always be accepted as an assurance that the bioptome is safely within the confine of the right ventricular wall, as the procedure intends.

Myocytolysis, or vacuolar degeneration (Fig. 6), occurs in both the contractile myocardium and conduction fibers of the heart. The vacuoles do not react with histochemical stains for glycogen, fat, or mucopolysaccharides; the nature of their content is not known. Myocytolysis is a nonspecific histological finding that is most commonly attributed to nonlethal chronic ischemic injury to cardiac myocytes. It is often seen in the subendocardium and at the margin of recent infarcts, but myocytolysis also occurs in a variety of seemingly unrelated conditions, including experimental hypoxia, adrenal injection, myxedema, and hyperthyroidism.[71] Its appearance may also closely resemble the spider or balloon cells of a cardiac rhabdomyoma.

Basophilic (mucinous) degeneration refers to the accumulation of basophilic, periodic acid Schiff (PaS)-positive, finely granular material in the cytoplasm of individual cardiac myocytes (Fig. 7a). Little is known of the mechanism of formation, chemical composition, and clinical significance of basophilic degeneration.[64,72] Kosek and Angell[36] and Roy[66] described ultrastructure and histochemical features of basophilic degeneration to resemble those of central nervous system corpora amylacea and Lafora bodies. Although it may affect any chamber of the heart, it occurs most frequently in the left ventricular and ventricular septal myocardium. Its reported incidence is variable but has been quoted to be as high as 70 percent in 75 hearts[72] and 89 percent in 135 hearts.[64] It is probably a nonspecific marker of myocardial injury or senescent change in the cardiac myocytes.

Both metastatic and dystrophic *calcifications* occur in the myocardium, but the latter is more common. In dystrophic calcification, calcium is deposited in degenerated and devitalized tissue, such as necrotic myocardium. It tends to occur in patients who have had recent open heart surgery and, especially, in children and the elderly.[74] Calcification may affect individual or a group of myocardial fibers, often invoking a striking inflammatory reaction (Fig. 7b). The occurrence of dystrophic or metastatic myocardial calcification bears no relationship to calcification of the annulus fibrosus in senescent hearts.[43]

ISCHEMIC HEART DISEASE

In the United States, ischemic heart disease accounts for just over 70 percent of all deaths due to heart disease and just under 30 percent of all mortality, according to the most recently available vital statistics.[57] Ischemic heart disease with atypical presentation, especially in younger persons, may mimic other forms of heart disease, notably myocarditis, and vice versa. With increased use of open and endomyocardial biopsy in clinical practice, histological diagnosis of ischemic heart disease has emerged from the closet of a mortuary to test the acumen of unsuspecting surgical pathologists.

The pathologist is often confronted with the problem of detecting or confirming the presence of acute myocardial infarction in patients suspected to have ischemic heart disease. Recognition of *early* myocardial infarction on the

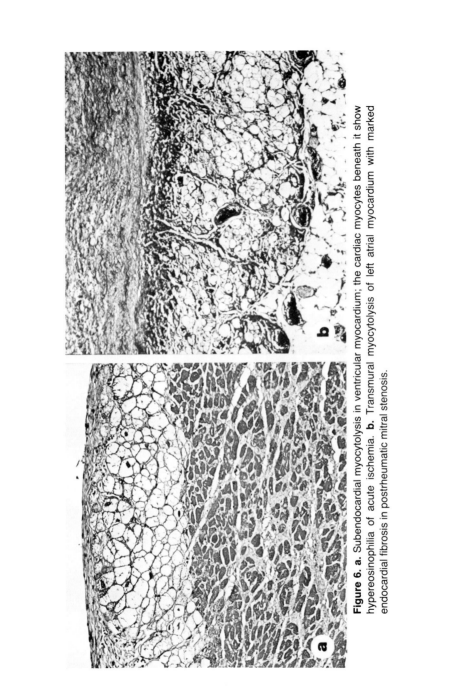

Figure 6. a. Subendocardial myocytolysis in ventricular myocardium; the cardiac myocytes beneath it show hypereosinophilia of acute ischemia. **b.** Transmural myocytolysis of left atrial myocardium with marked endocardial fibrosis in postrheumatic mitral stenosis.

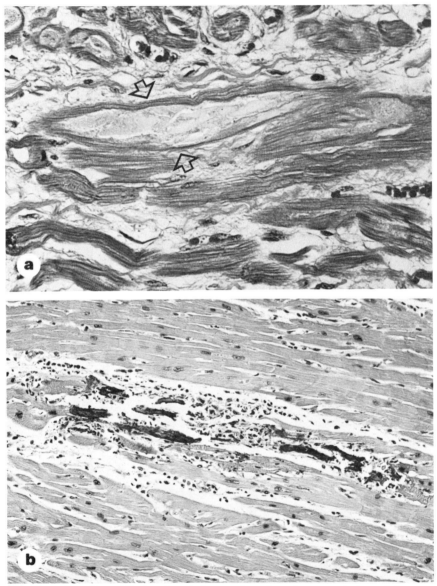

Figure 7. a. Basophilic (mucinous) degeneration of cardiac myocyte (*arrow*). **b.** Dystrophic calcification of necrotic cardiac myocytes with associated inflammatory reaction.

basis of gross and light microscopic observations is often plagued with uncertainty because appreciable changes become manifest only several hours after the onset of irreversible ischemia (Table 1).

A number of histochemical and fluorescence microscopy methods have been used by investigators to detect early myocardial infarcts with variable success.[13,44,45,67] The earliest histological diagnosis of myocardial infarction is possible at about 6 to 12 hours after the onset of ischemia. This is at a stage before the telltale polymorphonuclear infiltration of infarcted myocardium. In well-stained H&E sections, hypereosinophilia (or fuchsinorrhagia),[46] contraction band necrosis (or myofibrillar degeneration),[32] and wavy, attenuated fibers[11] are three sensitive, but individually nonspecific, histological markers of earlier myocar-

TABLE 1. DATING OF MYOCARDIAL INFARCTION BY PATHOLOGIC CRITERIA

Age of Infarct	Gross Features[a]	Light Microscopy[b]
< 4–6 hr	None detectable	None detectable consistently
6–12 hr	None detectable	Developing hypereosinophilia of fibers
12–24 hr	Subtle pallor or some mottling appearance of cut surface of myocardium	More clearcut hypereosinophilia and dense (opaque) appearance of fibers, with concomitant but variable degrees of contraction band necrosis, stretched-out attenuated or wavy fibers, edema, and very few intravascular or interstitial polymorphonuclear leukocytes
2–5 days	More clearcut pallor or a tan discoloration of affected myocardium	Above plus increasing number of polymorphs, but intensity of infiltrate may vary greatly from one area to another
5–10 days	Unequivocal and well-demarcated zone of grayish-yellow, dry, necrotic myocardium with hyperemic border	Above plus karyorrhexis of polymorphs, basophilic debris, anuclear necrotic myocardial fibers with accentuated sarcomere markings, early appearance of lymphomononuclear cells, pigment-containing macrophages, and phagocytosis of necrotic myocytes
10–14 days	Same as above with discernible retraction and depressed zone of infarct	Formation of vascular granulation tissue, fibroblast proliferation, increased phagocytosis of necrotic myocytes, and a reversed ratio of polymorphs (fewer) and lymphomononuclear cell (greater number) infiltrate
2–4 wk	More obvious retraction and depressed infarct zone, gelatinous and hemorrhagic	Formation of a young scar tissue with neovascularization, early collagen deposition and persistence of chronic inflammatory infiltrate. Islands of mummified necrotic myocytes may remain
> 4 wk	Firm, grayish-white retracting scar with wall thinning	Formation of a mature scar tissue with increased collagen deposition and persistence of vascularization and decreasing number of chronic inflammatory infiltrate

[a]The gross features are better defined and more easily discernible when a heart slice is held and viewed under the surface of a clear water bath.
[b]As seen in well-stained H&E sections.

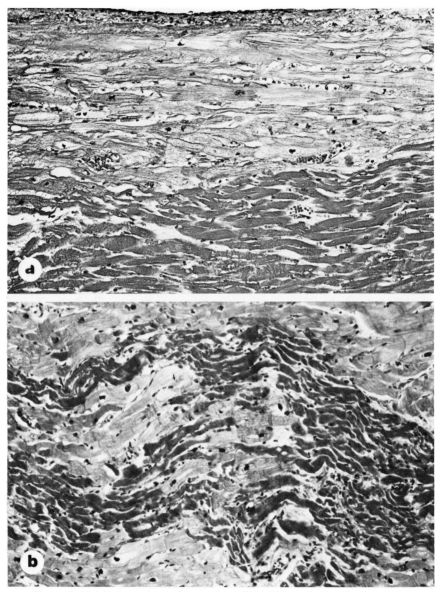

Figure 8. Histologic markers of early phase (6 to 24 hours) of acute myocardial infarction (before polymorphonuclear infiltration). **a.** Subendocardial hypereosinophilia and myofibrillar degeneration (contraction band necrosis). **b.** Wavy fibers with hypereosinophilia and contraction band necrosis.

dial infarction (Fig. 8). The specificity for diagnosis of early infarction approaches 100 percent when all three features are present and co-exist. They may persist for 24 to 48 hours thereafter when diagnostic changes of a definite or established myocardial infarction become apparent (Fig. 9).

None of the cumbersome enzyme histochemical techniques proposed to date offer any real advantage over a well-stained H&E section for conventional light microscopic diagnosis of early myocardial infarction.[44] However, two easily performed fluorescence microscopy techniques[13,67] can be recommended as useful adjuncts for the detection of acute myocardial ischemia. Myocardial sections stained with acridine orange[67] show apple-green fluorescence of tissue obtained within 30 minutes of coronary artery ligation in experimental animals[17]; the fluorescence observed is quite distinct from the golden brown color of the surrounding non-ischemic myocardium. Bright yellow autofluorescence of H&E sections of myocardium in ultraviolet light becomes detectable 60 minutes to 6 hours after the onset of myocardial infarction.[13,17] The fluorescent areas correspond to the hypereosinophilic ischemic myofibers observed by H&E staining (Fig. 10).

ANITSCHKOW CELLS, ASCHOFF BODIES, RHEUMATIC DISEASES, AND MYOCARDITIS

Anitschkow Cells, Aschoff Bodies, and Rheumatic Diseases

Anitschkow cells and Aschoff bodies are two venerable enigmatic structures found uniquely in the heart. Both are of uncertain histogenesis, but they may possibly be related.[16,49,61,62,84]

Anitschkow cells are small and oblong shaped with poorly defined cell borders and scanty cytoplasm. Their most distinguishing feature is the nuclei, which contain a centrally located bar of chromatin with a serrated edge, which is separated from the nuclear membrane by a clear zone on all sides (Fig. 11). Cell nuclei showing this morphology are known as Anitschkow-type nuclei, caterpillar nuclei, or owl-eye nuclei.[61,62,84] This nuclear morphology can be found in cardiac myocytes, endothelial cells, smooth muscle cells, Schwann cells, and cells of Aschoff bodies (Fig. 12). It has also been seen in cells of intracardiac metastases but not in the coresponding primary tumors.[62]

Anitschkow cells are present focally in small numbers of normal hearts but are more numerous and widespread in a variety of pathologic conditions.[61,62,84] Ultrastructurally, Anitschkow cells resemble fibroblasts. Their cytoplasm contains a few fibrosomes, cisterns of rough-surfaced endoplasmic reticulum, and mitochondria. Cytoplasmic filaments are of the cytoskeletal type, and dense bodies such as seen in smooth muscle cells are absent as is an external lamina.[61] Thus, it is no longer correct to refer to (as in the old literature) Anitschkow cells as Anitschkow "myocytes." They are probably activated myocardial fibroblasts, fibroblast-like mesenchymal cells of the heart, or myocardial histiocytes.[84]

An Aschoff body is a proliferation of myocardial histiocytes, which may be

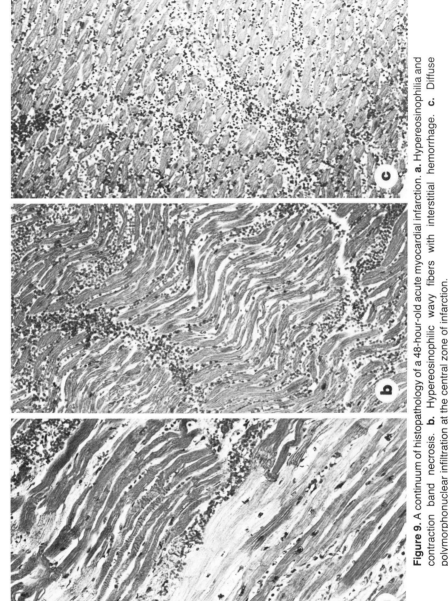

Figure 9. A continuum of histopathology of a 48-hour-old acute myocardial infarction. **a.** Hypereosinophilia and contraction band necrosis. **b.** Hypereosinophilic wavy fibers with interstitial hemorrhage. **c.** Diffuse polymorphonuclear infiltration at the central zone of infarction.

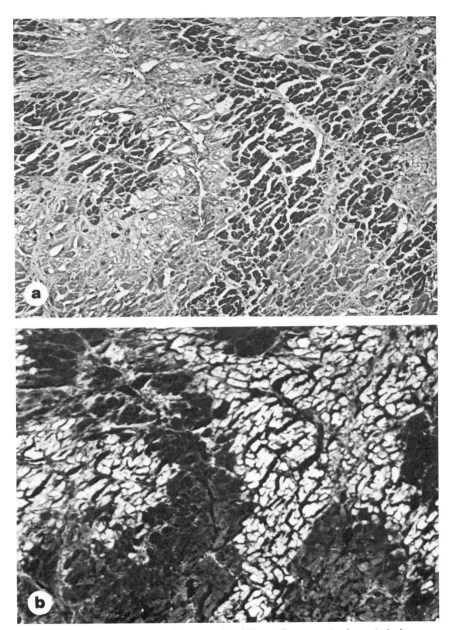

Figure 10. a. Patchy areas of hypereosinophilic cardiac myocytes in acute ische-mia. **b.** Corresponding areas of autofluorescence when the same H&E section is examined under ultraviolet light.

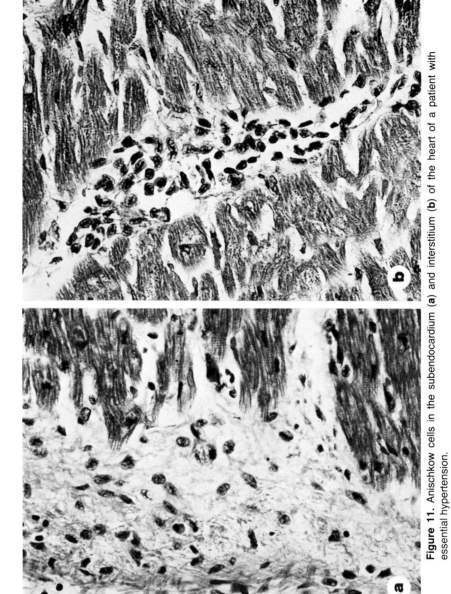

Figure 11. Anischkow cells in the subendocardium (**a**) and interstitium (**b**) of the heart of a patient with essential hypertension.

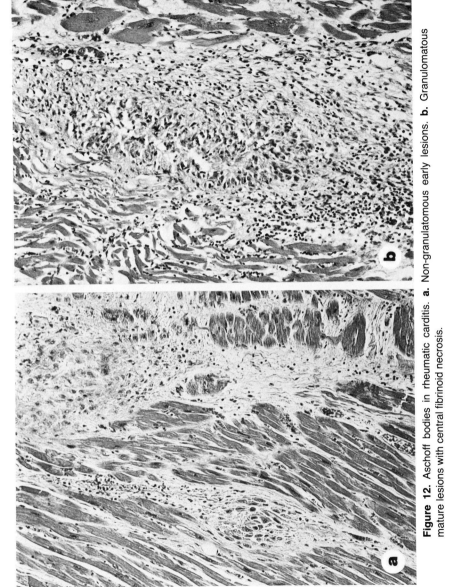

Figure 12. Aschoff bodies in rheumatic carditis. **a.** Non-granulatomous early lesions. **b.** Granulomatous mature lesions with central fibrinoid necrosis.

non-granulomatous (early lesions) or granulomatous (mature lesions), with or without central fibrinoid necrosis, and is usually subendocardial or perivascular in distribution (Fig. 12). Aschoff bodies are a unique histological marker of rheumatic carditis, especially in younger patients. They occur in no other diseases and in no other organs.[70] Although this is generally accepted, there is still some controversy as to the origin of Aschoff bodies; cells comprising Aschoff bodies have been claimed to be derived from cardiac myocytes, smooth muscle, connective tissue, endothelial cells, lymphatics, nerves, and fibroblasts.[16] The results of cell marker studies by the immunoperoxidase technique show that Aschoff bodies and Anitschkow cells label with specific antibodies suggesting a common derivation of both from a mesenchymal or histiocytic origin rather than the previously presumed histogenesis from smooth or cardiac muscle, nerve or nerve sheath, and lymphatic or vascular endothelium.[49] The reported incidence of Aschoff bodies identified in surgical and autopsy cardiac specimens from patients with valvular heart disease varies widely, from 9 to 84 percent.[63] The detection of Aschoff bodies in these settings probably represent inactive or obsolescent rheumatic disease of past rather than current or recrudescent carditis.[18]

There is some disparity between the clinical and pathologic evidence of involvement of the heart in rheumatic arthritis.[38] Clinically, only 10 to 20 percent of patients develop cardiac symptoms that are causally attributable to rheumatoid arthritis, but pericarditis and myocarditis have been observed in 30 to 40 percent of patients in several autopsy series.[14,37,38,77] A myocarditis in patients with rheumatoid arthritis may be either nonspecific or granulomatous. The nonspecific form consists of interstitial infiltrates of lymphocytes, plasma cells, and histiocytes in the myocardium, with only occasional cardiac myocyte necrosis. The specific lesions include the presence of rheumatoid (necrobiotic) nodules in any part of the affected heart and a granulomatous myocarditis with histiocytic components that resemble Aschoff bodies (Fig. 13). A central zone of fibrinoid necrosis is common in this specific form of rheumatoid heart disease. Some of these patients may also have rheumatoid vasculitis affecting large and small blood vessels.

In other connective tissue diseases, a nonspecific type of myocarditis occurs in about 20 to 30 percent of patients with systemic lupus erythematosus or polymyositis,[21] and more infrequently in scleroderma and mixed connective tissue disease, juvenile rheumatoid arthritis,[55] adult Still's disease,[3] Behçet's disease,[41] and Lyme disease.[79]

Definition and Prevalence of Myocarditis

The term *myocarditis* should strictly apply to a true inflammatory disease of cardiac myocytes from a variety of causes, known or unknown (Table 2), and is not to be used for inflammatory reaction of injuries to cardiac myocytes, such as an acute myocardial infarction. This approach was adopted by a Working Group[2] who defined myocarditis as "a process characterized by an inflammatory

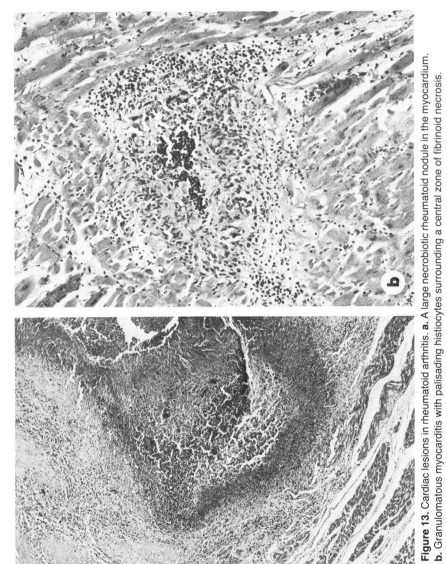

Figure 13. Cardiac lesions in rheumatoid arthritis. **a.** A large necrobiotic rheumatoid nodule in the myocardium. **b.** Granulomatous myocarditis with palisading histiocytes surrounding a central zone of fibrinoid necrosis.

TABLE 2. CLASSIFICATION OF MYOCARDITIS

Primary (idiopathic) myocarditis
  Isolated interstitial myocarditis (of Fiedler)
  Granulomatous (giant cell) myocarditis
  Cardiac sarcoidosis
  Eosinophilic myocarditis
  Lymphocytic myocarditis
Secondary (nonspecific) myocarditis
  Infective myocarditis (with or without endocarditis)
    Bacterial
    Fungal
    Viral
    Rickettsial
    Protozoal
  Noninfective myocarditis (associated with systemic disease)
    Chemical-induced and drug hypersensitivity
    Rheumatic and other connective tissue diseases
    Associated with other systemic diseases
    Radiation
    Spurious

infiltrate of the myocardium with necrosis and/or degeneration of adjacent myocytes not typical of the ischemic damage associated with coronary artery disease."

Myocarditis of any type is a relatively uncommon form of heart disease and, until recently, has seldom been correctly diagnosed before postmortem examination of the heart. In the preantibiotics era, an autopsy incidence of 2.9 percent and 4.3 percent were reported by Gore and Saphir[27] and Saphir,[69] respectively. The reported prevalence of myocarditis in the postantibiotics era was even lower. Whitehead[85] described 18 cases in 12,815 autopsies (0.14 percent) in a general hospital practice. Myocarditis has no diagnostic clinical features or laboratory test results. In young patients, myocarditis can clinically mimic acute myocardial infarction, the most common form of heart disease.[54] It is, therefore, not surprising that clinicians rely heavily on endomyocardial biopsy for the diagnosis of suspected myocarditis but, unfortunately, this diagnostic procedure is plagued with intrinsic sampling problems and observer errors in interpretation.[42]

Histological Diagnosis of Myocarditis

The histological diagnosis of myocarditis in endomyocardial biopsies is subjective. It is fraught with an unacceptably high interobserver variability in regard to such seemingly straightforward morphological features as the presence or absence of fibrosis, hypertrophy, nuclear changes, and abnormal lymphocyte counts.[42] Caution should be exercised in the interpretation of inflammatory cells in the myocardium, and the pathologist must resist the temptation of overdiagnosing myocarditis if clinical credibility is to be maintained. Focal

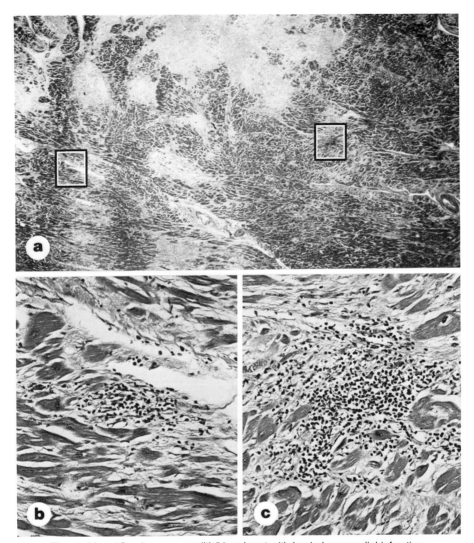

Figure 14. a. "Spurious myocarditis" in a heart with healed myocardial infarction. The left-hand side and right-hand side boxed areas of focal collection of lymphocytes are shown at higher magnification in **b** and **c,** respectively.

collections of inflammatory cells are found not infrequently in a routine section of the heart with healed myocardial infarction (Fig. 14), in accident victims presumed to have been healthy, in patients under stress of catecholamine excess or vasopressor agents, as well as in patients with the clinical diagnosis of idiopathic dilated cardiomyopathy.[8]

Virtually all normal and abnormal endomyocardial biopsies have contraction band (myofibrillar degeneration) artifact (Fig. 15). The formation of contrac-

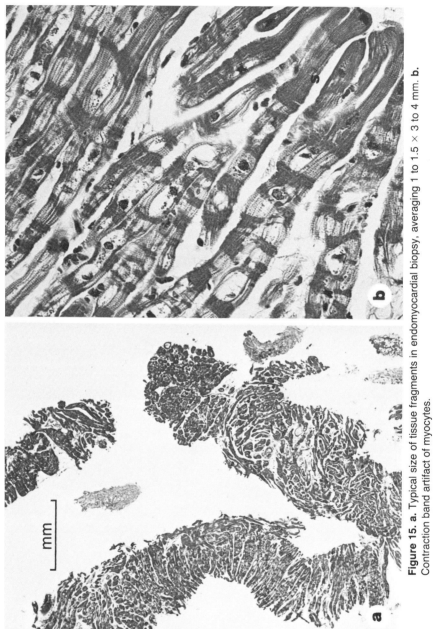

Figure 15. a. Typical size of tissue fragments in endomyocardial biopsy, averaging 1 to 1.5 × 3 to 4 mm. **b.** Contraction band artifact of myocytes.

tion bands are due to depolarization of cardiac myocytes by the biopsy procedure resulting in activation of contractile apparatus together with unopposed sarcomere hypercontraction.[1] Contraction bands, despite their versatility as a sensitive marker of myocardial injuries,[31,32] cannot be relied upon as a morphological marker of cardiac pathology in biopsies.

The correct timing of the endomyocardial biopsy from the onset of disease and sequential biopsies are crucial to the diagnosis of myocarditis and for assessment of spontaneous resolution or response to treatment. Lessons learned from studies of experimental viral myocarditis[86,87] suggest that the timing of biopsy determines the likeliness of detecting changes in the cell type and intensity of inflammatory infiltrates, macrophage and fibroblast proliferation, and scar formation.

Granulocytic, Eosinophilic and Lymphocyte Myocarditis

Bacterial or fungal pyogenic infection is the most common form of *neutrophil granulocytic myocarditis*. While a well-formed microabscess (Fig. 16a) could hardly be missed by even a casual observer, the diagnosis may not be so apparent with a more indefinite cell type and less intense inflammatory infiltrate in the myocardium (Fig. 16b).

Eosinophilic myocarditis (Fig. 17) has many causes, including Löffler's disease, idiopathic hypereosinophilic syndrome, parasitic infection, drug hypersensitivity, and Churg–Strauss syndrome. Only Löffler's disease leads to significant mural thrombosis and restrictive endomyocardial fibrosis.[40,78,81]

Lymphocytic myocarditis, with or without demonstrable cardiac myocyte necrosis, is probably the most common variety of myocarditis diagnosed by endomyocardial biopsy,[73] and it is also the most inconsistently diagnosed entity with its reported prevalence in patients with unexplained heart failure ranging from zero[65] to 80 percent.[19] The problem exists because of the intrinsic limitations of endomyocardial biopsy as a diagnostic tool and imprecise histological criteria for myocarditis applied by different investigators.[42]

The assumption that most idiopathic lymphocytic myocarditis is postviral is based on experimental data, clinical and epidemiologic observations. Animal models have shown that viral infection of the heart can result in a morphological pattern of injury resembling lymphocytic myocarditis, and eventually in a dilated cardiomyopathy with immunologic markers suggestive of an autoimmune disease.[35,50] In man, various aberrations of immune responses also have been documented in patients with idiopathic myocarditis and dilated cardiomyopathy.[22] In clinical practice, a postviral myocarditis may be diffuse with widespread cardiac myocyte necrosis, histologically indistinguishable from a case of drug hypersensitivity myocarditis (Fig. 18). Or it may be very focal with only isolated individual myocyte necrosis (Fig. 19) that an endomyocardial biopsy may fail to detect. Even if detected, there may be difficulty in interpreting its significance.

278

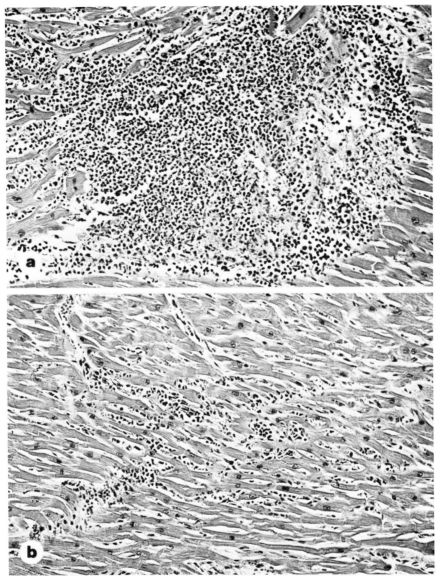

Figure 16. Neutrophil granulocytic myocarditis in disseminated candidiasis. **a.** A microabscess. **b.** Sparse interstitial infiltrate with intact myocytes in an area adjacent to the microabscess less than 4 mm away.

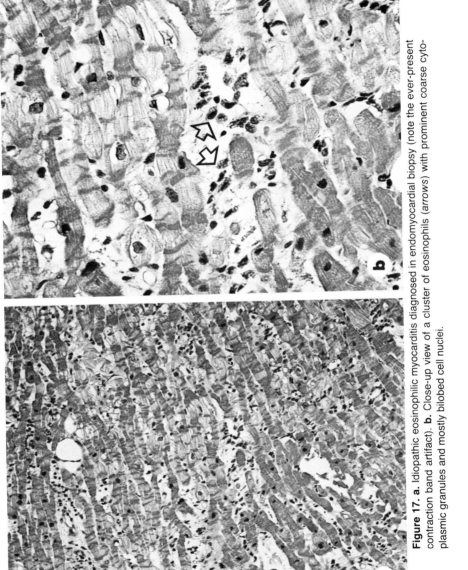

Figure 17. a. Idiopathic eosinophilic myocarditis diagnosed in endomyocardial biopsy (note the ever-present contraction band artifact). **b.** Close-up view of a cluster of eosinophils (arrows) with prominent coarse cytoplasmic granules and mostly bilobed cell nuclei.

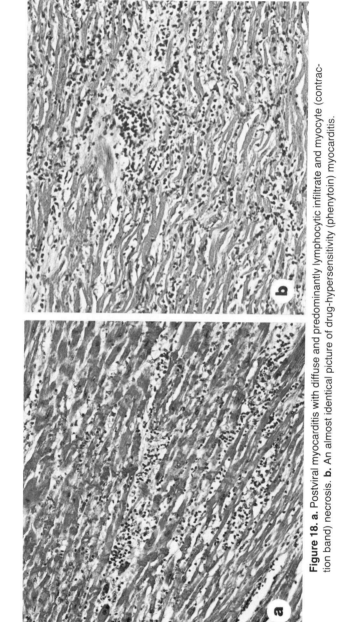

Figure 18. a. Postviral myocarditis with diffuse and predominantly lymphocytic infiltrate and myocyte (contraction band) necrosis. **b.** An almost identical picture of drug-hypersensitivity (phenytoin) myocarditis.

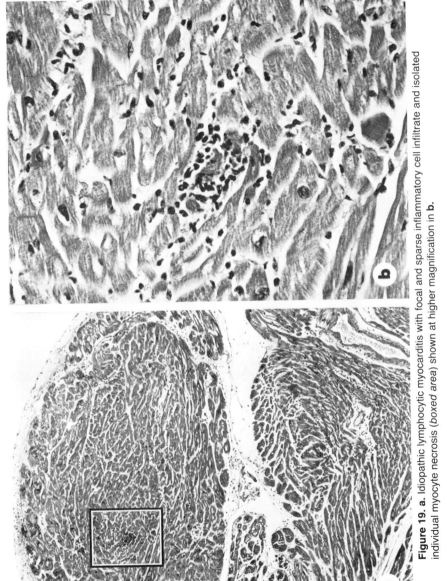

Figure 19. a. Idiopathic lymphocytic myocarditis with focal and sparse inflammatory cell infiltrate and isolated individual myocyte necrosis (*boxed area*) shown at higher magnification in **b.**

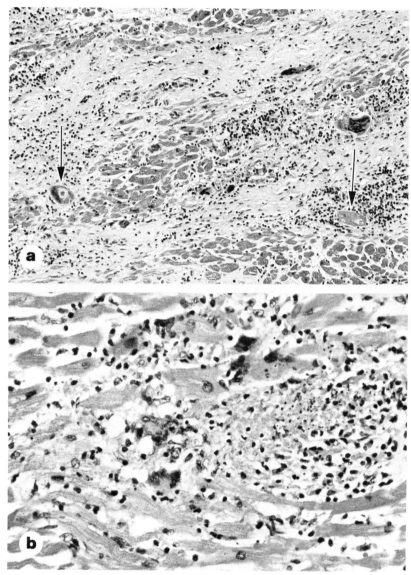

Figure 20. a. Granulomatous myocarditis with interstitial fibrosis in cardiac sarcoidosis; note the multinucleated giant cells with inclusion bodies (*arrows*). **b.** Idiopathic giant cell myocarditis with cardiac myocyte necrosis; the giant cells are thought to be either myogenic or histiocytic in origin.

Cardiac Sarcoidosis and Giant Cell Myocarditis

Cardiac sarcoidosis and giant cell myocarditis (Fig. 20) can now be diagnosed in living patients by endomyocardial biopsy and both conditions respond favorably to treatment with corticosteroids.[48,51] However, the pathologist should be reminded that because of the sampling problem, cardiac sarcoidosis in endomyocardial biopsies may appear as a lymphocytic myocarditis with prominent inter-stitial fibrosis without the telltale granulomas and giant cells.

Cardiac sarcoidosis has been, until recently, a neglected entity. Clinicians are hardly aware of cardiac involvement, and it is seldom diagnosed before death.[24] Arrhythmia, heart blocks, and sudden death are common, and they are often the initial manifestations of unsuspected cardiac sarcoidosis.[45] Subclinical involvement of the heart in sarcoidosis almost certainly occurs more often than it is generally recognized. In a review of autopsy cases, cardiac granulomas were found in 23 of 84 patients (27 percent) dying of systemic sarcoidosis, but in 8 of the 23 patients (35 percent) the cardiac sarcoidosis was clinically silent.[75]

Idiopathic giant cell myocarditis is a distinct clinicopathologic entity. It resembles cardiac sarcoidosis, but can be distinguished histologically (Fig. 20). It is characterized by a granulomatous inflammation of the myocardium with multinucleated giant cells in the infiltrate and, usually, widespread cardiac myocyte necrosis.[20,29] The disease occurs predominantly in young to middle-aged adults and the clinical course is rapidly fatal with sudden onset of symp-toms.[20] Implicit in the definition of idiopathic giant cell myocarditis is the notion that the lesion is limited to the heart. However, giant cell myocarditis with multiple organ involvement, including the blood vessels, has also been reported, as has the association of myocarditis with thymic tumors, thyroiditis, rheumatic diseases, and ulcerative colitis.[20,34,52,60]The derivation of the multinu-cleated giant cells in myocarditis remains controversial and, according to recent studies,[82,83] supports for either a myogenic or macrophage–histiocytic origin are divided.

CARDIAC ALLOGRAFT REJECTION

It was the successful use of the procedure for the management of cardiac allograft rejection first proposed in 1973 to 1974[15] that launched endomyocardial biopsy as a diagnostic tool for the investigation of myocardial disease. After a decade of experience,[7] diagnosis of cardiac rejection by endomyocardial biopsy has been continually fine tuned and modified.[28,53] The subject has been discussed in detail elsewhere, recently,[33] and will not be duplicated in this chapter.

CARDIOMYOPATHIES

Idiopathic or primary cardiomyopathies, defined as heart muscle diseases of unknown cause, comprise three distinct groups: (1) hypertrophic, (2) dilated (previously congestive), and (3) restrictive. These exclude all other conditions in which the myocardial disorder is part of a general systemic disease.[26]

Endomyocardial biopsy has been roundly advocated for the diagnosis of cardiomyopathies,[25,73] but the results to date have been quite disappoint-ing.[5,42,80] Neither idiopathic hypertrophic nor dilated cardiomyopathy have pathognomonic histological features that can be captured by endomyocardial biopsies. The pathologist's conclusion of an endomyocardial biopsy that reads "if ischemic, valvular, or hypertensive heart disease can be excluded, the findings are compatible with idiopathic dilated (or hypertrophic) cardiomyopathy" is an acknowledgment of the inadequacy of the procedure (biopsy) as a diagnostic tool for the disease (cardiomyopathy) in question.[5]

Hypertrophic Cardiomyopathy

The cardiologist does not need nor should he or she rely on an endomyocardial biopsy to diagnose hypertrophy cardiomyopathy. Myocardial fiber disarray is a histological feature of hypertrophy cardiomyopathy but it lacks specificity without a quantitative assessment,[80] which an endomyocardial biopsy cannot offer. Furthermore, myocardial fiber disarray is usually not found immediately subendocardial, within the reach of the bioptome; and a random focus of subendocardial fiber disarray may be a normal occurrence (see Fig. 3a) and not indicative of hypertrophic cardiomyopathy. An isolated focus of fiber disarray can be found quite frequently in normal and abnormal hearts and has no diagnostic value whatsoever (Fig. 21). Other characteristic, but nonspecific, histological features of hypertrophic cardiomyopathy include thick-walled occlusive small vessel disease of the myocardium and contraction band myofibrillar degeneration (Fig. 22). The latter also occurs in ischemic contracture of the hypertrophied heart, or "stone heart."[4,47,88]

Dilated Cardiomyopathy

Because of the absence of specific histological features in dilated cardiomyopathy, the role of endomyocardial biopsies in diagnosis and management of this primary myocardial disease is questionable.[5] When a biopsy is performed to rule out idiopathic lymphocytic myocarditis in patients with unexplained congestive heart failure, the success rate is so disparate and unpredictable that no valid conclusion is possible.[42]

The histological findings in dilated cardiomyopathy are largely determined by the time course of the disease. The cardiac myocytes may show no detectable light microscopic abnormalities early in the evolution of the disease. Toward the end stage of the disease, a biopsy may show varying degrees of myocyte hypertrophy, vacuolar degeneration, fiber dropout, and interstitial fibrosis. None of these is specific and all, when fully developed, may be indistinguishable from changes of anthracycline cardiotoxicity (Fig. 23).[9] Clinically, anthracycline cardiotoxicity usually manifests as dilated (congestive) cardiomyopathy,[5] but a more recent study[56] suggests that pronounced endocardial fibrosis may occur and result in the development of restrictive endomyocardial disease.

Restrictive Cardiomyopathy

Restrictive cardiomyopathy is characterized hemodynamically by impaired ventricular compliance with normal systolic function.[6] Idiopathic endomyocardial fibrosis is the only "pure" type of restrictive cardiomyopathy. Tropical and

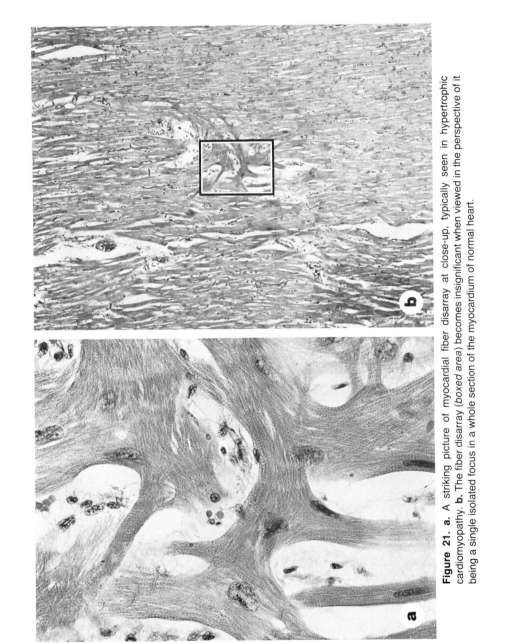

Figure 21. a. A striking picture of myocardial fiber disarray at close-up, typically seen in hypertrophic cardiomyopathy. **b.** The fiber disarray (*boxed area*) becomes insignificant when viewed in the perspective of it being a single isolated focus in a whole section of the myocardium of normal heart.

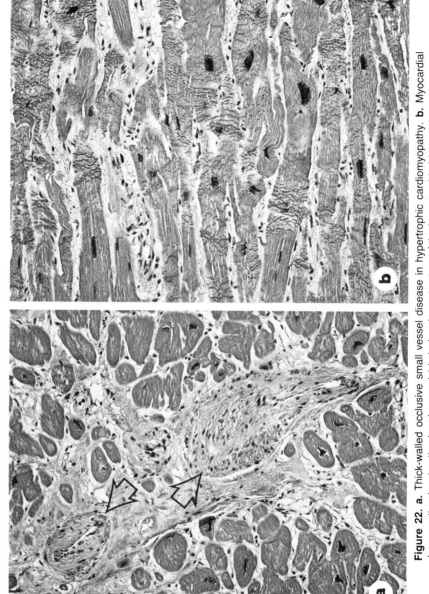

Figure 22. a. Thick-walled occlusive small vessel disease in hypertrophic cardiomyopathy. **b.** Myocardial degeneration (contraction band necrosis) in ischemic contracture of the hypertrophied (stone) heart.

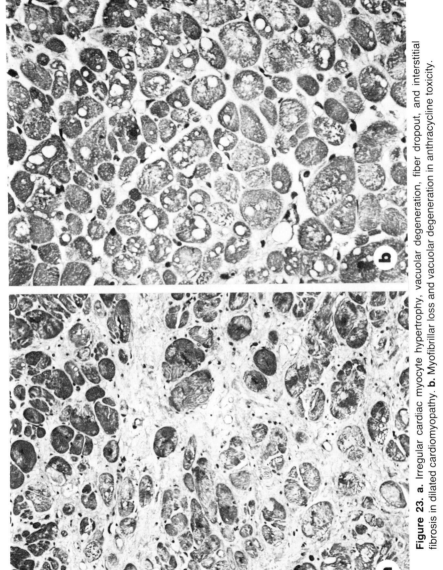

Figure 23. a. Irregular cardiac myocyte hypertrophy, vacuolar degeneration, fiber dropout, and interstitial fibrosis in dilated cardiomyopathy. **b.** Myofibrillar loss and vacuolar degeneration in anthracycline toxicity.

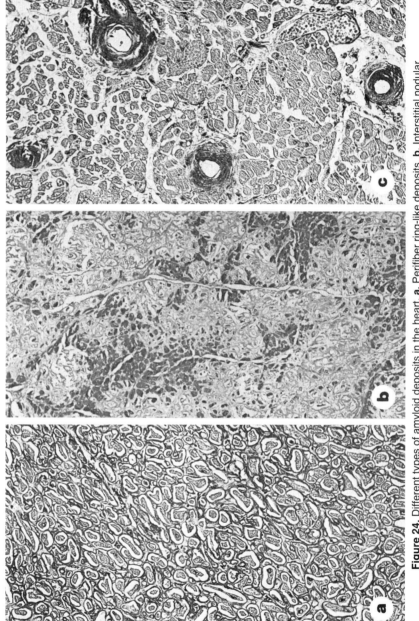

Figure 24. Different types of amyloid deposits in the heart. **a.** Perifiber ring-like deposits. **b.** Interstitial nodular deposits. **c.** Vascular deposits with little or no involvement of cardiac myocytes.

temporate climate types of endomyocardial fibrosis are one and the same disease, and both begin as an eosinophilic myocarditis.[58,78]

Cardiac amyloidosis was originally classified as a restrictive cardiomyopathy. Inasmuch as amyloidosis may occur in organs other than the heart, even when the heart is the predominant site of involvement,[39,76] it should be classified as a *specific heart muscle disease*.[5,26] Functionally, cardiac amyloidosis has many features in common with the diastolic abnormalities in restrictive and hypertrophic cardiomyopathies, but end-stage cardiac amyloidosis with progressive loss of systolic function may simulate dilated cardiomyopathy or even chronic ischemic heart disease.[12] The pattern of amyloid deposition in the heart may be predominantly perifiber, interstitial, or vascular (Fig. 24), and each has its own clinical significance. Perifiber and interstitial deposits are more common in senile cardiac amyloidosis, whereas vascular deposits predominate in primary systemic amyloidosis.[39,76]

CONCLUSION

Heart disease is the leading cause of death. The growing clinical application of endomyocardial biopsy has heightened the need of pathologists for greater proficiency in diagnostic cardiac histology. This review offers a pictorial survey of normal and abnormal cardiac histology as an aid to pathologists in the diagnosis of common and uncommon forms of heart disease. It focuses on the typical histological findings as well as highlighting the subtleties and pitfalls for which one needs to be watchful. Major categories of cardiac histopathology surveyed in this chapter include normal histology, variations, and artifacts; ischemic heart disease; myocarditis; and cardiomyopathies.

REFERENCES

1. Adomian GE, Laks MM, Billingham ME: The incidence and significance of contraction bands in endomyocardial biopsies from normal human hearts. Am Heart J 95:348, 1978
2. Aretz HT, Billingham ME, Edwards WD, et al: Myocarditis: A histopathologic definition and classification. Am J Cardiovasc Pathol 1:3, 1986
3. Bank I, Marboe CC, Redberg RF, Jacobs J: Myocarditis in adult Still's disease. Arthritis Rheum 28:452, 1985
4. Baroldi G, Milam JD, Wukasch DC, et al: Myocardial cell damage in "stone hearts." J Mol Cell Cardiol 6:395, 1974
5. Becker AE: Pathology of cardiomyopathies. Cardiovasc Clin 19(1):9, 1988
6. Benotti JR, Grossman W, Cohn PF: Clinical profile of restrictive cardiomyopathy. Circulation 61:1206, 1980
7. Billingham ME: Diagnosis of cardiac rejection by endomyocardial biopsy. Heart Transplant 1:25, 1982
8. Billingham ME: Acute myocarditis: A diagnostic dilemma. Br Heart J 56:6, 1987

9. Billingham ME, Mason JW, Bristow MR, Daniel JR: Anthracycline cardiomyopathy monitored by morphologic changes. Cancer Treat Rep 62:865, 1978

10. Bloom W, Fawcett DW: A Textbook of Histology. Philadelphia: Saunders, 1968, pp. 285–300

11. Bouchardy B, Majuo G: Histopathology of early myocardial infarcts. Am J Pathol 74:301, 1974

12. Brigden W: Cardiac amyloidosis. Prog Cardiovasc Dis 7:142, 1964

13. Carle BN: Autofluorescence in the identification of myocardial infarcts. Hum Pathol 12:643, 1981

14. Cathcart ES, Spodick DH: Rheumatoid heart disease: A study of the incidence and nature of cardiac lesions in rheumatoid arthritis. N Engl J Med 266:959, 1962

15. Caves PK, Billingham ME, Stinson EB, Shumway NE: Serial transvenous biopsy of the transplant human heart: Improved management of acute rejection episodes. Lancet 1:821, 1974

16. Chopra P: Origin of Aschoff nodule: An ultrastructural, light microscopic and histochemical evaluation. Jap Heart J 26:227, 1985

17. Chopra P, Sabherwal U: Histochemical and fluorescent techniques for detection of early myocardial ischemia following experimental coronary artery occlusion: A comparative and quantitative study. Angiology 39:132, 1988

18. Dalldorf FG, Murphy GE: Relationship of Aschoff bodies in cardiac atrial appendages to the natural history of rheumatic heart disease. Am J Pathol 37:507, 1960

19. Daly K, Richardson PJ, Olsen EGJ, et al: Acute myocarditis: Role of histological and virological examination in the diagnosis and assessment of immunosuppressive treatment. Br Heart J 51:30, 1984

20. Davies MJ, Pomerance A, Teare RD: Idiopathic giant cell myocarditis: A distinctive clinicopathological entity. Br Heart J 37:192, 1975

21. Denbow CE, Lie JT, Tancredi RG, Bunch TW: Cardiac involvement in polymyositis: A clinical pathologic study of 20 autopsied patients. Arthritis Rheum 22:1088, 1979

22. Eckstein R, Mempel W, Bolte HD: Reduced suppressor cell activity in congestive cardiomyopathy and myocarditis. Circulation 65:1224, 1982

23. Fenoglio JJ, Pham TD, Hordof A, et al: Right atrial ultrastructure in congenital heart disease. Am J Cardiol 43:820, 1979

24. Fleming HA: Sarcoid heart disease: A review and an appeal. Thorax 35:641, 1980

25. Fowles RE, Mason JW: Endomyocardial biopsy. Ann Intern Med 97:885, 1982

26. Goodwin JF: Overview and classification of the cardiomyopathies. Cardiovasc Clin 19(1):1, 1988

27. Gore I, Saphir O: Myocarditis: A classification of 1402 cases. Arch Pathol Lab Med 34:827, 1947

28. Graham AR, Paplanus SH: Fluorescence of damaged myocardium in endomyocardial biopsy specimen for the evaluation of cardiac transplantation. Hum Pathol 16:1110, 1985

29. Johansen A: Isolated myocarditis versus myocardial sarcoidosis. Acta Pathol Microbiol Scandinav 67:15, 1966

30. Jordan HE, Bardin J: The relation of the intercalated discs to the so-called "segmentation" and "fragmentation" of heart muscle. Anat Anz 43:612, 1913

31. Karch SB: The pathology of the heart in near drowning. Arch Pathol Lab Med 109:176, 1985

32. Karch SB, Billingham ME: Myocardial contraction bands revisited. Hum Pathol 17:9, 1986
33. Kemnitz J, Cohnert T, Schäfers HJ, et al: A classification of cardiac allograft rejection: A modification of the classification by Billingham. Am J Surg Pathol 11:503, 1987
34. Kennedy LJ, Mitchinson MJ: Giant cell arteritis with myositis and myocarditis. Calif Med 115:84, 1971
35. Kitaura Y: Experimental Coxsackie virus myocarditis in mice: 18-month histologic and virologic study. Jpn Heart J 45:47, 1981
36. Kosek JC, Angell W: Fine structure of basophilic myocardial degeneration. Arch Pathol Lab Med 89:491, 1970
37. Lebowitz WB: The heart in rheumatoid arthritis (rheumatoid disease). A clinical and pathological study of sixty-two cases. Ann Intern Med 58:102, 1963
38. Lie JT: Rheumatoid arthritis and heart disease. Primary Cardiol 8(10):137, 1982
39. Lie JT: Pathology of amyloidosis and amyloid heart disease. Applied Pathol 2:341, 1984
40. Lie JT: The classification of vasculitis and a reappraisal of allergic granulomatosis and angiitis (Churg–Strauss syndrome). Mount Sinai J Med 53:429, 1986
41. Lie JT: Cardiac and pulmonary manifestations of Behçet's syndrome. Pathol Res Pract 183:347, 1988
42. Lie JT: Myocarditis and endomyocardial biopsy in unexplained heart failure: A diagnosis in search of a disease. Ann Intern Med 109:525, 1988
43. Lie JT, Hammond PI: Pathology of the senescent heart: Anatomic observations on 237 autopsy studies of patients 90 to 105 years old. Mayo Clin Proc 63:552, 1988
44. Lie JT, Holley KE, Kampa WR, Titus JL: New histochemical method for morphologic diagnosis of early stages of myocardial ischemia. Mayo Clin Proc 46:319, 1971
45. Lie JT, Hunt D, Valentine PA: Sudden death from cardiac sarcoidosis with involvement of conduction system. Am J Med Sci 267:123, 1974
46. Lie JT, Pairolero PC, Holley KE, Titus JE: Macroscopic enzyme-mapping verification of large, homogeneous experimental myocardial infarcts of predictable size and location in dogs. J Thorac Cardiovasc Surg 69:599, 1975
47. Lie JT, Sun SC: Ultrastructure of ischemic contracture of the left ventricle ("stone heart"). Mayo Clin Proc 51:785, 1976
48. Lorell B, Alderman EL, Mason JW: Cardiac sarcoidosis: Diagnosis with endomyocardial biopsy and treatment with corticosteroids. Am J Cardio 42:143, 1978
49. Love GL, Restrepo C: Aschoff bodies of rheumatic carditis are granulomatous lesions of histiocytic origin. Modern Pathol 1:256, 1988
50. Matsumori A, Kawai C: An experimental model for congestive heart failure after encephalomyocarditis virus myocarditis in mice. Circulation 65:1230, 1982
51. McFalls EO, Hosenpud JD, McAnulty JH, et al: Granulomatous myocarditis: Diagnosis by endomyocardial biopsy and response to corticosteroids in two patients. Chest 89:509, 1986
52. McKeon J, Haagsma B, Bett JHN, Boyle CM: Fatal giant cell myocarditis after colectomy for ulcerative colitis. Am Heart J 111:1208, 1986
53. Meda K, Baumgartner WA, Beschorner WE, et al: Histologic pattern of early heart allograft rejection under cyclosporine treatment. Heart Transplant 4:296, 1985
54. Miklozek CL, Crumpacker CS, Royal HD, et al: Myocarditis presenting as acute myocardial infarction. Am Heart J 115:768, 1988

55. Miller JJ III, French JW: Myocarditis in juvenile rheumatoid arthritis. Am J Dis Child 131:205, 1977

56. Mortensen SA, Olsen HS, Baandrup U: Chronic anthracycline cardiotoxicity: Haemodynamic and histopathological manifestations suggesting a restrictive endomyocardial disease. Br Heart J 55:274, 1986

57. National Center for Health Statistics: Vital Statistics of the United States, 1984. Washington DC, Public Health Service 1987; DHHS publication (PHS)87–1122

58. Odek-Ogunde M: Myocardial capillary density in hypertensive rats. Lab Invest 46:54, 1982

59. Olsen EGJ, Spray CJF: The pathogenesis of Löffler's endomyocardial disease, and its relationship to endomyocardial fibrosis. Prog Cardiol 8:281, 1979

60. Palmer HP, Michael IE: Giant cell myocarditis with multiple organ involvement. Arch Intern Med 116:444, 1965

61. Pienaar JG, Price HM: Ultrastructure and origin of the Anitschkow cell. Am J Pathol 1063, 1967

62. Ragsdale BD: Anitschkow nuclear structure in cardiac metastases. Am J Clin Pathol 59:798, 1973

63. Roberts WC, Virmani R: Aschoff bodies at necropsy in valvular heart disease. Circulation 57:803, 1978

64. Rosai J, Lascano EF: Basophilic (mucoid) degeneration of myocardium: A disorder of glycogen metabolism. Am J Pathol 61:99, 1970

65. Rose AG, Fraser RC, Beck W: Absence of evidence of myocarditis in endomyocardial biopsy specimens from patients with dilated (congestive) cardiomyopathy. S Afr Med J 66:871, 1984

66. Roy PE: Basophilic degeneration of myocardium: An ultrastructural study. Lab Invest 32:729, 1975

67. Sahai VB, Knight B: The postmortem detection of early myocardial infarction by a simple fluorescent method. Med Sci Law 16:17, 1976

68. Saphir O: Anatomic evidence of functional disorders of the heart. Arch Pathol Lab Med 16:315, 1933

69. Saphir O: Myocarditis: A general review, with an analysis of two hundred and forty cases. Arch Pathol Lab Med 32:1000, 1941 and 33:88, 1942

70. Saphir O: The Aschoff nodule. Am J Clin Pathol 31:534, 1959

71. Schlesinger MJ, Reiner L: Focal myocytolysis of the heart. Am J Pathol 31:443, 1955

72. Scotti TM: Basophilic (mucinous) degeneration of the myocardium. Am J Clin Pathol 25:994, 1955

73. Sekiguchi M, Olsen EGJ, Goodwin JF (eds): Myocarditis and related disorders. Heart Vessels 1(suppl):58, 1985

74. Shapiro J: Calcification of the Heart. Springfield: Chas. C Thomas, 1963

75. Silverman KH, Hutchins GM, Bulkley BH: Cardiac sarcoidosis: A clinicopathologic study of 84 unselected patients with systemic sarcoidosis. Circulation 58:1204, 1978

76. Smith TJ, Kyle RA, Lie JT: Clinical significance of histopathologic patterns of cardiac amyloidosis. Mayo Clin Proc 59:547, 1984

77. Sokoloff L: The heart in rheumatoid arthritis. Am Heart J 45:635, 1953

78. Spry CJF: The hypereosinophilic syndrome: Clinical features, laboratory findings and treatment. Allergy 47:539, 1982

79. Steere AC, Batsford WP, Weinberg M, et al: Lyme carditis: Cardiac abnormalities of Lyme disease. Ann Intern Med 93:8, 1980

80. Sutton MG StJ, Lie JT, Anderson KR, et al: Histopathologic specificity of hypertro-

phic obstructive cardiomyopathy: Myocardial fiber disarray and myocardial fibrosis. Br Heart J 44:433, 1980

81. Taliercio CP, Olney BA, Lie JT: Myocarditis related to drug hypersensitivity. Mayo Clin Proc 60:463, 1985
82. Tanaka M, Ichinohasama R, Kawahara Y, et al: Acute idiopathic interstitial myocarditis: Case report with special reference to morphological characteristics of giant cells. J Clin Pathol 39:1209, 1986
83. Theaker JM, Gatter KC, Brown DC, et al: An investigation into the nature of giant cells in cardiac and skeletal muscle. Hum Pathol 19:974, 1988
84. Wagner BM, Siew S: Studies in rheumatic fever. V. Significance of human Anitschkow cell. Hum Pathol 1:45, 1970
85. Whitehead R: Isolated myocarditis. Br Heart J 27:220, 1965
86. Wilson FM, Miranda Q, Chason J, Lerner AM: Residual pathologic changes following murine Coxsackie A and B myocarditis. Am J Pathol 55:153, 1969
87. Woodruff JF: Viral myocarditis: A review. Am J Pathol 101:427, 1980
88. Wukasch DC, Reul GJ, Milam JD, Cooley DA: The "stone heart" syndrome. Surgery 72:1071, 1972

Lesions of the Breast in Children Exclusive of Typical Fibroadenoma and Gynecomastia
A Clinicopathologic Study of 113 Cases

Guido Pettinato, Juan Carlos Manivel, David R. Kelly, Lester E. Wold, and Louis P. Dehner

Breast enlargement and its clinical significance in a child must be judged according to the age, sex, hormonal status, and other physical findings. For instance, minor breast prominence is normal at birth and even into the first year of life. Breast development in a prepubertal male or female, however, may be a sign of precocious pseudopuberty secondary to a functioning gonadal or adrenal neoplasm. Later in childhood, around the time of puberty, some degree of gynecomastia is very common and, in females, breast maturation occurs through the five Tanner's phases.[1] The process of breast development is asymmetrical in some cases; normal occurrence of asymmetry or premature thelarche has resulted in unfortunate surgical intervention.[2]

Not surprisingly, for those who are familiar with pediatric pathology in general, the clinical and morphological spectrum of breast lesions is very different in children and adolescents when compared to the common adult experience of middle age to older females with fibrocystic changes and carcinomas. In the pediatric age population, fibroadenoma and gynecomastia together account for more than 70 percent of all diagnoses. Most of the published series with a few exceptions have included only adolescent females (Table 1).[3-8] Our study was undertaken to focus and amplify upon the group of breast lesions which, because of their small representations in a single institutional experience, we often relegate to a few brief comments. In order to produce a large enough sample size, the experiences of three institutions were reviewed. A particularly

*Dr. Pettinato was a research fellow at the University of Minnesota through a grant from the Associazione Italiana per la Ricerca sul Cancro, Milan, Italy.

TABLE 1. TYPES OF BREAST LESIONS IN CHILDREN AND ADOLESCENTS: REVIEW OF SIX PUBLISHED SERIES

	Bower et al[3]	Stone et al[4]	Farrow and Ashikari[5]	Simpson and Barson[6]	Hein et al[7]	Jimenez et al[8]	Total	(%)
Fibroadenoma	84	104	181	5	71	13	458	70
Gynecomastia	23	—	—	—	—	15	38	6
Cyst and fibrocystic changes	3	9	33	—	9	—	54	8
Inflammation	9	4	2	—	11	—	26	4
Intraductal papillomatosis	1	4	13	1	—	—	19	3
Hyperplasia	—	17	—	—	—	—	17	3
Cystosarcoma phyllodes	—	2	—	—	2	3[a]	7	1
Fat necrosis	1	—	5	—	—	—	6	1
Pubertal hypertrophy	4	—	—	—	—	2	6	1
Hemangioma	—	—	—	2	—	—	2	< 1
Rhabdomyosarcoma	1	—	2	—	—	—	3	< 1
Adenocarcinoma	—	1	1	1	—	—	3	< 1
Lipoma	1	—	—	—	2	—	3	< 1
Fibrosis	—	2	—	—	—	—	2	< 1
Granular cell tumor	—	1	—	—	—	—	1	< 1
Supernumerary nipple	2	—	—	—	—	—	2	< 1
Axillary breast tissue	1	—	—	—	—	—	1	< 1
Other	4	1	—	—	—	—	5	< 1
Total	134	145	237	9	95	33	653	100

[a]Two benign cystosarcoma phyllodes

worrisome variant of fibroadenoma, the juvenile cellular fibroadenoma, and pubertal or juvenile hypertrophy were the two most common lesions in our survey. However, there were several examples of "small round cell neoplasms," a familiar category of highly malignant tumors of childhood, which are typically found in sites other than the breast.[9] Approximately 11 percent of all breast tumors in this composite review were malignant, which is probably in excess of the overall frequency due to the referral nature of our institutions.

MATERIALS AND METHODS

One hundred and thirteen cases of breast lesions which presented either as diffuse enlargement or as a discrete mass in patients 20 years of age or less at diagnosis were retrieved for study. These cases were accessioned in the files of the Division of Surgical Pathology, University of Minnesota Hospital and Clinics, Minneapolis, Minnesota; the Department of Pathology and Laboratory Medicine, The Children's Hospital, Birmingham, Alabama; and the Department of Surgical Pathology, Mayo Clinic, Rochester, Minnesota.

Slides and reports were reviewed and referring physicians were contacted for clinical follow-up. Only fibroadenomas showing prominent stromal cellularity to qualify as a "cellular fibroadenoma" or benign phyllodes tumor were included,[2] whereas the usual, uncomplicated fibroadenomas and cases of gynecomastia were excluded from the study. Hematoxylin and eosin (H&E) stained sections were available in each case; in selected cases, mucicarmine, periodic acid Schiff (PAS), trichrome and Fontana–Masson stains were also available. In cases of small-cell malignancies and in some vascular tumors, immunohistochemical studies were performed. Paraffin-embedded sections were treated with antibodies against the following antigens: leukocyte common antigen (LCA, DakoPatts, Santa Barbara, CA, 1:40); vimentin (BioGenex Co., Dublin CA, 1:8000); desmin (BioGenex Co., 1:2); muscle-specific actin (Enzo-Biochem., New York, NY, 1:4000); epithelial membrane antigen (EMA, DakoPatts, 1:1000); cytokeratins AE1/AE3 (CK, Hybritech Inc., San Diego, CA, 1:150); neuron-specific enolase (NSE, BioGenex Co., 1:300); neurofilaments (NF, BioGenex Co., 1:200); synaptophysin (SP, Boehringer-Manheim Biochemicals, Indianapolis, IN, 1:75); S-100 protein (DakoPatts, 1:600); and Factor VIII-related antigen (DakoPatts, 1:80). Affinity for *Ulex europaeus I* agglutinin (UEA, Vector, Burlingame, CA, 1:2000; rabbit anti-Ulex, Dako-Patts, 1:2000) was also assessed. Immunoperoxidase procedures were performed as previously described using peroxidase–antiperoxidase (PAP) and avidin–biotin–peroxidase complex (ABC) methods.[10,11] Appropriate positive and negative controls were included. In two cases of peripheral neuroectodermal tumor and two cases of rhabdomyosarcoma, tissue was fixed in 2 percent glutaraldehyde for electron microscopy.

TABLE 2. DEMOGRAPHIC FEATURES, SITE, AND TYPE OF BREAST INVOLVEMENT

Age	Range	4 mo–20 yr
	Mean	13.5 yr
	Median	14.5 yr
	< 1 yr	6 (5%)
	< 10 yr	19 (17%)
	< 15 yr	85 (75%)
Sex	Females	102 (90%)
	Males	11 (10%)
Race	White	60 (54%)
	Black	53 (47%)
Site	Right	40
	Left	38
	Bilateral	23 (21 (s); 2 (m))[a]
	Multiple	5 (3 left, 2 right)
	Unknown	12

[a]s = synchronous; m = metachronous.

RESULTS

Table 2 summarizes the clinical findings of the 113 patients. The ages at diagnosis ranged from 4 months to 20 years (mean, 13.5 years; median, 14.5 years). Six patients (5.3 percent) were 1 year old or less, 19 (16.9 percent) were 10 years or less, and 85 (75.2 percent) were 15 years or less. There were 102 females and 11 males. Sixty patients were Caucasian and 53 were black; the latter were almost exclusively from The Children's Hospital, Birmingham, Alabama. Twenty-three patients had bilateral masses (21 synchronous and 2 metachronous) and 5 patients had multiple lesions in the same breast. There were 13 malignancies (11.5 percent), 5 of which were primary and 8 metastatic. The lesions were divided into five principal pathologic categories (Table 3).

Congenital and Developmental Anomalies

Ten cases (8.8 percent) represented one or another expression of congenital or anomalous development. A supernumerary nipple was excised in two girls, ages 10 and 12 years; and histologically, all components of the normal nipple including fibromuscular tissues and ductal structures were identified. A congenital breast nodule measuring 0.4 cm presented in the subareolar region of an infant female. Microscopically, it consisted of diminutive lobules and dilated ducts, moderately hyperplastic epithelium, and luminal secretions. Seven adolescent females (mean age, 14 years) presented with a moderately firm axillary mass measuring from 3 to 6 cm in greatest dimension. Grossly, the excised specimen consisted of fibrous and fatty tissue with an ellipse of skin. Histologically, each mass was composed of breast tissue in the lower dermis and subcutaneous tissue, and was characterized by discrete fibroepithelial nodules without lobular differentiation. An inflammatory infiltrate within the accessory breast tissue explained the clinical impression of hydradenitis suppurativa in one case.

TABLE 3. LESIONS OF THE BREAST IN CHILDREN AND ADOLESCENTS: AGES, SEX DISTRIBUTION, AND PATHOLOGIC TYPES IN 113 CASES

			No. of Cases	Sex M	Sex F	Age
A.	Congenital and developmental anomalies:					
	Accessory breast tissue		7	0	7	11–15 yr
	Supernumerary nipple		2	0	2	10, 12 yr
	Congenital hypertrophy		1	0	1	Newborn
		Total	10 (9%)			
B.	Inflammatory conditions:					
	Acute and chronic mastitis		13	0	13	11–16 yr
	Fat necrosis		3	0	3	8–14 yr
		Total	16 (14%)			
C.	Cysts and fibrocystic changes:					
	Fibrous mastopathy		6	1	5	14–17 yr
	Galactocele		3	3	0	1–6 yr
	Fibrocystic changes		2	0	2	16, 20 yr
	Fibroadenomatosis		2	0	2	18, 19 yr
	Keratin cyst of nipple		2	1	1	9, 13 yr
	Solitary cyst		2	1	1	11, 13 yr
		Total	17 (15%)			
D.	Tumor-like lesions:					
	Juvenile hypertrophy		20	0	20	8–17 yr
	Juvenile papillomatosis		5	0	5	15–19 yr
		Total	25 (22%)			
E.	Neoplasms:					
	Juvenile cellular fibroadenoma		18	0	18	11–19 yr
	Vascular tumors		9	3	6	4 mo–17 yr
	Metastatic tumors		8	0	8	13–20 yr
	Lipoma		3	2	1	3–13 yr
	Adenoma of nipple		2	0	2	10, 14 yr
	Cystosarcoma phyllodes		2	0	2	12, 17 yr
	Fibromatosis		1	0	1	11 mo
	Malignant lymphoma (primary)		1	0	1	12 yr
	Rhabdomyosarcoma (primary)		1	0	1	12 yr
		Total	45 (40%)			
			113 (100%)			

Inflammatory Conditions

Sixteen cases in this category included 13 patients (11.5 percent) with a unilateral breast mass, mainly subareolar, and each had the histological features of mastitis. The age at diagnosis varied from 11 to 16 years (mean, 13 years). In five years, the histological findings confirmed the presence of an abscess; in the remaining cases, an acute and chronic inflammatory infiltrate was present in the stroma. *Staphylococcus aureus* was the principal pathogen in those cases with positive bacteriologic cultures. In one case, granulomatous inflammation with giant cells was the predominant feature. Special stains failed to identify acid-fast organisms or fungi. Fat necrosis was encountered in three patients, ages 8, 13, and 14 years. Lipophages, inflammatory cells, fibrosis, and dystrophic calcifications were the histological findings. The etiology of the fat necrosis was not apparent from the clinical history.

Cysts and Fibrocystic Changes

Seventeen patients comprised this group. Fibrocystic changes including apocrine metaplasia, cystic dilation of ducts, intraductal hyperplasia, and sclerosing adenosis were observed in two patients ages 16 and 20 years (Fig. 1). One of these patients had a maternal history of breast cancer. Two patients, 18 and 19 years old, had fibroadenomatosis or fibroadenomatoid hyperplasia, a composite lesion with fibrocystic features intermingled with fibroadenomatous foci (Figs. 2 and 3).[12] Six patients, ages 14 to 17 years, had fibrous mastopathy; they presented with a firm, mobile breast mass most commonly located in the upper outer quadrant. Histologically, a moderately cellular to dense stroma with scattered islands of terminal duct–lobular units was noted (Fig. 4). In two patients, the only abnormality in the biopsy was a solitary cyst lined by apocrine epithelium. Also included in this group were three galactoceles, all occurring in males, 12 months, 21 months, and 6 years of age. These lesions presented as a solitary nodule that measured from 3 to 6.5 cm in diameter. The contents of the lesion were milky fluid, and histologically, a cuboidal-to-columnar epithelium

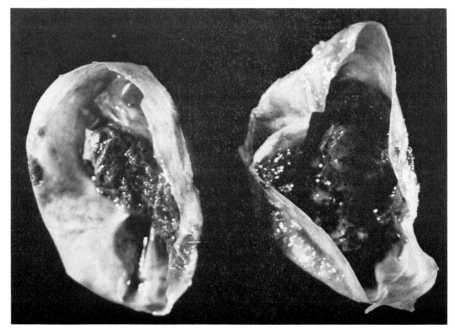

Figure 1. Fibrocystic changes. A 3-cm cyst containing partially clotted blood was excised from a 16-year-old female.

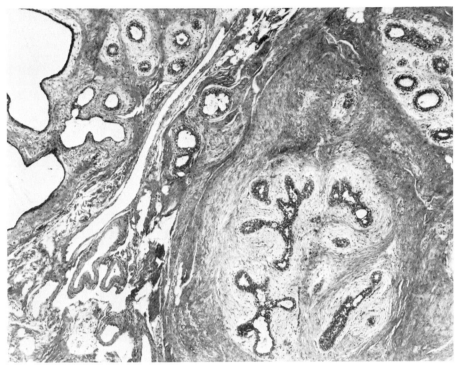

Figure 2. Fibroadenomatosis in 18-year-old female. Cystic ducts are seen on the left, fibroadenomatous tissue is on the right. (H&E ×50)

with apocrine features was identified. Two of these cases showed lactational-like secretory changes in adjacent mammary tissue (Fig. 5). None of the three young males had endocrinologic abnormalities. Two patients, 9 and 13 years of age, had keratinous (epidermal inclusion) cysts of the nipple; in one case the lesion was bilateral. Histologically, an inflammatory reaction with foreign-body granulomas to keratinous debris and squamous epithelium was observed.

Tumor-Like Lesions

There were 25 cases in this category. Twenty patients (17.6 percent) between the ages of 8 and 17 years (mean, 13.5 years) had so-called juvenile hypertrophy (pubertal hypertrophy, macromastia). In all cases, a disproportionate enlargement of one or both breasts occurred over a relatively short period of a few weeks to months. The lesions were bilateral in ten patients, and the enlargement was asymmetrical in six instances. A history of irregular menses was recorded in five patients. Reduction mammoplasty was performed in eight patients and the remainder had biopsies only. The excised tissue weighed from 71 to 5481 grams (mean, 630 grams). The cut surface was homogeneous,

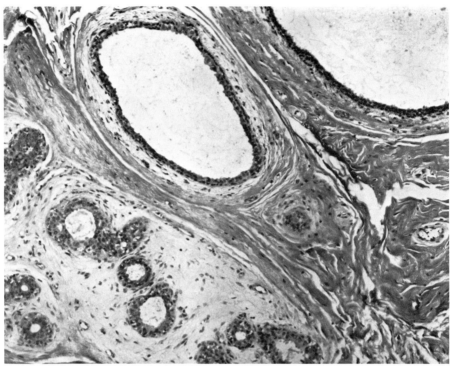

Figure 3. Fibroadenomatosis. Dilated ducts in a fibrous stroma (*upper right*) are seen adjacent to fibroadenomatous tissue (*lower left*). (H&E ×100)

grayish-tan to yellow. A diffuse, uniform, dense fibrous stroma with irregularly distributed ducts was the histological appearance (Fig. 6). Varying degrees of intraductal hyperplasia and cystic dilation of the ducts without lobular accentuation were present. A periductal zone of edema and a very mild chronic inflammatory infiltrate were reminiscent of gynecomastia.

Five patients (4.5 percent), ages 15 to 19 years, had juvenile papillomatosis ("swiss-cheese disease"); they presented with a firm and freely mobile mass. Grossly, a poorly demarcated mass measuring 2.5 to 3.0 cm in greatest dimension with multiple cysts was observed; in some cases, ill-defined fibrous tissue merged with the multicystic areas (Fig. 7). Microscopically, dilated ducts and cysts, marked papillomatosis, papillary apocrine metaplasia, sclerosing adenosis, ductal ectasia, scattered inflammatory cells, and mild cytological atypia were constant features (Figs. 8 and 9). Necrosis was not seen, but prominent mitotic activity was present in two cases. Follow-up biopsy of the ipsilateral breast in one patient 6 years later, at 21 years of age, revealed fibrocystic changes of a low risk type and sclerosing papillary proliferations.[13] The remaining four patients with follow-up to 11 years have had no local recurrences nor developed breast cancer.

Neoplasms

Forty-five cases were neoplasms and represented the most diverse pathologic group of lesions in the study. Nipple duct adenoma (florid papillomatosis of the nipple, subareolar papillomatosis) was observed in two girls, ages 10 and 14 years; they presented with a unilateral subareolar mass measuring 1 and 2 cm in diameter, respectively. Both patients had a history of a rapidly enlarging nodule of the nipple with erosion of the overlying skin. Microscopically, one lesion showed a sclerosing papillomatous growth with syringomatous features, and the other a florid papillomatosis pattern without sclerosis. Both tumors showed a complex glandular pattern with extension of the glands to the ulcerated surface, hyperplasia of the residual surface epithelium, squamous-lined cysts at the superficial ends of the ducts, scattered mitotic figures, and chronic inflammation (Fig. 10). Neither apocrine changes nor necrosis were noted. Simple excision was curative in both cases.

Eighteen females (15.9 percent) had juvenile cellular fibroadenomas; they ranged in age from 11 to 19 years (mean, 14.5 years). Sixteen patients were black. A history of rapid growth over a period of a few weeks to months was provided in a majority of patients. The tumors ranged from 1 to 11 cm in size,

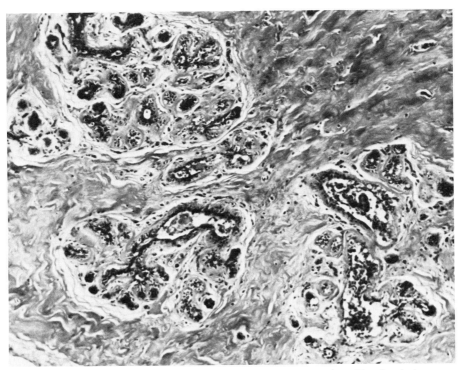

Figure 4. Fibrous mastopathy in a 14-year-old female presenting with a firm fusiform mass. Lobules are surrounded by dense hypocellular collagen. (H&E ×100)

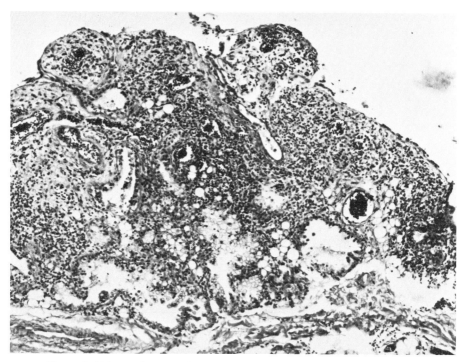

Figure 5. Galactocele presenting as a 6.5-cm cyst in a 12-month-old male. The cyst wall is inflammed and secretory changes are observed in the glandular structures (*lower, center*). (H&E ×60)

with a mean of 2.9 cm (5 < 2 cm, 13 between 2 and 5 cm). Five patients had multiple unilateral masses and six had bilateral tumors. One patient with a history of irregular menses had the changes of juvenile hypertrophy in the contralateral breast. Grossly, the tumors were all well circumscribed with bosselated external surfaces. The cut surface was gray to pink and multinodular (Fig. 11). Some tumors had cleft-like depressions and minute cysts. Histologically, these tumors were all characterized by prominent cellularity of the periductal stroma (Fig. 12). A spindle-cell proliferation was associated with pericanalicular and intracanalicular patterns of growth; the latter produced a phyllodes-like appearance. The periductal stromal spindle cells showed no atypia; mitotic activity was inconspicuous in each instance. A consistent microscopic feature was the presence of scattered areas with decreased stromal cellularity and fibrosis. A moderate to even marked degree of ductal epithelial hyperplasia was present in approximately 50 percent of the tumors. None of the patients contacted to 5 years developed breast cancer.

Cystosarcoma phyllodes was diagnosed in two females, 12 and 17 years of age, who presented with a solitary mass of several months' duration. In one patient, an encapsulated 7-cm tumor was excised with surrounding normal-appearing breast tissue. A small, round cell neoplasm with the features of embryonal rhabdomyosarcoma virtually replaced the remnants of the cytosarcoma phyllodes. The patient died within a year of diagnosis with widespread metastases to the bones, lungs, and liver. The other patient had a circumscribed but non-encapsulated tumor measuring 9 × 6 cm and weighing 75 grams. The cut surface was gray-tan to yellow, with cyst-like structures and clefts. Histologically, branching epithelial structures were surrounded by atypical vacuolated cells with the features of lipoblasts (Fig. 13). Following a diagnosis of cytosarcoma phyllodes with liposarcomatous stroma, the patient underwent simple mastectomy. She remains well 1 year later.

A single case of fibromatosis of the breast was seen in this group. The patient was an 11-month-old female with an ill-defined firm mass. Histologically, dense cellular fibroblastic tissue surrounded the normal glandular structures of the breast (Fig. 14). The spindle-cell proliferation formed irregular bundles and contained rare mitotic figures.

Three examples of lipoma were identified in patients 3 to 13 years of age.

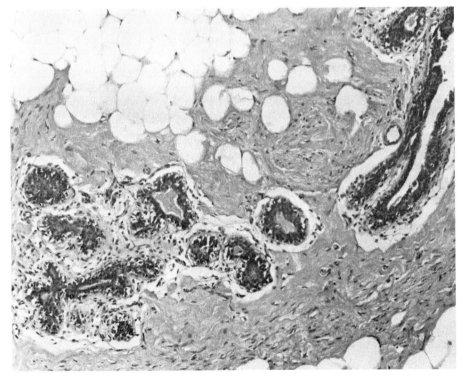

Figure 6. Juvenile hypertrophy in a 12-year-old female with bilateral, diffuse breast enlargement. Ducts are surrounded by dense connective tissue. Note periductal clear areas due to edema or stromal retraction. (H&E ×100)

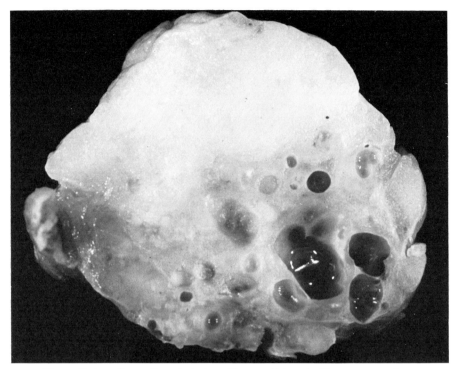

Figure 7. Juvenile papillomatosis in a 17-year-old female. The gross specimen consists of multiple cysts and dense fibrous stroma.

The encapsulated tumors ranged from 2.4 to 8.2 cm in diameter; they were bilateral in one patient. No recurrences were observed after simple excision.

Nine patients (7.9 percent) with vascular tumors ranged in age from 4 months to 17 years (mean, 6.2 years; median, 1.4 years). Diffuse capillary hemangioma, the most common vascular neoplasm, occurred in four children, 4 to 12 months of age, as subareolar solitary nodules measuring 2 to 3 cm. One child had a similar lesion on the scalp. Histologically, a meshwork of capillary-sized vessels with a multinodular configuration intermingled with the lobular and terminal duct units (Fig. 15). One case of cavernous hemangioma was observed in a 4-year-old male. Microscopically, the lesion was poorly circumscribed, and was composed of dilated and congested cavernous blood vessels. In two patients, ages 14 and 17 years, the vascular lesions consisted of thin- and thick-walled vessels infiltrating deep fibromuscular and adipose tissue of the breast and chest wall. These lesions were interpreted as infiltrating hemangiomas of possible non-parenchymal origin.[14] All patients were free of disease after simple excision. A 16-month-old male, with a slowly growing subareolar mass, had a histiocytoid hemangioma (epithelioid hemangioma, angiolymphoid hyperplasia with eosinophilia). This lesion was composed of tightly arranged diminutive vascular spaces lined by plump endothelial cells, surrounded by lymphocytes and eosinophils. Solid sheets of endothelial cells with vacuolated cytoplasm infiltrated the stroma between the ductal structures (Fig. 16). Positive immunoreactivity for Factor VIII-related antigen and affinity for *Ulex europaeus I* agglutinin confirmed the endothelial nature of this lesion. This patient has not experienced a recurrence 3 years after excision. One example of angiosarcoma was included in this series; the patient was a 17-year-old female who presented with a left breast mass. The biopsy consisted of soft hemorrhagic tissue and histologically, anastomosing vascular channels with hyperchromatic and atypical endothelial cells, papillary projections, numerous mitoses, necrosis, and hemorrhage were the features. The patient underwent mastectomy, and she died 4 years later with osseous and pulmonary metastases.

Ten other malignant tumors were included in this study (Table 4). Among the four rhabdomyosarcomas (RMS), there was one primary tumor presenting as a solitary breast mass in a 12-year-old female. The neoplasm was composed of poorly differentiated small cells (Fig. 17). Although ultrastructural evidence for rhabdomyogenic differentiation was lacking, immunoperoxidase studies showed reactivity of individual tumor cells for desmin and muscle-specific actin (Fig. 17,

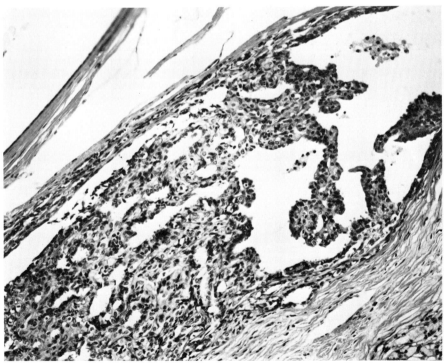

Figure 8. Juvenile papillomatosis. A complex papillary epithelial proliferation characterizes this lesion. (H&E ×160)

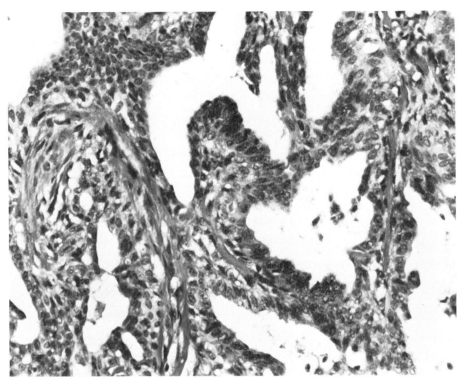

Figure 9. Juvenile papillomatosis. Papillary fronds with hyperplastic epithelium supported by delicate fibrovascular stroma. (H&E ×250)

TABLE 4. MALIGNANT TUMORS OF THE BREAST

| | Sex | | |
	M	F	Age (yr)
Primary			
Cystosarcoma phyllodes	2	0	2	12, 17
Angiosarcoma	1	0	1	17
Rhabdomyosarcoma	1	0	1	12
Lymphoma (non-Hodgkin's type)	1	0	1	12
Secondary			
Rhabdomyosarcoma	3	0	3	14–20
Peripheral neuroectodermal tumor	2	0	2	13, 16
Classic neuroblastoma	1	0	1	13
Malignant melanoma	1	0	1	20
Hodgkin's disease	1	0	1	19
Total	13 (11.5% of total series)			

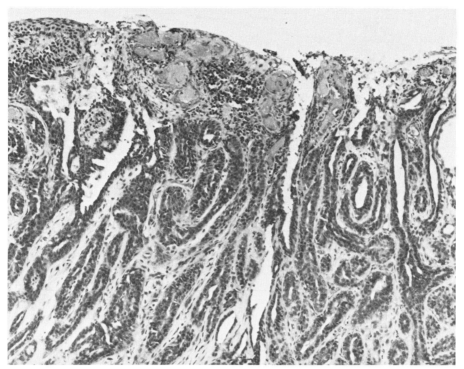

Figure 10. Nipple duct adenoma in a 14-year-old female. A complex glandular proliferation extends to the overlying ulcerated skin. (H&E ×160)

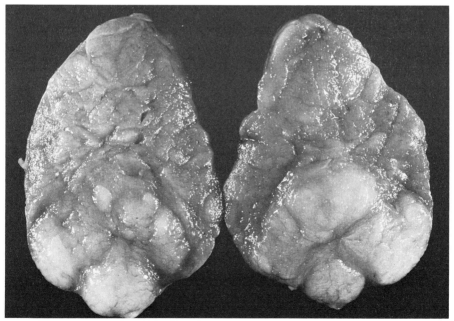

Figure 11. Juvenile cellular fibroadenoma presenting as a rapidly enlarging mass in a 14-year-old female. Note the multinodular appearance of the cut surface.

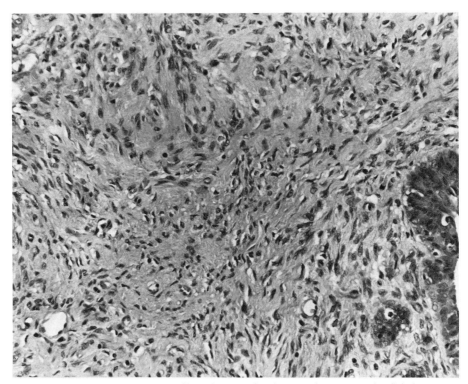

Figure 12. Juvenile cellular fibroadenoma showing prominent stromal cellularity and ducts lined by bland-appearing epithelium. (H&E ×160)

inset). Metastatic RMS presented as multiple bilateral nodules in three females, 14, 17, and 20 years of age. Microscopically, an alveolar pattern with multinucleated giant cells was observed in one case, and an embryonal pattern in the other two. In one case, ultrastructural examination showed a dense network of intermediate filaments in the cytoplasm, but myofilaments and sarcomeric differentiation were absent. Immunoperoxidase staining of this tumor for myoglobin and desmin showed focal reactivity.

Metastatic neuroblastoma presented as multiple unilateral breast nodules in a 13-year-old female who died a few months later with cerebral and bone metastases. The urinary catecholamine levels were strikingly elevated in this patient. Two cases of peripheral neuroectodermal tumor presented as breast masses. A 13-year-old female had multiple, bilateral breast nodules of 1 month's duration. Roentgenographic examination disclosed bilateral ovarian masses and filling defects in the liver. The second patient was a 16-year-old female who presented with a rapidly growing left breast mass developing over a 1-month period. An abdominal tumor was identified by computed tomography (CT) scan. After the breast biopsy, a large mass in the mesentery was resected. In both patients, urinary catecholamines were within normal limits. Histologically, the neoplasms infiltrated the stroma of the breast in a pseudoalveolar pattern of small hyperchromatic cells lining the fibrovascular connective tissue. A striking feature in one case was the presence of numerous Homer–Wright rosettes with central neurofibrillary processes (Fig. 18). In both cases, electron microscopy revealed numerous interdigitating cytoplasmic processes with microtubules and intermediate filaments. Secretory granules were identified in one case (Fig. 19). Immunoperoxidase stain for neuron-specific enolase was positive, whereas stains for actin, desmin, neurofilaments, synaptophysin, and S-100 protein were negative.

Metastatic malignant melanoma was found in the breast of a 20-year-old female who had a history of a skin lesion on the back resected 6 years before, which was interpreted as a benign nevocytic lesion. She also had enlarged axillary nodes. Immunoperoxidase reactivity for S-100 protein was helpful in the differential diagnosis of this case.

Two cases of malignant lymphoma involving the breast were observed. A 19-year-old female presented with stage III Hodgkin's disease. She underwent combined radiation and chemotherapy; 6 months later she developed a breast mass that histologically proved to be Hodgkin's disease. The other patient was a

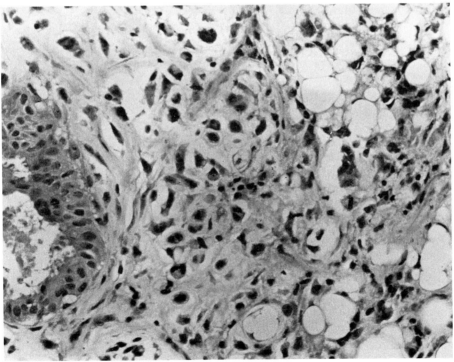

Figure 13. Cystosarcoma phyllodes in a 17-year-old female. The stroma is composed of neoplastic lipoblasts. (H&E ×200)

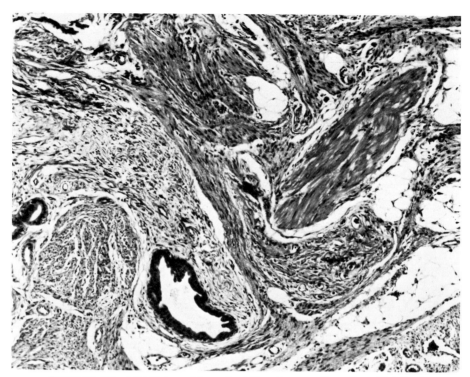

Figure 14. Fibromatosis in an 11-month-old female presenting with an ill-defined breast mass. Irregular bundles of uniform spindle cells surround and entrap mammary lobules. (H&E ×60)

12-year-old female in whom the initial and exclusive site of the disease was the breast. Histologically, a non-Hodgkin's lymphoma, diffuse, large cell type replaced the breast parenchyma and infiltrated into the fatty tissues (Fig. 20).

DISCUSSION

A decade has passed since Oberman last reviewed the topic of pathologic lesions in the breasts of young patients.[15] Reviews have emphasized the pathology of the adolescent female breast since the majority of cases present in this age group.[3,4,7,16] Our study focuses upon breast-related lesions other than the usual fibroadenoma and gynecomastia, including individuals in the first 2 decades of life with a variety of developmental, inflammatory, and neoplastic epithelial and/or mesenchymal lesions. No claims are made about the incidence or frequency of certain types of lesions from this study. It is our purpose only to amplify information on lesions which have sometimes been relegated to the "other" or "miscellaneous" category in comprehensive overviews.

Even though the clinician and pathologist may be confident that a discrete mass or diffuse enlargement of the breast(s) beyond what is generally regarded as normal in a child or adolescent is very likely benign, some anxiety on the part of the patient and family is not unexpected. Overall, less than 2 percent of all breast lesions in the pediatric age group are malignant. In the cases of malignant lymphoma or rhabdomyosarcoma, breast involvement is more often a sign of widely disseminated disease with a few exceptions. For the overwhelming majority of young adolescent females, a mass is a fibroadenoma with the typical pathologic features. In a minority of cases, marked epithelial hyperplasia, lactational changes, or a number of unusual mesenchymal alterations are recognized.[17–21] One of the more disturbing of the mesenchymal changes is the presence of stromal cellularity with or without a phyllodes pattern (wide clefts, cysts).[22,23] It was this specific type of fibroadenoma which was included in our review.

Gynecomastia is undoubtedly more common in adolescent males than the fibroadenoma is in females of the same age. There is little need in most cases of gynecomastia to biopsy or excise breast tissue except in a minority of boys who

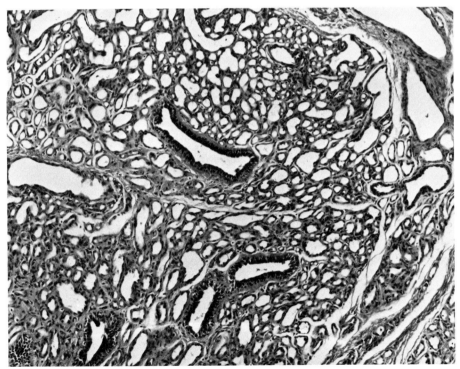

Figure 15. Capillary hemangioma presenting as a subareolar nodule in a 7-month-old female. The lesion is composed of a meshwork of small vascular spaces entrapping ductal structures. (H&E ×160)

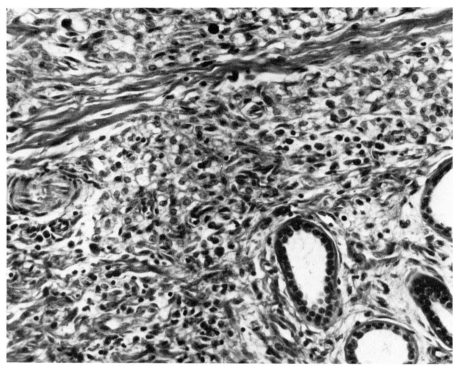

Figure 16. Histiocytoid hemangioma in a 16-month-old male. Mammary ducts are surrounded by inflammatory cells and sheets of vacuolated endothelial cells. Factor VIII-related antigen and *Ulex europaeus* were positive. (H&E ×250)

may require a reduction mammoplasty. The ductal epithelium may display dramatic proliferative changes.[2,24]

Congenital changes or developmental anomalies of the breast are either incidental and clinically inconsequential or may portend more serious problems.[1,2] For instance, subareolar breast tissue may be prominent as bilateral nodules in the newborn; this constitutes a normal congenital change and the nodules may persist throughout the first year of life.[25,26] One such case in our study was biopsied, which in retrospect was an error with the risk of excising a major portion of the developing breast. Premature thelarche may present as a unilateral subareolar nodule in a prepubertal female. Failure to appreciate the nature of the change may result in the excision of normal but asymmetrically developing breast tissue.[2] In our study, accessory mammary tissue presenting as an axillary mass was the most common developmental anomaly. There is at least one report of two generations in one family with ectopic axillary breast tissue.[27] Inflammatory changes were present in one of our cases, whereas the others were recognized as fibroepithelial nodules in the subcutaneous tissues without a discernible relationship to the breast itself. Accessory or supernumerary nipples are the vestiges of the "milk line" and are found in 1 to 2.5 percent of infants.[28] There is a reported association between accessory nipples and renal anomalies in children.[29]

Acute and chronic inflammation of the breast occurs throughout life. In the pediatric age group, neonates and adolescents are especially vulnerable.[2,30] All of the patients in our series were older children or adolescents and none gave a history of a recent pregnancy nor were lactational changes recognized in the tissues. Despite that fact, acute mastitis with or without the formation of an abscess is often related to parturition and lactation.[2] The excision of breast tissue in these cases is often a part of the procedure to drain an abscess. Inflammatory and reparative changes may produce relatively few or marked alterations of the breast parenchyma. In the latter instance, the existing ducts are compressed, distorted, and rearranged so as to produce pseudocarcinomatous changes.[15]

There were three examples of fat necrosis in this study. Necrosis of the breast in a young individual usually is associated with pregnancy and lactation.

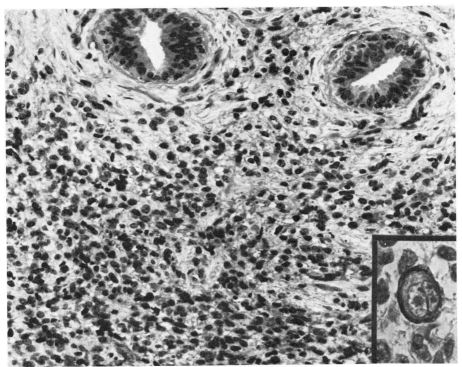

Figure 17. Primary rhabdomyosarcoma of the breast in a 12-year-old female. Small, round tumor cells infiltrate the stroma and surround mammary ducts. Cytoplasmic reactivity for desmin confirms the myogenic phenotype of this neoplasm (*inset*). (H&E: ×250, PAP: ×400)

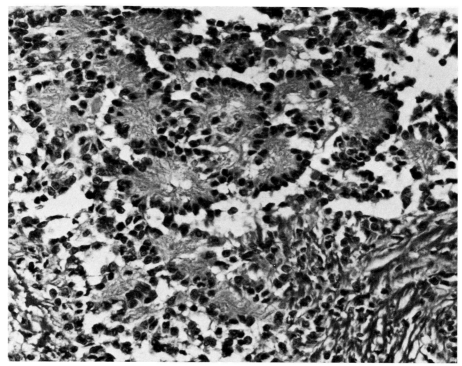

Figure 18. Metastatic peripheral neuroectodermal tumor in a 16-year-old female. Prominent Homer–Wright rosettes characterize this tumor. A normal duct is present at lower right. (H&E ×250)

It typically occurs in a fibroadenoma or lactating adenoma or occasionally as a localized finding in the parenchyma without an appreciable underlying lesion.[2] Infarction in a fibroadenoma is also seen as a spontaneous, primary event in an adolescent. In either case, an identifiable vascular occlusion is difficult to demonstrate. Our three cases were atypical in that the necrosis was confined to a focus of fat necrosis, a lesion which is more common in adult females with pendulous fatty breasts.[31] Because adipose tissue is a minor component in the adolescent female breast, there is a less vulnerable volume at risk for trauma. Although trauma was the suspected etiology for the fat necrosis in our cases, an appropriate history was not available.

Fibrocystic change (disease), also called mammary dysplasia, constitutes a group of benign cystic and proliferative lesions which are commonly encountered in breast biopsies from adult women.[31] A graded risk for the potential development of breast carcinoma has been correlated with the degree of atypia in the ductal and lobular hyperplasia.[13,32] These changes are almost exclusively confined to the adult breast, but some "no risk" lesions are recognized in the late adolescence and early adulthood. Approximately 10 percent of cases in our series represented one or another of the "no risk" lesions of fibrocystic change which compares to the 5 percent figure in the composite review of the literature (Table 1). Fibrosis or fibrous mastopathy was the most common lesion in the category of fibrocystic change, findings supported by Rivera Pomar et al.[33] More complex types of fibrocystic changes were essentially nonexistent in our study if one excludes juvenile papillomatosis or swiss cheese disease of the breast which has several features of fibrocystic change.[34] One other interesting lesion in the context of fibrocystic change is fibroadenomatosis or fibroadenomatous hyperplasia.[12] In contrast to the typical fibroadenoma with its circumscription, fibroadenomatosis is a more diffuse lesion which is composed of microscopic intra- and pericanalicular fibroadenomatoid foci and sclerosing adenosis, apocrine metaplasia, terminal duct hyperplasia, and simple cysts.

The cysts in our study were all solitary and lined by a simple cuboidal or squamous epithelium. A milky fluid was contained in the three galactoceles

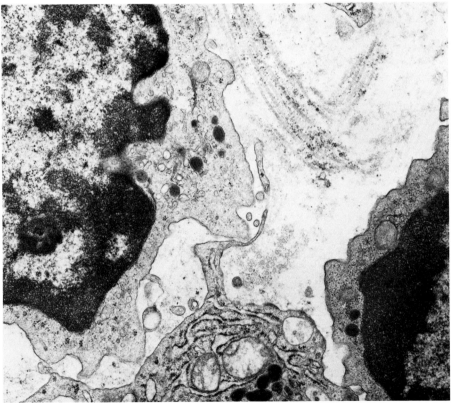

Figure 19. Metastatic peripheral neuroectodermal tumor showing electron dense neurosecretory-like granules in the cytoplasm. (Uranyl acetate and lead citrate ×9000)

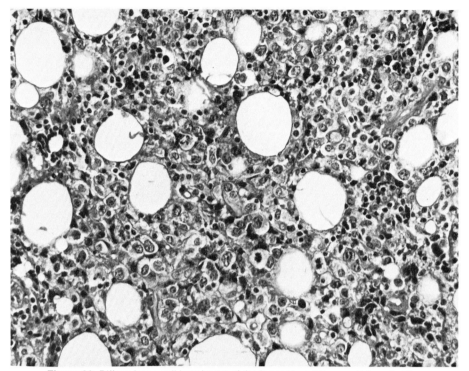

Figure 20. Diffuse large-cell lymphoma of the breast in a 12-year-old female. The fibro-fatty tissue is infiltrated by formless sheets of large lymphoid cells. (H&E ×250)

which occurred in young males unlike their usual presentation in lactating females.[35] Galactoceles are rarely seen in infants whose breast tissues have responded to maternal and placental hormones.[2] A facile pathogenetic explanation for the galactoceles in our cases was not forthcoming. The two examples of keratinous cysts were localized to the nipple.

Quasi-neoplastic and overtly neoplastic lesions accounted for over 60 percent of cases in our study (Table 2). Juvenile or diffuse hypertrophy was the most common tumor-like condition with a total of 20 cases. Although most of the pubertal and adolescent females had symmetrical enlargement of the breasts, there were examples of predominant involvement of one side. Essentially no insights were gained about the pathogenesis of juvenile hypertrophy from these cases since the patients were admitted for reduction mammoplasty and few studies beyond the very basics were performed before surgery. An end-organ hypersensitivity to estrogens is one hypothesis,[36] but estrogen receptor studies have not been performed to date on these cases to the best of our knowledge. There were no instances of abnormal breast enlargement after surgery in our cases, which is the experience of others.[15,36] There are many histopathologic similarities between hypertrophy and gynecomastia.

Juvenile papillomatosis (JP) was the only one of the papillary breast lesions represented in our series. The others include the solitary intraductal papilloma, papillomatosis exclusive of JP, and sclerosing papillomatosis. Rosen has applied the generic designation of papillary duct hyperplasia for the latter three lesions.[37] Because these papillary lesions share a number of histological features, there is the possibility of confusing one with the other. The question of intraductal papillary carcinoma should be anticipated even in this young age group with a highly complex papillary lesion and even focal necrosis in a minority of cases. In the specific context of JP, these findings are not regarded as evidence of malignancy.[34]

A type of florid papillomatosis in the breast of adolescent and young adult females was documented by Oberman, who in 1979 reported his experience with five patients between 15 and 17 years of age who had multiductal papillomatosis.[15] Whether all of Oberman's cases had JP per se is not entirely clear in light of the other types of papillary duct hyperplasia and papillomatosis in the breast of young females.[37] Papillary duct hyperplasia resembles JP in terms of the papillomatous growth, but it does not have the characteristic cystic changes, stasis, and apocrine metaplasia. At least one case with apocrine metaplasia among Oberman's five cases was most likely an example of JP.[15] The potential importance of the specific diagnosis of JP was evident in the follow-up studies of patients who were enrolled in the Juvenile Papillomatosis Registry.[38,39] In the initial study, the risk of breast carcinoma was not fully appreciated,[34] but with longer periods of clinical observation in a larger cohort of patients, several patients emerged who had a carcinoma of the breast concurrently or subsequently to JP. A family history of breast cancer in 26 percent of patients with JP was also higher than expected in the general population.[38] Careful clinical surveillance is strongly recommended in females with JP. Recently, the putative association of JP and secretory carcinoma of the breast was reported in a 4½-year-old girl, however, the description of the papillary tumor as "sclerosing" evoked some questions about the underlying benign lesion.[40] None of our five patients with JP has developed breast cancer to date, but a repeat biopsy on the ipsilateral side several years later in one patient showed "low risk" intraductal hyperplasia.

Among neoplasms, juvenile cellular fibroadenoma (JCF) and cystosarcoma phyllodes accounted for almost 50 percent of cases in this category in our series (Table 3). It is probably significant that 16 of 18 JCFs occurred in black females, all from the files of The Children's Hospital, Birmingham, Alabama with population demographics very different from the two Minnesota institutions. However, the fact remains that fibroadenomas in the young, predominantly white females at the Mayo Clinic and University of Minnesota were not characterized by unusual degrees of stromal and epithelial cellularity. One notable finding in blacks was the presence of multiple ipsilateral tumors in five patients and bilateral masses in six other patients. There is epidemiologic evidence that fibroadenomas in young black females are more often multiple and bilateral, and that the overall incidence is higher than in comparably aged young white females.[41,42] Because the JCFs are often large (greater than 5 cm), prominently cellular, and may have the branching phyllodes pattern, these tumors have been diagnosed in the past as benign cystosarcoma phyllodes, giant fibroadenoma, phyllodes tumor, or simply cystosarcoma phyllodes.[43-48] The designation of JCF is preferred for these neoplasms with a mitotically poor cellular stroma and minimal cytological atypia. Stromal overgrowth at the expense of the epithelial components should be viewed with concern about a bona fide cystosarcoma phyllodes with the potential for metastases. Stromal atypia and mitoses as a rule accompany the overgrowth of the spindle cells.[49-53] The epithelium in both the JCF and cystosarcoma phyllodes may be exuberantly hyperplastic.[18] There is no prognostic importance to the florid epithelial changes in either one of these tumors.

The diagnosis of cystosarcoma phyllodes (CP) was reserved in this study for those mixed epithelial and stromal neoplasms with sarcomatous changes indicative of the potential for local invasion, recurrence, and even metastasis in a minority of cases. If neoplasms alone are considered, CP constitutes approximately 5 percent of all breast tumors in children but only 1 percent of all breast lesions in this age group (Table 1). There are well-documented examples of locally recurring and metastasizing CP in young females.[54-57] A review of 44 CPs in adolescent females indicated that only 14 percent were malignant and even this figure may be inflated.[58-61] Thus the overall prognosis for those neoplasms diagnosed as CP in pediatric patients is more favorable than its presumed counterpart in adults.[49,50,52] However, the argument becomes somewhat tautological if there is no agreement that most CPs in adolescents are juvenile cellular fibroadenomas. Phyllodes tumor is an acceptable alternative in those cases with equivocal pathological findings and therefore an indeterminate prognosis. Both CPs in the present study had a definite sarcomatous component. One of the cases was previously reported by Jimenez et al.[8] Barnes and Pietruszka[62] have described a case of rhabdomyosarcoma originating in a CP but their patient was a 45-year-old female. The majority of CPs have a spindle-cell stroma whose sarcomatous nature is either more or less apparent, based upon the pathologic features.[49-51]

Nipple adenoma was the only pure benign epithelial neoplasm among our cases.[63] No tubular or lactating adenomas were seen. Tubular and lactating adenomas are generally diagnosed in the third and fourth decades whereas it is a decade later for nipple duct adenomas.[64-66] The age range at presentation of the nipple duct adenoma is quite broad as evidenced by the initial appearance at birth through the late adult years.[66] Swelling with enlargement of the nipple often accompanied by superficial ulceration is the principal clinical finding. The microscopic features are often unsettling with complex glandular and papillomatous patterns, cytological atypia, and a spindle-cell stroma possibly on the basis of tissue repair secondary to the ulceration. However, the low power appearance is one of architectural orderliness and circumscription. Rosen and Caicco have described three histological patterns based upon the predominance and mixture of papillary, adenomatous, and sclerosing features.[66]

Somewhat surprisingly, from the sizes of our institutions, there were no cases of carcinoma, which is one measure of the extreme rarity of breast cancer in the first 2 decades of life.[15,16] One type of breast carcinoma, juvenile or secretory carcinoma, was initially reported only in children[67]; however, it has since come to be recognized in adults. For this reason, secretory carcinoma is considered the more appropriate appellation. Some of the earlier reports on invasive breast cancer in children have raised questions about the original diagnosis. One example is the report of an 11-year-old female with a small-cell malignancy in the breast who also had diffuse lymphadenopathy and osseous and pulmonary metastases.[68] She died within 9 months of presentation. A hematolymphoid malignancy or rhabdomyosarcoma would look and behave in a similar manner. Secretory carcinoma is one of a small group of invasive ductal carcinomas with a favorable prognosis. It infrequently spreads beyond the breast to regional lymph nodes or has hematogenous dissemination.[69] Approximately 17 cases of secretory carcinoma have been reported in children between the ages of 3 and 17 years with a median of 10 years.[70] Three of the 17 cases occurred in males. Grossly, the tumor infrequently measures greater than 3.0 cm in greatest dimension and its circumscribed, glistening appearance on cut surface resembles the fibroadenoma. This tumor may also have the macroscopic features of the usual infiltrating duct carcinoma. Sheets and nests of glandular and papillary profiles consisting of vacuolated or clear cells with minimal cytological atypia are the principal histological features. The intracellular vacuoles and extracellular secretions are sulfomucins.

Conventional infiltrating duct carcinoma and even medullary carcinoma are encountered on rare occasions in women in the early third decade of life and, in some cases, the diagnosis is made during or shortly after pregnancy. One possible source of error in the pathologic diagnosis is the failure to recognize the infiltrating, round cell neoplasm as a rhabdomyosarcoma or hematolymphoid malignancy rather than an infiltrating ductal or lobular carcinoma. An appreciation of these other, even more likely diagnostic considerations can be pursued with appropriate cell marker and immunohistochemical studies.

Most malignancies in the present series reflected the general diagnostic problem of "small round cell neoplasms" of children and adolescents.[9] Primary rhabdomyosarcoma (RMS) of the breast is very rare. A review of the literature revealed only 25 cases and most of these occurred in adults.[62,71] On the other hand, approximately 6 percent of children with diagnosed RMS develop breast metastases, and the majority of these patients have a primary alveolar RMS of the extremity.[72] Very uncommonly, the patient, usually an adolescent, presents with widely disseminated tumor with one or several masses in the breast(s) and with other sites of involvement including the bones, bone marrow, and lymph nodes. The primary site may be difficult to establish and because of the distribution of disease, malignant lymphoma, or acute leukemia is strongly suspected clinically. Usually the pattern of nodal and/or bone marrow involvement is the first indication of a metastatic small-cell neoplasm exclusive of a hematolymphoid malignancy. The three patients with metastatic RMS in our series had prior confirmed diagnoses at the time of their presentation with multiple nodules in the breast. A solitary breast mass was the clinical presentation of the 12-year-old female with the only example of a primary RMS. Solid, formless cohesive sheets or smaller nests of monomorphic round cells may not immediately suggest the diagnosis of RMS, especially the alveolar type in the absence of the loosely arranged cellular aggregates interspersed with larger, anaplastic cells with eosinophilic cytoplasm. The strategy or approach to all round cell neoplasms in the child or adolescent regardless of the peculiarity of the clinical presentation, even a breast mass, is to exclude an RMS.

Neuroectodermal or neuroendocrine neoplasms of the breast are very rare in children.[2] The so-called neuroendocrine carcinoma of the breast which has been the subject of numerous clinicopathologic and immunohistochemical studies in the past is a tumor exclusively of adult women. One of us (LPD) has seen an apparent metastatic neuroendocrine carcinoma in a 15-year-old female who presented with multiple subcutaneous nodules in and around the breast (not included in this study). Three examples of primitive neuroectodermal tumors (PNET), one classic neuroblastoma and two peripheral PNETs, were included in our multi-institutional survey. All three were presumably metastatic. The basic distinction between a peripheral PNET and classic neuroblastoma was predicated in part upon elevated urinary catecholamines in the one patient and normal values in the other two adolescent females.[73,74] Homer–Wright rosettes were particularly striking in one of the non-catecholamine-associated PNETs. The histopathologic appearance of the other two tumors was essentially a small-cell neoplasm with very few diagnostic microscopic clues. Ultrastructurally, both tumors had the characteristic features of PNETs with complex interdigitating cytoplasm processes and microtubules.[9]

One final example of a neural crest-derived neoplasm with a breast metastasis in our series was a malignant melanoma occurring in a 20-year-old female who had a pigmented skin lesion excised from the back 6 years earlier. In retrospect, the original diagnosis of a benign nevocytic lesion was incorrect. Axillary lymph nodes on the ipsilateral side of the breast lesion also contained metastatic melanoma. Since malignant melanoma is uncommon in children and adolescents (less than 5 percent of all melanomas), it is unlikely that a clinician or pathologist will encounter a case like this. In the adult age group, malignant melanoma is among the most common malignancies to metastasize to the breast,[75] and oat cell carcinoma of the lung may rarely present as a breast mass.[76]

Leukemias of various lineages and malignant lymphomas of non-Hodgkin's and Hodgkin's types are well documented in the literature as the cause of a mass(es) in the breast(s) of children and adults.[77–81] Acute myelogenous leukemia may initially present with bilaterally enlarged breasts in a young patient. Multiple masses in both breasts of an adolescent female may be the first sign of malignant lymphoma, small non-cleaved cell type (Burkitt's lymphoma).[82,83] Approximately 50 percent of all malignant lymphomas of the breast have the B-cell phenotype and cytomorphology of small non-cleaved lymphocytes.[79,80] Our two examples are somewhat atypical in that one patient had a primary diffuse large-cell lymphoma of the breast, and the other patient had advanced Hodgkin's disease with dissemination to the breast. Virtually all young patients with Burkitt's lymphoma involving the breast have stage IV disease and those with extramedullary leukemia have bone marrow infiltration or will develop it within days or weeks of presentation.[2]

Tumors of the soft tissues exclusive of the 4 rhabdomyosarcomas accounted for a total of 13 cases of fibrous (myofibroblastic), lipomatous, and vascular derivation. Despite the fact that the fibromatoses are among the most common soft tissue tumors of childhood, the presentation in the breast is more frequent in adults than in children.[84,85] The pathologic findings and the recurrent, locally aggressive behavior are the same features in the breast as elsewhere in the soft tissues. Lipoma of the breast is possibly as uncommon in children as fibromatosis. Interestingly, one of our three cases presented with multiple lipomatous masses. A careful examination of a lipomatous tumor in a child regardless of site may reveal residual features of a lipoblastoma.[2]

Vascular neoplasms of the skin and soft tissues are generally considered the most frequent mesenchymal tumors in the pediatric age group.[86] It is widely appreciated by pathologists and clinicians alike that the majority of vascular neoplasms (65 to 70 percent) in adults are angiosarcomas.[87] Some of the anguish associated with vascular tumors of the breast has been relieved by the studies of Rosen who has carefully documented the occurrence of various benign vascular neoplasms and also the prognostic importance of size and pathologic grading of angiosarcomas.[87,88] Although most angiosarcomas of the breast present in adults, our one case and the several other examples in the literature clearly establish its presence in the prepubertal or adolescent patient.[87,89] The high grade angiosarcoma behaved as anticipated in our case. Five infants in our study presented with a subareolar mass which consisted of closely arranged vascular lobules surrounding the mammary ducts.[88] The tumor in each case had the appearance of a typical juvenile or cellular hemangioma which is seen in the skin, soft tissues, and occasionally organs (liver, parotid, intestinal tract) of infants. There was a single example of a histiocytoid or epithelioid hemangioma in a 16-month-old female. This lesion is well described in sites other than the breast.[90] Because of the vacuolated, histiocytoid, or epithelioid appearance of the endothelial cells, this lesion may be confused with an infiltrating epithelial neoplasm. Immunoreactivity for Factor VIII-related antigen and affinity for the *Ulex europaeus* agglutinin are confirmatory of the endothelial phenotype of the tumor. With the exception of the angiosarcoma, simple excision is the treatment of choice, and as much potential breast tissue as possible should be spared, especially in a female infant.

SUMMARY

This large series of cases demonstrates that the breast of the child or adolescent is the potential site for a number of interesting lesions exclusive of fibroadenoma and gynecomastia. Adenoma of the nipple, juvenile papillomatosis, and juvenile or cellular fibroadenoma should be correctly diagnosed to insure conservative surgical management and appropriate clinical follow-up. The results of the Juvenile Papillomatosis Registry suggest that this lesion is a morphological marker of potentially more serious breast disease in the future. Recognition of a cellular fibroepithelial neoplasm, especially in young black females, as a cellular fibroadenoma will hopefully eliminate the need for the diagnosis of "benign" cytosarcoma phyllodes. On occasion, the equivocal case may be labeled a "phyllodes tumor of indeterminate biologic behavior." Those neoplasms with stromal atypia and mitotic activity, overgrowth of stroma with epithelial dissociation, and sarcomatous elements are appropriately designated as cytosarcoma phyllodes. In contrast to vascular tumors of the breast in adults, the majority of vascular lesions in the child's breast are benign and represent either a capillary or a histiocytoid hemangioma. Our experience and reports in the literature support the conclusion that most malignancies of the breast in children are metastatic. Rhabdomyosarcoma was the most common example in our study, but secondary involvement by acute leukemia or malignant lymphoma also occurs.

REFERENCES

1. Vorherr H: The Breast. Morphology, Physiology, and Lactation. New York, Academic Press, 1974, pp. 1–19
2. Dehner LP: Pediatric Surgical Pathology, 2nd ed. Baltimore, Williams & Wilkins, 1987, pp. 104–119
3. Bower R, Bell MJ, Ternberg JL: Management of breast lesions in children and adolescents. J Pediatr Surg 11:337, 1976
4. Stone AM, Shenker IR, McCarthy K: Adolescent breast masses. Am J Surg 134:275, 1977
5. Farrow JH, Ashikari H: Breast lesions in young girls. Surg Clin North Am 49:261, 1969
6. Simpson JS, Barson AJ: Breast tumors in infants and children: A 40-year review of cases at a children's hospital. Can Med Assoc J 101:100, 1969
7. Hein K, Dell R, Cohen MI: Self-detection of a breast mass in adolescent females. J Adolesc Health Care 3:15, 1982
8. Jimenez JF, Gloster ES, Perrot LJ, et al: Liposarcoma arising within a cytosarcoma phyllodes. J Surg Oncol 31:294, 1986
9. Triche TJ, Askin FB, Kissane JM: Neuroblastoma, Ewing's sarcoma, and the differential diagnosis of small-, round-, blue-cell tumors. In Finegold M (ed): Pathology of Neoplasia in Children and Adolescents. Philadelphia: Saunders, 1986, pp 145–195
10. Hsu S-M, Rain L, Fanger H: Use of avidin-biotin-peroxidase complex (ABC) in immunoperoxidase techniques: A comparison between ABC and unlabeled antibody (PAP) procedures. J Histochem Cytochem 29:577, 1981
11. Sternberger LA: Immunohistochemistry, 3rd ed. New York, Wiley, 1986, pp 90–114
12. Hanson CA, Snover DC, Dehner LP: Fibroadenomatosis (fibroadenomatoid masto-

pathy): A benign breast lesion with composite pathologic features. Pathology 19:393, 1987

13. Is "fibrocystic disease" of the breast precancerous? (Consensus Meeting, October 3–5, 1985, New York). Arch Pathol Lab Med 110:171, 1986

14. Rosen PP: Vascular tumors of the breast. V. Non-parenchymal hemangiomas of mammary subcutaneous tissues. Am J Surg Pathol 9:723, 1985

15. Oberman HA: Breast lesions in the adolescent female. Pathol Annu 14 (Pt. 1):175, 1979

16. Dehner LP: Pathology of the breast in the first two decades of life. In Najarian JS, Delaney JP (eds): Advances in Breast and Endocrine Surgery. Chicago, Year Book Med Pub, 1986, pp 63–81

17. Ashikari R, Farrow JH, O'Hara J: Fibroadenomas in the breast of juvenile. Surg Gynecol Obstet 132:259, 1971

18. Mies C, Rosen PP: Juvenile fibroadenoma with atypical epithelial hyperplasia. Am J Surg Pathol 11:184, 1987

19. Azzopardi JG: Problems in Breast Pathology. London, Saunders, 1979, pp 39–55

20. Ohtani H, Sasano N: Stromal cells of the fibroadenoma of the human breast. An immunohistochemical and ultrastructural study. Virchows Arch [A] 404:7, 1984

21. Nielsen BB, Ladefoged C: Fibroadenoma of the female breast with multinucleated giant cells. Pathol Res Pract 180:721, 1985

22. Pike AM, Oberman HA: Juvenile (cellular) adenofibromas. A clinicopathologic study. Am J Surg Pathol 9:730, 1985

23. Fekete P, Petrek J, Majmudar B, et al: Fibroadenomas with stromal cellularity. A clinicopathologic study of 21 patients. Arch Pathol Lab Med 111:427, 1987

24. Bannayan GA, Hajdu SI: Gynecomastia: Clinicopathologic study of 351 cases. Am J Clin Pathol 57:431, 1972

25. McKiernan J, Hull D: Breast development in the newborn. Arch Dis Child 56:525, 1981

26. McKiernan J, Coyne J, Cahalane S: Histology of breast development in early life. Arch Dis Child 63:136, 1988

27. Weinberg SK, Motulsky AG: Aberrant axillary breast tissue: A report of a family with six affected women in two generations. Clin Genet 10:325, 1976

28. Mimouni F, Merlob P, Reisner SH: Occurrence of supernumerary nipples in newborns. Am J Dis Child 137:952, 1983

29. Meggyessy V, Méhes K: Association of supernumerary nipples with renal anomalies. J Pediatr 111:412, 1987

30. Rudoy RC, Nelson JD: Breast abscess during the neonatal period. A review. Am J Dis Child 129:1031, 1975

31. Love SM, Connolly JL, Schnitt SJ, Shirley RL: Benign breast disorders. In Harris JR, Hellman S, Henderson IC, Kinne DW (eds): Breast Diseases. Philadelphia, Lippincott, 1987, pp 15–53

32. Dupont WD, Page DL: Risk factor for breast cancer in women with proliferative breast disease. N Engl J Med 312:146, 1945

33. Rivera Pomar JM, Vilanova JR, Burgos Bretones JJ, Arocena G: Focal fibrous disease of breast. A common entity in young women. Virchows Arch [A] 386:59, 1980

34. Rosen PP, Cantrell B, Mullen DL, De Palo A: Juvenile papillomatosis (swiss cheese disease) of the breast. Am J Surg Pathol 4:3, 1980

35. Golden GT, Wangensteen SL: Galactocele of the breast. Am J Surg 123:271, 1972

36. Hollingsworth DR, Archer R: Massive virginal breast hypertrophy at puberty. Am J Dis Child 125:293, 1973
37. Rosen PP: Papillary duct hyperplasia of the breast in children and young adults. Cancer 56:1611, 1985
38. Rosen PP, Lyngholm B, Kinne DW, Beattie EJ: Juvenile papillomatosis of the breast and family history of breast carcinoma. Cancer 49:2591, 1982
39. Rosen PP, Holmes G, Lesser ML, et al: Juvenile papillomatosis and breast carcinoma. Cancer 55:1345, 1985
40. Ferguson BT, McCarty KS, Filston HC: Juvenile secretory carcinoma and juvenile papillomatosis: Diagnosis and treatment. J Pediatr Surg 22:637, 1987
41. Oluwole SF, Freeman HP: Analysis of benign breast lesions in blacks. Am J Surg 137:786, 1979
42. Morris JA, Kelly JF: Multiple bilateral breast adenomata in identical adolescent Negro twins. Histopathology 6:539, 1982
43. Gogas J, Sechas M, Skalkeas G: Surgical management of diseases of the adolescent female breast. A clinicopathologic study. Am J Surg 137:634, 1979
44. Devitt JE: Juvenile giant fibroadenoma of the breast. Can J Surg 17:205, 1974
45. Simpson TE, Van Dervoort RL, Lynn HB: Giant fibroadenoma (benign cytosarcoma phyllodes): Report of case in 13-year-old girl. Surgery 65:341, 1969
46. Raganoonan C, Fairbairn JK, Williams S, Hughes LE: Giant breast tumours of adolescence. Aust NZ J Surg 57:243, 1987
47. Daniel WA, Mathews MD: Tumors of the breast in adolescent females. Pediatrics 41:743, 1968
48. Iverson RE, Hegg SI: Cystosarcoma phyllodes presenting as massive unilateral breast hypertrophy in an adolescent. Ann Plast Surg 4:315, 1980
49. Norris HJ, Taylor HB: Relationship of the histologic appearance to behavior of cystosarcoma phyllodes: Analysis of ninety-four cases. Cancer 20:2090, 1967
50. Pietruszka M, Barnes L: Cystosarcoma phyllodes. A clinicopathologic analysis of 42 cases. Cancer 41:1974, 1978
51. Hart WR, Bauer RC, Oberman HA: Cystosarcoma phyllodes. A clinicopathologic study of twenty-six hypercellular periductal stromal tumors of the breast. Am J Clin Pathol 70:211, 1978
52. Ward RM, Evans HL: Cystosarcoma phyllodes. A clinicopathologic study of 26 cases. Cancer 58:2282, 1986
53. Hines JR, Murad TM, Beal JM: Prognostic indicators in cystosarcoma phyllodes. Am J Surg 153:276, 1987
54. Amerson JR: Cystosarcoma phyllodes in adolescent females: A report of seven patients. Ann Surg 171:847, 1979
55. Turalba CIC, El-Mahdl AM, Lagada L: Fatal metastatic cystosarcoma phyllodes in an adolescent female: Case report and review of treatment approaches. J Surg Oncol 33:176, 1986
56. Adami HOG, Hakelius L, Rimsten A, Willen R: Malignant, locally recurring cystosarcoma phyllodes in an adolescent female. A case report. Acta Chir Scand 150:93, 1984
57. Hoover HC, Trestioreanu A, Ketcham AS: Metastatic cystosarcoma phyllodes in an adolescent girl: An unusually malignant tumor. Ann Surg 181:279, 1975
58. Stromberg BV, Gollady ES: Cystosarcoma phyllodes in the adolescent female. J Pediatr Surg 13:423, 1978

59. Andersson A, Bergdahl L: Cystosarcoma phyllodes in young women. Arch Surg 113:742, 1978
60. Briggs RM, Walters M, Rosenthal D: Cystosarcoma phyllodes in adolescent female patients. Am J Surg 146:712, 1983
61. Mollitt DL, Golladay ES, Gloster ES, Jimenez JF: Cystosarcoma phyllodes in the adolescent female. J Pediatr Surg 22:907, 1987
62. Barnes L, Pietruszka M: Rhabdomyosarcoma arising within a cystosarcoma phyllodes. Case report and review of the literature. Am J Surg Pathol 2:423, 1978
63. Hertel BF, Zaloudek C, Kempson RL: Breast adenomas. Cancer 37:2891, 1976
64. Perzin KH, Lattes R: Papillary adenoma of the nipple (florid papillomatosis, adenoma, adenomatosis). A clinicopathologic study. Cancer 29:996, 1972
65. Smith EJ, Jones EW: Erosive adenomatosis of the nipple. Clin Exper Dermatol 2:79, 1977
66. Rosen PP, Caicco JA: Florid papillomatosis of the nipple. A study of 51 patients, including nine with mammary carcinoma. Am J Surg Pathol 10:87, 1986
67. McDivitt KW, Stewart FW: Breast carcinoma in children. JAMA 195:388, 1966
68. Ramirez G, Ansfield FJ: Carcinoma of the breast in children. Arch Surg 96:222, 1968
69. Tavassoli FA, Norris HJ: Secretory carcinoma of the breast. Cancer 45:2404, 1980
70. Karl SR, Ballantine TVN, Zaino R: Juvenile secretory carcinoma of the breast. J Pediatr Surg 20:368, 1985
71. Woodard BH, Farnham R, Mossler JA, et al: Rhabdomyosarcoma of the breast (letter). Arch Pathol Lab Med 104:445, 1980
72. Howarth CB, Cases JN, Pratt C: Breast metastases in children with rhabdomyosarcoma. Cancer 46:2520, 1980
73. Dehner LP: Peripheral and central primitive neuroectodermal tumors. A nosologic concept seeking a consensus. Arch Pathol Lab Med 110:997, 1986
74. Hashimoto H, Enjoji M, Nakajima T, et al: Malignant neuroepithelioma (peripheral neuroblastoma). A clinicopathologic study of 15 cases. Am J Surg Pathol 7:309, 1983
75. Boddie AW Jr, Smith JL Jr, McBride CM: Malignant melanoma in children and young adults: Effect of diagnostic criteria on staging and end results. South Med J 71:1074, 1978
76. Kelly C, Henderson D, Corris P: Breast lumps: Rare presentation of oat cell carcinoma of lung. J Clin Pathol 41:171, 1988
77. Lamovec J, Jancar J: Primary malignant lymphoma of the breast. Lymphoma of the mucosa-associated lymphoid tissue. Cancer 60:3033, 1987
78. Smith MR, Brustein S, Straus DJ: Localized non-Hodgkin's lymphoma of the breast. Cancer 59:351, 1987
79. Mambo NC, Burke JS, Butler JJ: Primary malignant lymphomas of the breast. Cancer 39:2033, 1977
80. Telesinghe PU, Anthony PP: Primary lymphoma of the breast. Histopathology 9:297, 1985
81. Meis JM, Butler JJ, Osborne BM: Hodgkin's disease involving the breast and chest wall. Cancer 57:1859, 1986
82. Garthenhaus WS, Mir R, Pliskin A: Granulocytic sarcoma of the breast: A leukemic bilateral matachronous presentation and literature review. Med Pediatr Oncol 13:22, 1985

83. Hubner KF, Littlefield LG: Burkitt lymphoma in three American children. Clinical and cytogenetic observations. Am J Dis Child 129:1219, 1975

84. Rosen Y, Papasozomenos SC, Gardner D: Fibromatosis of the breast. Cancer 41:1409, 1978

85. Wargotz ES, Norris HJ, Austin RM, Enzinger FM: Fibromatosis of the breast: A clinical and pathological study of 28 cases. Am J Surg Pathol 11:38, 1987

86. Harms D, Schmidt D: Classification of solid tumors in children: The Kiel Pediatric Tumor Registry. Monogr Paediatr 18:1, 1986

87. Donnel RM, Rosen PP, Lieberman PH, et al: Angiosarcoma and other vascular tumors of the breast. Am J Surg Pathol 5:629, 1981

88. Jozefczyk MA, Rosen PP: Vascular tumors of the breast. II. Perilobular hemangiomas and hemangiomas. Am J Surg Pathol 9:491, 1985

89. Merino MJ, Carter D, Berman M: Angiosarcoma of the breast. Am J Surg Pathol 7:53, 1983

90. Rosai J, Gold J, Landy R: The histiocytoid hemangioma: A unifying concept embracing several previously described entities of skin, soft tissue, large vessels, bone and heart. Hum Pathol 10:707, 1979

Index

Abscess, breast, 40
Acute myelogenous leukemia, 322
Adenocarcinoma
  Arias–Stella changes vs., 201
  breast, 27, 29, 32–36, 42
    fibroadenomas vs., 32–36
    inflammatory lesions vs., 36
    radiation changes vs., 37–38, 42
    well-differentiated, 27, 29
  colorectal. *See* Colorectal
        adenocarcinomas
  endocervical, 182
  endometrial, 182, 183
  in situ, Arias–Stella changes vs., 201
  inflammatory lesions vs., 36
  mesonephric, 209
  minimal deviation, 203
Adenoid cystic carcinoma of breast, 237–
        251
  age, 241, 249
  bloody nipple discharge, 242
  breast-conserving therapy, 250
  clinical features, 242, 249–250
  clinical presentation, 242
  collagenous spherulosis (adenoid cystic
        hyperplasia) vs., 251, 252
  differential diagnosis, 250–251
  fibroadenoma, 242
  follow-up, 247
  grading, 251
  gross pathology, 237–238
  growth patterns, 250
  high grade, 240–241, 246, 248
    alveolar growth, 248
    cribriform pattern, 246

hormone receptor analysis, 242, 249
laterality, 241–242
locality in breast, 241–242
low grade, 237–238, 239, 240, 241
  three patterns of in situ growth, 244,
        245
mastectomy, 249
microscopic pathology, 238–241
misclassified, 250
pathology, 250–251
prognosis, 249
radiotherapy as adjunct, 250
recurrence, 249
sexual gender, 249
size, 237–238
subclassification, 250–251
syringomatous features, 243
treatment, 247, 249, 250
Adenoid cystic hyperplasia, 251, 252
Adenoma, 37, 303, 309, 320
  nipple, 303, 309, 320
    children, 320
    nipple duct, 303, 309
  tubular, 37
Adenoma malignum, 203, 209–211
Adenomatous hyperplasia, 205
Adenosis, vaginal papillary, 200, 202
Adult T-cell leukemia-lymphoma, IL-2 re-
        ceptor expression in, 151–154
Age
  adenoid cystic carcinoma of breast, 241,
        249
  endosalpingiosis, 1
  serous borderline neoplasia of perito-
        neum, 5